RESEARCHING
HEALTH

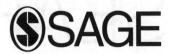

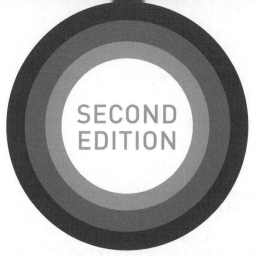

SECOND
EDITION

RESEARCHING
HEALTH

QUALITATIVE, QUANTITATIVE AND MIXED METHODS

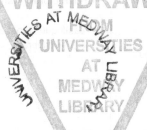

EDITED BY
MIKE SAKS AND
JUDITH ALLSOP

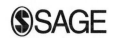

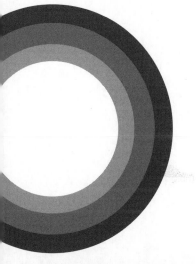

Los Angeles | London | New Delhi
Singapore | Washington DC

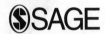

Los Angeles | London | New Delhi
Singapore | Washington DC

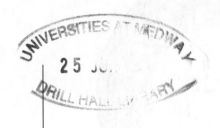

SAGE Publications Ltd
1 Oliver's Yard
55 City Road
London EC1Y 1SP

SAGE Publications Inc.
2455 Teller Road
Thousand Oaks, California 91320

SAGE Publications India Pvt Ltd
B 1/I 1 Mohan Cooperative Industrial Area
Mathura Road
New Delhi 110 044

SAGE Publications Asia-Pacific Pte Ltd
3 Church Street
#10-04 Samsung Hub
Singapore 049483

Editor: Alison Poyner
Assistant editor: Emma Milman
Production editor: Katie Forsythe
Copyeditor: Sharon Cawood
Proofreader: Mary Dalton
Marketing manager: Tamara Navaratnam
Cover design: Lisa Harper
Typeset by: C&M Digitals (P) Ltd, Chennai, India
Printed by Ashford Colour Press Ltd

Library of Congress Control Number: 2012938025

British Library Cataloguing in Publication data

A catalogue record for this book is available from
the British Library

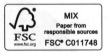

MIX
Paper from
responsible sources
FSC® C011748

ISBN 978-1-4462-5226-0
ISBN 978-1-4462-5227-7 (pbk)

Contents

List of Contributors

Andy Alaszewski
Emiritus Professor of Health Studies and Director of the Centre for Health Services Studies at the University of Kent, UK.

Priscilla Alderson
Professor of Childhood Studies in the Social Sciences Research Unit at the Institute of Education, University of London, UK.

Judith Allsop
Professor of Health Policy at the University of Lincoln, UK, and Visiting Professor at University Campus Suffolk, UK.

Ellen Annandale
Professor of Sociology at the University of York, UK.

George Argyrous
Senior Lecturer in ANSZOG Evidence-based Decision-making at the University of New South Wales, Australia.

Peter Bradley
Director of Public Health for Wales and Visiting Senior Fellow at University Campus Suffolk, UK.

Viola Burau
Associate Professor in the Department of Political Science at the University of Aarhus, Denmark.

Michael Calnan
Professor of Medical Sociology in the School of Social Policy, Sociology and Social Research at the University of Kent, UK, and Visiting Professor at University Campus Suffolk, UK.

Penny Cavenagh
Director of Research and Enterprise at University Campus Suffolk, UK, and Visiting Professor at the University of East Anglia, UK.

Peter Davis
Professor of Health and Well-being and Director of the COMPASS Research Centre at the University of Auckland, New Zealand.

Stephen Gillam
Professor in the Department of Public Health at the University of Cambridge, UK.

Judith Green
Reader in Sociology of Health at the London School of Hygiene and Tropical Medicine, UK.

Sophie Hill
Head of Centre for Health Communication and Participation at La Trobe University, Australia.

David Hughes
Professor of Health Policy at the University of Wales, UK.

Mark R.D. Johnson
Professor of Diversity in Health and Social Care at the Mary Seacole Research Centre in the Faculty of Health and Life Sciences at De Montfort University, UK.

Kathryn Jones
Senior Research Fellow in the Department of Public Policy at De Montfort University, UK.

Ellen Kuhlmann
Visiting Professor at University Campus Suffolk, UK, and Research Fellow at the Instituteof Economy, Labour and Culture at Goethe University, Frankfurt, Germany.

George Lewith
Professor of Health Research, Primary Care and Population Sciences in the School of Medicine at the University of Southampton, UK.

Paul Little
Professor of Primary Care in the Faculty of Medicine at the University of Southampton, UK.

Jacqueline Low
Professor in the Department of Sociology at the University of New Brunswick, Canada.

Alan Maynard
Professor of Health Economics at the University of York, UK.

Martin von Randow
Data manager and analyst at the University of Auckland, New Zealand.

Janet Richardson
Professor of Health Service Research in the School of Nursing and Midwifery at the University of Plymouth, UK.

Mike Saks
Professor of Health and Community Studies and Provost at University Campus Suffolk, UK, and Visiting Professor at the University of Essex and the University of Lincoln, UK.

Alastair Scott
Professor in the Department of Sociology at the University of Auckland, New Zealand.

A. Niroshan Siriwardena
Professor of Primary and Pre-Hospital Health Care at the University of Lincoln, UK.

Jonathan Tritter
Professorial Fellow in the Institute of Governance and Public Management in the Business School at Warwick University, UK.

Heather Waterman
Professor of Nursing and Ophthalmology in the School of Nursing, Midwifery and Social Work at the University of Manchester, UK.

About the Companion Website

Visit the companion website at www.sagepub.co.uk/saks_allsop2e to find a range of teaching and learning material for lecturers and students, including the following:

For lecturers:

- **Teaching notes:** Password-protected teaching notes with chapter overviews, core themes and seminar topics for discussion.
- **PowerPoint slides:** Slides for each chapter for use in teaching.

For students:

- **Editor online video**: Professor Mike Sake gives an introduction to the book.
- **Chapter overviews**: Short chapter overviews with learning outcomes and key themes.
- **Key concepts**: Essential concepts from the Glossary for each chapter.
- **Web links**: Links to related websites for each chapter.
- **SAGE online readings**: Free access to two journal articles for each chapter.
- **Study skills**: Free chapters to support readers in completing their research project.

The editors wish to thank Dr Kathryn Jones and Katherine Hooper for their assistance in compiling this website.

PART I

Conducting Health Research

1

Introduction: The Context for Researching Health

MIKE SAKS AND JUDITH ALLSOP

The second edition of this book aims to provide an extended and updated guide to the range of ways in which readers may approach researching health. The volume contains a number of key enhancements. There are new chapters on gender and health research and public health research, and all the chapters have been updated with new material. There is more emphasis on mixed methods in health research and on research ethics. The chapters on qualitative and quantitative methods also now all contain sections on how to read and critically appraise published work using the methods concerned. This is in addition to other updates to the high quality chapters from the first edition of *Researching Health*.

After the opening chapters in Part I of the book on how to conduct health research, Part II examines how qualitative methods have been used to research health, illness and the delivery of services in health care settings. In Part III, the quantitative methods used in health research to investigate health, illness and treatment for disease, and to assess the costs and benefits of interventions in health care, are discussed. In both these sections, the aim is to describe the use of various methods in practice; the type of questions each method is intended to address; and the strengths and weaknesses of each approach. This is followed by a consideration of the challenges likely to be encountered in carrying out research.

The book then turns in Part IV to consider selected issues in the field of health research that have emerged as under-researched areas, such as the health of minority groups and issues of gender, and where current research practice has faced a critical challenge, leading to ongoing debate. Questions of how to ensure ethical research practice and how to involve those who use health care in the research process have become more central to health research, but are areas where opinion is divided. The interests of researchers may conflict with those people who are the subjects of research. Even if there is agreement that ethics is a central issue in health research, and that a partnership between researchers and health care users offers a way forward, there are still practical problems about how this can best be achieved.

The concluding chapters in Part V focus on applying health research, addressing specifically the issues of mixed methods and multidisciplinary research; the research process and writing up health research; and disseminating and using such research. Throughout the book, we have aimed to engage with the practical problems of conducting research. In so doing, each chapter provides examples of health research in practice – including those from the authors' own research where appropriate – to aid readers in carrying out their own research project and/or in using the research of others in their work.

We continue to take the view as editors that two principles underlie all research. First, research is about producing new insights and new knowledge by setting answerable research questions; collecting data in a systematic way; analysing research questions intelligently and rigorously; and identifying patterns and establishing associations. In this way, researchers may contribute to a greater understanding of individual health and collective health behaviour; the role and impact of health providers; and the options for delivering health services to communities. In putting together the book, we believe that:

> Research is about illumination. If we don't succeed in that we have failed. If a person reads something and doesn't feel any wiser, then why was it done? Research should fire curiosity and the imagination ... If people feel research illuminates their understanding and gets into their thinking, then it's of use. (cited in Richardson et al. 1990: 75)

The second principle is that the findings produced by research are always contingent on the context in which the research is carried out; the methods used; and how the data have been analysed and interpreted. We therefore think that it is incumbent upon the researcher to be explicit and transparent about these elements in the research process. New knowledge or insights occur in small steps. Often, studies need to be replicated and/or reanalysed and revisited before findings can be said to be soundly based. All research results are subject to reinterpretation and review. In this sense, the production of new knowledge is a collective enterprise and each researcher, even if working alone, is part of a wider research community. Although there is no single organization that covers all researchers in health and/or other fields, there are both formal and informal rules that govern research. These are outlined and assessed in the various chapters in this volume.

What Is Health Research?

What, though, is 'research' in the health context? At its most general level, the conventions of health research can be viewed as work conducted to develop knowledge based on available evidence, following certain rules and procedures. However, as Henn et al. (2006) point out, what is to count as knowledge and how we acquire that knowledge is a contested area. Most significantly, there are different paradigms or clusters of beliefs and assumptions that shape what is studied, how research is conducted, what methods are used to ground knowledge and how results are interpreted. It is fundamental to understand these as they frame how we view the world and lead to many different types of research. They are more fully discussed in Chapter 2.

At a macro level, there is a division between research in the natural sciences in areas such as anatomy, biology, chemistry, physiology and physics, on which the more clinical areas of health research tend to be based (see, for example, Foss and Farine 2007), and research in the social sciences like history, policy, politics, psychology and sociology that explore patterns of health and illness and the social meanings surrounding these (see, for instance, Garner and Christiansen 2008). At a micro level, it is important to note that there are also distinctive approaches both between, and within, such disciplines and sub-disciplines (Daly et al. 1992).

There are distinctions too between the various methods used in health research that are divided broadly between qualitative research (as illustrated by Bourgeault et al. 2010) and quantitative research (as exemplified by Bruce et al. 2008). Classically, these are based on paradigms that provide a philosophical and methodological context for such work in the health field (Dyson and Brown 2006). However, as a number of the chapters in this book highlight, many research projects are now carried out using a mixture of methods (Andrew and Halcomb 2009). In these circumstances, it is vital for the researcher to understand what kind of knowledge each type of method produces; what kind of evidence supports the interpretation of findings from research data; and how different kinds of evidence may or may not be linked together to determine how a particular piece of research adds to knowledge.

According to Richardson et al. (1990), within the broader frame of reference delineated by paradigms, health research itself can take many different forms depending on the purpose of the research and its subject matter. As can be seen from Box 1.1 below, these principally include the following types: contextual/descriptive, diagnostic/analytical, strategic, evaluative, developmental and methodological.

These types of research have different audiences. To highlight this, contextual research has broad appeal to academic and other communities, while strategic research is of most interest to those concerned with policy and practice. The varying forms of research also relate to various stages of a research project. Thus, for example, methodological research is usually involved in establishing foundations for further research. Evaluative research, in contrast, typically looks back on programmes already developed – and by definition provides evaluations of them. In the health sphere, the methods employed to collect data within these various types of research are wide ranging – from surveys to observational techniques. A fuller account can be found in Jenkinson (1997).

Box 1.1   Different types of research: A summary

Contextual/descriptive: providing current information or intelligence on a problem – for example, the prevalence of Alzheimer's disease.

Diagnostic/analytical: attempting an explanation of phenomena based on a notion of cause and effect – such as accounting for changes in the birth rate.

Strategic: discovering implications, assessing alternatives and finding solutions – as, for instance, in the analysis of those at risk from a universal vaccination programme.

Evaluative: assessing the benefits and costs of a specific programme or course of action to those directly concerned or the wider community – as illustrated by the testing of a new drug.

Developmental: studying the implementation of programmes to feedback information to enable change – for example, on an anti-smoking campaign.

Methodological: assessing methods and techniques and developing new ones – as in the case of finding new means to diagnose particular diseases.

Source: Richardson et al. (1990)

Conceptualizing Health: The Social and Natural Sciences

The notion of 'health' itself has been conceptualized in many ways. Turner (2003) charts the manner in which the concepts of health and illness have changed historically, from primitive societies where they were linked to spiritual notions of purity and danger, to the dominant biomedical, scientific and professional definitions that focus on disease and pathology that affects the body and body parts. In the modern context, though, as he notes, there are still many debates about interpretation. Typically, social scientists view health as a moral norm defining a socially constructed, prescriptive standard that tends towards an ideal of well-being or social functioning – although we know that people in different social groups also define health very differently depending on such variables as social class, gender, ethnic group and age (Scambler 2008). Within this perspective, illness is usually conceptualized as the obverse of health. Social scientists have conceptualized illness as subjectively defined, socially sanctioned and legitimated. It is also socially patterned through the interpretations of individuals themselves and significant others, such as family, friends and health providers (see, for instance, Calnan 1987).

From a social science perspective, the types of study that have been carried out in the health arena from various theoretical viewpoints are very wide ranging. Psychologists, for example, who tend to focus on individuals and small groups, have considered subjects such as the hierarchy of needs (Maslow 1954), health and value systems (Herzlich 1973), psycho-social factors and health (Cassileth et al. 1984), stress and health (Lovallo 2005), health practitioner–client interaction (Purtilo 2007) and the role of psychology in specific health conditions (Straub 2011). Sociologists, on the other hand, who focus more on the broader study of social groups in society, have classically examined such topics as the sick role (Parsons 1951), stigma and adjustment (Goffman 1968), the impact of wider structures of power on health and illness (Navarro 1986), health and lifestyles (Blaxter 1990), inequalities in health (Bartley 2003), the relationship between orthodox and alternative medicine (Saks 2003) and health policy and governance (Kuhlmann and Saks 2008).

From a natural scientific viewpoint, there has been a greater emphasis on the identification and classification of disease categories (see, for instance, Neighbors and Tannehill-Jones 2009), and on the causes of mortality and morbidity, based on objective clinical pathology (as illustrated by Damjanov 2012). Such work focuses less on personal and social contexts of health and more on the biomedical frame of reference – in subjects ranging from infectious diseases (Török et al. 2009) to the implications of genetic structures for the disease process (Panno 2010). Aside from enhancing our understanding of disease and pathology, this has led to considerations of how particular interventions and technologies can best treat disease in individuals (see, among others, Jass 1999) and to the epidemiological study of the incidence and prevalence of particular diseases in groups and communities, not least to facilitate prevention (see, for example, Buettner and Muller 2012) – a subject which is covered in more detail later in this book.

The sciences as more broadly defined, including areas such as economics and statistics as well as more overtly clinical science subjects defining outcomes, significantly underpin health service research that looks at the relationship between the provision, effectiveness and efficiency of health services – as, for example, in relation to surgical interventions for coronary heart disease (Bowling 2009). However, like epidemiology, health service research is genuinely multidisciplinary and is also based on the social sciences. This is well illustrated in terms of health outcome measures. These have traditionally tended to be centred on indicators of morbidity and mortality and physical functioning, drawn from the biomedical sciences. Increasingly now, however, they are focused on wider indicators, such as social functioning, patient-perceived health status and quality of life (Kane and Radosevich 2011).

This outline indicates that research on health, illness and disease can be focused at many different levels in the historic and contemporary context: from the individual to the community, from the activities of patients as health producers to the contribution of informal carers, and from health care assistants with brief training to fully fledged health professionals in the labour force. It can be critically challenging of the higher level structures surrounding health care, as well as being supportive of positive client-centred change on the ground in practice. As such, those concerned with health care may operate in a local, national and/or international context. This is reflected in the range of research undertaken in the health field, as well as in its applicability to different layers of government policy.

Research for Policy

From this viewpoint, we would emphasize that health research using a range of methods may be undertaken not only to gain an understanding of health, illness and disease in contemporary society, but also to contribute to policy development. In this regard, there has been a major change in the culture of health services in the developed world. Not only have clinical interventions become more evidence based, but policy makers too may be more inclined to pivot their policies on interventions that are most efficacious (Kuhlmann and Saks 2008). Recently, clinical science centred on a biomedical model of disease has made a considerable contribution to developing evidence for treatment based on clinical trials and experimental methods. This is witnessed by the Cochrane Collaboration, for example, which since its establishment has driven the growth of international centres for preparing, maintaining and disseminating systematic reviews in health care, typically based on randomized controlled trials (RCTs) (Lancaster et al. 1997).

In the UK specifically, governments over the past 15–20 years have put an emphasis on the maxim: 'what counts is what works' (Rawnsley 2001). In the clinical care arena, this is illustrated by such developments as the National Institute for Clinical Excellence (NICE) that produces clinical guidelines based on research evidence and the National Service Frameworks (NSFs) that seek to develop a firmer foundation for clinical interventions (Brown et al. 2003). NICE includes a remit to reconsider the funding of interventions that are not effective. For balance, it also has a Patients' Council with representatives of consumers and there is a network to support health consumer groups to submit evidence. NSFs, on the other hand, have set the parameters for a framework of policy priorities, in terms of which disease and illness should have priority for funding, along with what are considered to be the most efficacious interventions.

Both clinical and policy research in recent decades have benefited from unprecedented levels of research funding to evaluate interventions and to carry out pilot projects. The National Institute of Health Research (NIHR) Research and Development Programme, directed by the Department of Health, has made substantial research funds available for work on policy priorities such as the cause, care, cure and prevention of dementia and surgical interventions. However, there has been considerable debate and controversy about the validity and utility of the evidence base for clinical and policy guidelines on the efficacy of treatments and the appropriateness of the services provided; evolution has been fast, but not all developments have been based on sound research evidence (Brown et al. 2003). There have also been differences of opinion about the balance between clinical and more social science-oriented research and the role of lay people in providing a perspective and form of knowledge distinct from those of health professionals – as well as about the ethical issues raised in health research explored in Chapter 15. What is apparent is that both nationally and internationally, work on policy issues such as professional governance can be as important for health care users as clinical research itself, although the two are clearly interrelated.

However, we note that the contribution of research has developed unevenly in practice. The prime beneficiary of funds for evidence-based research in the health service in the UK at least has been conventional hospital-based acute care, following the establishment and expansion of scientific medicine (Le Fanu 2011). In contrast, many areas from nursing (Witz and Annandale 2006) and primary care (Saks et al. 2000) to complementary and alternative medicine (Saks 2005) and mental health (Heller et al. 2000) have until recently been Cinderella areas. Nonetheless, this balance in the UK and elsewhere is beginning to change as governments worldwide invest more extensively in health research and associated health policies.

The Readership, Aims and Focus of the Book

In this context, the main readership of this book is intended to be health researchers, academics working in the health field, health care managers, and health practitioners from doctors, nurses and midwives to pharmacists and physiotherapists – together with students on health programmes. In this latter regard, it is designed especially to appeal to those working on courses at a higher undergraduate and postgraduate level who are interested in health research. Although based predominantly on research undertaken in the UK, the aim has been to give the book an international dimension with contributors from other English-speaking countries such as Australia, New Zealand and Canada, as well as from a wider European context. This provides the reader with access to examples of health research undertaken in other countries. It also underlines the trend towards the globalization of health research, which has developed across national boundaries. We have acknowledged this as editors by including Chapter 21, which is dedicated to exploring how to conduct comparative health research by looking at single issues across countries. Although the comparative method presents many challenges, there is much to be learnt from policy and practice in other countries – not least in the health area where research can reveal that what appears immutable in any one country may be context-specific, and far from best practice.

The book has been planned to be clear, accessible and oriented to practice. It provides a distinctive overview in a critical, but constructive, manner of research in the health field. This differentiates it from more general research texts (as exemplified by Argyrous 2005; Bryman 2008; Silverman 2010). Unlike many texts in the health research field, the book also does not focus on a closely defined set of qualitative or quantitative research methods (see, for instance, Green and Thorogood 2004; Scott and Mazhindu 2005; Bruce et al. 2008); specific groups of health practitioners (see, for example, McSherry et al. 2001; Ernst 2006; Gerrish and Lacey 2010); or particular practice contexts such as clinical hospital-based medicine or primary care (as illustrated by Wilson et al. 2000; Earl-Slater 2002; Cosby et al. 2006). Instead, it discusses more expansively how health research methods can be applied more generally and the issues that they raise.

Despite its length, no single book can of course cover in detail all areas of health research. The references in each chapter, therefore, act as a guide to additional study, complementing the focused recommended further reading lists for each chapter. Contributors not only cover the technical issues related to their areas, but also illustrate their accounts with reference to their own personal experience of conducting health research, highlighting its pleasures and pitfalls. The subsequent chapters also contain case studies and conclude with a problem-solving exercise to encourage readers to demonstrate how theory, methods and data interrelate. In addition, chapters are cross-referenced to each other to assist readers in navigating the text.

As an edited collection with a consistent format, the book has the added advantage of drawing on a range of contributions from leading experts in the field. It is therefore distinct from, but complementary to, widely used texts by Bowling (2009) and Bowling and Ebrahim (2005), which take a multidisciplinary approach to health research. In putting this volume together, the editors bring much experience of both writing and editing books on many aspects of health, applying research methods to health and receiving funding from bodies such as the Department of Health, the Economic and Social Research Council and the European Union. Research projects in which they have engaged mutually or separately include using research methods in primary care, professional regulation, orthodox and alternative medicine, consumers in health care, quality assurance in health care and comparative health care (see, for example, Saks et al. 2000; Allsop and Saks 2002; Saks 2003; Baggott et al. 2005; Kuhlmann and Saks 2008; Kuhlmann et al. 2009). They also bring experience of examining doctoral research nationally and internationally, commissioning research and reviewing research protocols, and evaluating research reports through their membership of a range of government policy and research committees. Their experience is complemented by that of the broad span of nationally/internationally recognized specialists in different forms of health research who have written the specific chapters that make up this text.

The Organization of the Book

The book has been organized into parts. The first part starts with contributions on Conducting Health Research. Aside from Chapter 1 on the context for researching health by the editors, Mike Saks and Judith Allsop, it also contains two further building-block chapters relevant to conducting all health research. Chapter 2 is written by Judith Allsop on competing paradigms and health research, which examines different methodological paradigms in the process of the production of research knowledge – with a focus on outlining and evaluating the various dimensions of the more quantitative positivist and more qualitative interpretivist approaches. Chapter 3, on undertaking literature reviews in health, is by Kathryn Jones, who considers the two main types of literature review – the narrative and the systematic review – before going on to describe techniques for undertaking a comprehensive search, and giving guidance on how best to present an analysis of the literature.

Authors in the next two parts on Qualitative Methods and Health and Quantitative Methods and Health were asked to give attention to why the specific research methods concerned should be employed: what kind of research questions could be addressed by the methods and how the data would be gathered using them – including data coding, analysis and presentation. The main areas that authors were requested to address in each chapter on research methods were as follows:

- Definition/elaboration of the research method to be considered.
- The rationale for employing the type of research method concerned.
- Examples of employing the research method in practice.
- Strengths and weaknesses of the research method in question.
- Resources required to apply the method in practice.
- Issues involved in the coding/analysis of data using the research method.
- The identification, writing up and presentation of the findings.
- Questions appropriate to critically appraise the method.
- How to evaluate the findings of research studies that use the method.
- Ethics issues related to the method concerned.

Within this framework, the second part of the book on Qualitative Methods and Health covers a broad span of chapters on research methods written by seasoned qualitative researchers in the field. Andy Alaszewski starts by examining in Chapter 4 the ways in which documents have been and can be used for health research. He describes the nature of documentary research, identifying the resource base needed, assessing the research issues for which it is most appropriate and considering how documentary data can best be analysed. In Chapter 5, Jacqueline Low looks at parallel issues related to the increasing use of unstructured interviews including their advantages and disadvantages, the recruitment of participants and the techniques of both carrying them out and assessing and presenting the data that they produce. While a range of observational methods, including unobtrusive measures, are used in researching health, David Hughes in Chapter 6 provides a specific outline of, and justification for, the extensive use of participant observation in health research. Judith Green in Chapter 7 then considers the use of focus groups in research into health, examining various aspects of the employment of such groups, from their strengths and weaknesses to the resources they require and the ethical issues that they raise. The more general theme of action research in health is addressed by Heather Waterman in Chapter 8, who discusses some of the challenges of action research and how these difficulties can be overcome with positive effects on health and health care.

The third part on Quantitative Methods and Health also draws on the experience of a range of well-established authors, this time in the quantitative area. It begins with Chapter 9 from Peter Davis, Alastair Scott and Martin von Randow, which sets out the fundamental aspects of health sampling methods, with primary reference to probability sampling, drawing on a number of examples from the health field. Michael Calnan in Chapter 10 explains the nature of quantitative survey methods in health research, and describes how to go about using such methods. This chapter is linked to the previous one in so far as sampling is usually employed in conducting large-scale questionnaire surveys. George Argyrous in Chapter 11 clearly describes and evaluates a range of basic statistical methods to analyse the quantitative data deriving from these and other sources in researching health. The basic concepts and principles related to RCTs are then outlined by George Lewith and Paul Little in Chapter 12. Niroshan Siriwardena complements this contribution in Chapter 13 by selectively providing insights into experimental and quasi-experimental methods, which offer alternatives to the RCT in health research. Alan Maynard in Chapter 14 completes this section by writing on the use of economics in health research, in which he sets out a research framework for appraising evidence on cost and effectiveness to inform difficult rationing choices in health care.

The next part of the book deals with a selection of topical issues in health research. Contributors consider a number of contemporary challenges to researchers working in the health field. In the context of the wide range of research methods discussed, they were asked to:

- Define the issues involved.
- Consider the advantages and disadvantages of different approaches.
- Outline how the issues can best be addressed.
- Illustrate these points with examples of their own work in the area concerned.
- Discuss the politics of the process of applying research methods in health in their field.

Accordingly, the fourth part of the book on Contemporary Issues in Researching Health begins with a discussion in Chapter 15 of the increasingly important area of governance and ethics in health research by Priscilla Alderson, who considers the merits of various approaches to ethics review and governance, including how ethical issues can best be addressed in health research. Janet Richardson and Mike Saks in Chapter 16 then explore some of the issues involved in researching the controversial area of complementary and alternative medicine, as opposed to orthodox medicine, in which there is fast-rising public interest. In Chapter 17, Mark Johnson discusses in their wake issues of health research involving ethnic minority groups in a multicultural society. Ellen Kuhlmann and Ellen Annandale take further the analysis of minority groups in research by considering the role of gender in health research in Chapter 18. Stephen Gillam, Penny Cavenagh and Peter Bradley examine various aspects of public health research – including, epidemiology, health needs assessment and social marketing – in Chapter 19. Given the importance of users in lobbying for particular causes, it is most appropriate that Sophie Hill next examines the nature and characteristics of user engagement in health research in Chapter 20. This part of the text ends with Chapter 21 by Viola Burau on comparative health research, which points up the range of international challenges to health research and how these can be tackled.

Finally, the book finishes with an expanded fifth part on Applying Health Research. This begins with Chapter 22 by Jonathan Tritter which examines the advantages and disadvantages of mixed methods and multidisciplinary research in the health context, and also assesses their implications for research design and project management. Chapter 23 is then provided by the editors, Judith Allsop and Mike Saks, and centres on different phases of the research process and the skills involved in writing up a range of forms of health research. Finally, Chapter 24, also by Mike Saks and Judith Allsop, focuses on the central task of disseminating and using health research so that it can be effectively applied in practice, which provides one of the strongest rationales for undertaking research in this area in the first place.

Key Themes in Researching Health

In this volume, several strong substantive and interlinked contemporary themes emerge across the various chapters, in addition to the consideration of a range of quantitative and qualitative research methods. Two particular interrelated themes are highlighted here to illustrate the multidimensional nature of this volume. They include, first, the role of health care users, both patients and carers, in contributing to the research process and, second, the ethics of research in health. Health care users can contribute at all stages of the research process, from helping to determine topics for research to contributing to the publication and dissemination of research findings. They should be considered as participants and partners in health research and are drawn into research in different ways in different projects. There are now usually both institutions and rules to ensure that patients give their informed consent to taking part in research and that they understand what will be involved, as well as rules to protect confidentiality. Nevertheless, there are still underlying issues about power relationships in the research process and debates about whether research is done 'on' or 'for' health care users. There are therefore powerful arguments in favour of trying to ensure that users are active participants in health research, although their involvement poses a range of ethical, scientific and administrative problems that are discussed at different points in this book.

One major methodological theme that also runs through this text is that many current research projects use a mixture of methods and research and are consequently often interdisciplinary. This raises issues of how data collected using different methods can be analysed and integrated into the whole. In many respects, this kind of approach sits uneasily with the traditional model of lone researchers pursuing their own interest and making a career and reputation based on individual publications. The final part of the text will assist singleton researchers, among others, in developing and presenting their work. However, there is no doubt that undertaking research based on the work of teams is now a more typical setting for the career researcher. While this can often pose management problems, there are many benefits that flow from working collaboratively in a team – as the more general experience of inter-professional working in health and other fields amply demonstrates (see, for instance, Day 2007). The concluding part of the book and a number of other chapters comment on the implications of this more collective way of working.

Conclusion

Research in principle, with some caveats, benefits those involved with health, whether as provider, producer or user. This is a very good reason in its own right for conducting research into health. So too is the sheer exhilaration of engaging in health research that can further disciplinary and interdisciplinary knowledge, even where there is no obvious application. However, as we note above, the contribution of research in the health field has developed unevenly in practice.

We trust that this book will contribute in future to growth in both hitherto under-resourced areas of health research and health research more generally in this context. While opportunities for health research are increasing – notwithstanding the very challenging global economic climate – it is significant that the onus on researchers to produce robust results based on sound methods has never been greater (Kuhlmann and Saks 2008). Producing well considered and rigorous results will also be vital if researchers are to make a positive input to policy formation in the fast-changing health field locally, nationally and internationally, as discussed further in Chapter 24. We hope that this book on researching health will assist in this critical process, in shaping the health strategies and activities that lie ahead at all levels and across a wide range of settings.

Recommended Further Reading

Bowling, A. (2009) *Research Methods in Health: Investigating Health and Health Services*, 3rd edition. Maidenhead: Open University Press.
This gives a clear description of a range of selected research methods and has been produced in a third edition to reflect new methodological and other developments.

Bowling, A. and Ebrahim, S. (eds) (2005) *Handbook of Health Research Methods: Investigation, Measurement and Analysis*. Maidenhead: Open University Press.
This book contains a useful set of further readings, with the main aim of helping researchers from different disciplines work collaboratively in health research.

Dyson, S. and Brown, B. (2006) *Social Theory and Applied Health Research*. Maidenhead: Open University Press.
This introductory book highlights in an accessible manner the theoretical context underpinning applied research in the health care field.

Online Readings

Aldred, R. (2008) 'Ethical and political issues in contemporary research relationships', *Sociology*, 42: 887–903.
How do ethical guidelines underline research practice? According to the author what are the key issues that researchers must consider when undertaking research?

Hughner, R., Kleine, S. (2004) 'Views of health in the lay sector: a compilation and review of how individuals think about health', *Health*, 8: 395–422.
According to the authors what are the key ways in which lay people think about health? How does this resonate with your views on health and illness?

References

Allsop, J. and Saks, M. (eds) (2002) *Regulating the Health Professions*. London: Sage.

Andrew, S. and Halcomb, E.J. (eds) (2009) *Mixed Methods Research for Nursing and the Health Sciences*. Chichester: Wiley-Blackwell.

Argyrous, G. (2005) *Statistics for Research*, 2nd edition. London: Sage.

Baggott, R., Allsop, J. and Jones, K. (2005) *Speaking for Patients and Carers: Health Consumer Groups and the Policy Process*. Basingstoke: Palgrave.

Bartley, M. (2003) *Health Inequality: An Introduction to Concepts, Theories and Methods*. Cambridge: Polity Press.

Blaxter, M. (1990) *Health and Lifestyles*. London: Routledge.

Bourgeault, I., Dingwall, R. and de Vries, R. (eds) (2010) *The SAGE Handbook of Qualitative Methods in Health Research*. London: Sage.

Bowling, A. (2009) *Research Methods in Health: Investigating Health and Health Services*, 3rd edition. Maidenhead: Open University Press.

Bowling, A. and Ebrahim, S. (eds) (2005) *Handbook of Health Research Methods: Investigation, Measurement and Analysis*. Maidenhead: Open University Press.

Brown, B., Crawford, P. and Hicks, C. (2003) *Evidence-based Research: Dilemmas and Debates in Health Care*. Maidenhead: Open University Press.

Bruce, N., Pope, D. and Stanistreet, D. (2008) *Quantitative Methods for Health Research: A Practical Interactive Guide to Epidemiology and Statistics*. Chichester: Wiley & Sons.

Buettner, P. and Muller, R. (2012) *Epidemiology*. New York: Oxford University Press.

Bryman, A. (2008) *Social Research Methods*, 3rd edition. New York: Oxford University Press.

Calnan, M. (1987) *Health and Illness: The Lay Perspective*. London: Routledge.

Cassileth, B.R., Lusk, E.J., Strouse, T.B., Miller, D.S., Brown, L.L., Cross, P.A. and Tenaglia, A.N. (1984) 'Psycho-social status in chronic illness: a comparative analysis of six diagnostic groups', *New England Journal of Medicine*, 311: 506–11.

Cosby, R.A., DiClemente, R.J. and Salazar, L.F. (eds) (2006) *Research Methods in Health Promotion*. San Francisco, CA: Wiley.

Daly, J., McDonald, I. and Willis, E. (eds) (1992) *Researching Health Care: Designs, Dilemmas, Disciplines*. London: Routledge.

Damjanov, I. (2012) *Pathology for the Health Professions*, 4th edition. St Louis, MO: Elsevier Saunders.

Day, J. (2007) *Interprofessional Working: An Essential Guide for Health and Social Care Practitioners*. Andover: Cengage Learning.

Dyson, S. and Brown, B. (2006) *Social Theory and Applied Health Research*. Maidenhead: Open University Press.

Earl-Slater, A. (2002) *The Handbook of Clinical Trials and Other Research*. Abingdon: Radcliffe Medical Press.

Ernst, E. (2006) *The Desktop Guide to Complementary and Alternative Medicine: An Evidence-based Approach*. London: Mosby.

Foss, M. and Farine, T. (2007) *Science in Nursing and Health Care*. Harlow: Pearson Education.

Garner, J.B. and Christiansen, T.C. (2008) *Social Sciences in Health Care and Medicine*. Hauppauge, NY: Nova Publishers.

Gerrish, K. and Lacey, A. (2010) *The Research Process in Nursing*. Chichester: Wiley-Blackwell.

Goffman, E. (1968) *Stigma: Notes on the Management of Spoiled Identity*. Harmondsworth: Penguin.

Green, J. and Thorogood, N. (2004) *Qualitative Methods for Health Research*. London: Sage.

Heller, T., Reynolds, J., Gomm, R. and Muston, R. (eds) (2000) *Mental Health Matters: A Reader*. Basingstoke: Palgrave Macmillan.

Henn, M., Weinstein, M. and Foard, N. (2006) *A Short Introduction to Social Research*. London: Sage.

Herzlich, C. (1973) *Health and Illness: A Social Psychological Analysis*. New York: Academic Press.

Jass, J.R. (1999) *Understanding Pathology: From Disease Mechanisms to Clinical Practice*. Amsterdam: Harwood Academic Publishers.

Jenkinson, C. (1997) 'Assessment and evaluation of health and medical care: an introduction and overview', in C. Jenkinson (ed.), *Assessment and Evaluation of Health and Medical Care: A Methods Text*. Buckingham: Open University Press.

Kane, R.L. and Radosevich, D.M. (2011) *Conducting Health Outcomes Research*. London: Jones and Barlett Learning.

Kuhlmann, E., Allsop, J. and Saks, M. (2009) 'Professional governance and public control: a comparison of healthcare in the United Kingdom and Germany', *Current Sociology*, 57: 511–28.

Kuhlmann, E. and Saks, M. (eds) (2008) *Rethinking Professional Governance: International Directions in Healthcare*. Bristol: Policy Press.

Lancaster, T., Shepperd, S. and Silagy, C. (1997) 'Systematic reviews and meta-analysis', in C. Jenkinson (ed.), *Assessment and Evaluation of Health and Medical Care: A Methods Text*. Buckingham: Open University Press.

Le Fanu, J. (2011) *The Rise and Fall of Modern Medicine*, 2nd edition. London: Abacus.

Lovallo, W.R. (2005) *Stress and Health: Biological and Psychological Interactions*, 2nd edition. Thousand Oaks, CA: Sage.

Maslow, A. (1954) *Motivation and Personality*. New York: Harper and Row.

McSherry, R., Simmons, M. and Abbott, P. (eds) (2001) *Evidence-informed Nursing*. London: Routledge.

Navarro, V. (1986) *Crisis, Health and Medicine: A Social Critique*. New York: Tavistock.

Neighbors, M. and Tannehill-Jones, R. (2009) *Human Diseases*, 3rd edition. New York: Delmar Cengage Learning.

Panno, J. (2010) *Gene Therapy: Treatments and Cures for Genetic Diseases*, revised edition. New York: Facts on File.

Parsons, T. (1951) *The Social System*. Glencoe: Free Press.

Purtilo, R.B. (2007) *Health Professional and Patient Interaction*, 7th edition. Philadelphia, PA: Saunders.

Rawnsley, A. (2001) *Servants of the People: The Inside of New Labour*, 2nd edition. London: Hamish Hamilton.

Richardson, A., Jackson, C. and Sykes, W. (1990) *Taking Research Seriously: Means of Improving and Assessing the Use and Dissemination of Research*. London: HMSO.

Saks, M. (2003) *Orthodox and Alternative Medicine: Politics, Professionalization and Health Care*. London: Sage.

Saks, M. (2005) 'Improving the research base of complementary and alternative medicine', Editorial, *Complementary Therapies in Clinical Practice*, 11: 1–3.

Saks, M., Williams, M. and Hancock, B. (eds) (2000) *Developing Research in Primary Care*. Abingdon: Radcliffe Medical Press.

Scambler, G. (ed.) (2008) *Sociology as Applied to Medicine*, 6th edition. London: Elsevier.

Scott, I. and Mazhindu, D. (2005) *Statistics for Health Care Professionals*. London: Sage.

Silverman, D. (2010) *Qualitative Research: Theory, Method and Practice*, 3rd edition. London: Sage.

Straub, R.O. (2011) *Health Psychology: A Biopsychosocial Approach*, 3rd edition. New York: Worth Publishers.

Török, E., Moran, E. and Cooke, F. (2009) *Oxford Handbook of Infectious Diseases and Microbiology*. Oxford: Oxford University Press.

Turner, B.S. (2003) 'The history of the changing concepts of health and illness: outline of a general model of illness categories', in G.L. Albrecht, R. Fitzpatrick and S.C. Scrimshaw (eds), *The Handbook of Social Studies in Health and Medicine*. London: Sage.

Wilson, A., Williams, M. and Hancock, B. (eds) (2000) *Research Approaches to Primary Care*. Abingdon: Radcliffe Medical Press.

Witz, A. and Annandale, E. (2006) 'The challenge of nursing', in J. Gabe, D. Kelleher and G. Williams (eds), *Challenging Medicine*, 2nd edition. London: Routledge.

2

Competing Paradigms and Health Research: Design and Process

JUDITH ALLSOP

Introduction

- Health research plays an important role in public life and is part of popular culture through reports in the media and through web sources. A significant element of public and charity spending is devoted to health research, and health researchers are part of a global network of collaboration through professional and academic organizations and journals. Health research takes many forms, from basic scientific and social research to applied clinical research, as well as epidemiological research that investigates the causes of ill health, health economics that applies economic models to assess the costs and benefits of illness and health care, and translational research that converts research findings into products to be used in the treatment of patients.

- Underlying this diversity are two different philosophical approaches to 'knowing' about the world that guide research practice: the positivist and the interpretivist. Positivism aims to follow scientific principles and methodologies to produce evidence for a knowledge claim. Interpretivism is based on the principle that all knowledge derives from human perception and, therefore, research must take into account how human subjects understand the world. These two approaches to knowledge, or how we come to know about the world, provide a framework to be followed in research practice associated with methods appropriate to address specific research questions.

- In this chapter, the concept of 'paradigms' is used to explain the principles and guidelines embedded in positivist and interpretivist positions and the political and ideological stance they imply. One methodological paradigm is not necessarily better than another. This depends on the context, but the assumptions, or epistemological base of these two approaches, differ and so do the research questions they address. The positivist and interpretivist approaches produce different forms of 'truth-telling' about the social and natural world. The aim is to provide the reader with a critical understanding of the thinking behind each paradigm before engaging with the chapters on particular methods.

In the first section, two paradigms are discussed in turn to highlight the assumptions behind each approach: the implications for knowledge production; the advantages and disadvantages of each methodology; and the types of quantitative and qualitative methods associated with them. The second section discusses the trend in health research towards using a mix of methods. It is argued that the polarization between the two positions has been modified and they may be used in different combinations. This is pursued further in Chapter 22. The third section of the chapter discusses different forms of research design, while the final section discusses the research process and the more practical question of how to get started on a research project. Chapter 23 continues this discussion by following through the different stages of the research process and how to write up research reports and papers.

Positivism and Interpretivism: Contrasting Paradigms

Within the disciplines that contribute to the study of health, illness and disease, health policy and health services, there have been two major approaches to doing research: the positivist and interpretivist. These represent different research paradigms with a contrasting stance towards epistemology, methodology and methods for data collection.

- Epistemology refers to a theory or philosophy about the nature of knowledge and the stance we take on how we come to know what we know about the world.
- A paradigm is a framework for a set of beliefs about what should be studied, what methods should be used and how data should be interpreted for gaining knowledge of the natural or social world.

A paradigm for research is therefore a way of thinking about and doing research that rests on particular assumptions (Kuhn 1970). Paradigms have developed over time and may shift in the future. In 1660, the establishment of the Royal Society aided the development of scientific thinking. This marked the beginning of a paradigm shift towards positivism as a way of knowing and adding to knowledge, which gathered pace in the eighteenth century and by the mid-nineteenth century began to be applied to the practice of medicine (Porter 1997). Later developments in sociology and humanist philosophy in the twentieth century led to a contrasting paradigm for understanding the world that put greater emphasis on human subjectivity (Hughes 2002). Since each approach has a different understanding of the nature of knowledge, positivist and interpretivist approaches are associated with particular types of methodology – that is, particular guidelines and principles for gathering information and assessing evidence. Positivist methodologies tend to be linked to quantitative methods while researchers working within the interpretivist paradigm use qualitative research methods. Health researchers trained in particular disciplines may adopt either a positivist or interpretivist methodology and methods. The terms refer to ways of thinking about knowledge about the natural or social world, and not to disciplines which are substantive fields of study (De Vaus 2002).

Research in the positivist paradigm tends to proceed on the basis of a deductive form of reasoning. The researcher works from a particular body of theory and knowledge and deduces a hypothesis or proposition. This forms the basis for designing and planning a project to collect data that will test the hypothesis. Scientific enquiry was initially based on deductive logic (Williams and May 1996; De Vaus 2002; Bowling 2009). An alternative form of reasoning – inductive reasoning or theory building – starts with observation and/ or data collection, finds patterns or associations and develops theory, or explanations, on the basis of facts and evidence. Either approach can be used in a single health research study, although researchers within the positivist paradigm are more likely to be concerned with theory testing than with theory building, as they tend to begin with a more open research question. This can be represented diagrammatically as set out in Figure 2.1.

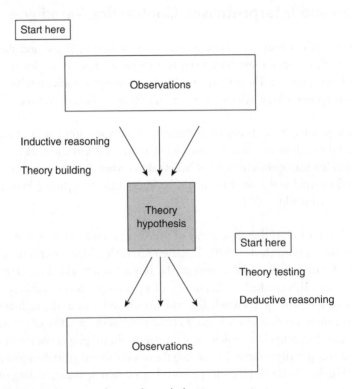

FIGURE 2.1 The positivist research paradigm: deductive reasoning
Source: De Vaus (2002: 6)

Researchers working within either the positivist or interpretivist tradition may use either or both forms of reasoning. For example, Darwin famously built his theories of evolution on his observations of the behaviour of species (Aydon 2002). Subsequently, scientists could use this body of theory to frame their research so as to validate or falsify the findings. For research students, the most important point is to distinguish between these different forms of reasoning and to be aware of how they are being used within their project. In practice, the research process is cyclical, with theory building followed by theory testing which in turn generates new theories to be tested.

The Positivist Paradigm

Most health research is carried out within the positivist paradigm. The various disciplines within the natural and social sciences that investigate the health field share a framework of assumptions and beliefs associated with the philosophical position known as positivism. They employ methodologies that are based on the principles of the scientific method and use methods that are quantitative. Positivism had its roots in the Enlightenment and the development of the natural sciences. The aim of scientists was to discover the general laws and objective facts in the natural world. These principles were taken up by nineteenth-century philosophers and sociologists, such as Comte, Spencer and Durkheim, who aimed to follow the premises of scientific enquiry in studying society (Giddens 1987). They believed that the role of the researcher was to collect and interpret social facts systematically and objectively to identify the laws that governed social life. Their aim was to develop concepts and theories and, by so doing, develop a 'science of man'.

Positivism has been the dominant force in both biomedical and social scientific research in health care to the present day. This is in part due to the rapid rate of development in the sciences in the twentieth century and the perceived success of positivist methods in establishing more evidence-based practice through protocols and guidelines for practice to improve treatment outcomes. In medicine, the book by Cochrane (1972), *Effectiveness and Efficiency: Random Reflections on Health Services*, drew attention to the lack of evidence on the outcomes of treatment interventions and the wide variations in what doctors recommended. The book was influential in focusing health research on establishing an evidence base for clinical interventions through randomized controlled trials (RCTs), seen as the most rigorous method for carrying out research and discussed in Chapter 12 (see also Brown et al. 2003; Greenhalgh 2010). Later, the Cochrane Centre in Oxford, England (www.ukcc.cochrane.org) was founded to act as the hub of a global network for carrying out systematic reviews of clinical trials worldwide. Most recently, patients have been included in an alliance to identify important gaps in knowledge about the effect of treatments. This is discussed further in Chapter 20.

A key assumption of positivist methodologies and methods, as applied in clinical research, is that the body and body parts are taken as objects for research, and that there is a similarity in the body's internal functioning and likely course of the disease process. Based on the biomedical model of disease, such studies approach the patient as a physical/mechanistic entity that can be measured, controlled and ultimately manipulated. Assumptions about the objectivity, neutrality and generalizability of data place most, but not all, biomedical research methods squarely within the positivist paradigm. Positivism in the social sciences is a tradition followed by certain social scientists who aim to follow the basic premises of scientific enquiry. It is assumed that the researcher is able to collect and interpret social facts objectively, and produce laws and models of behaviour from these social facts (De Vaus 2002). The objects for research are seen as external to the researcher, who identifies, observes, counts and measures, following the precepts in Box 2.1 below.

Box 2.1   The features of quantitative methods

- Positivism is linked to quantitative methodologies and methods. The researcher reduces the data collected to numbers and analyses these using statistical and mathematically based techniques.
- Knowledge is gained by discovering the scientific and social laws that govern the world through establishing the facts about the phenomena being studied and drawing causal inferences.
- Knowledge can be produced through the application of a rigorous methodology and methods.
- Researchers can take an objective stance in the research process as they are external to it. Knowledge is seen as cumulative. It is based on a body of theory derived from previous research and refined in the light of subsequent research findings.
- Phenomena exist in the natural and social world as fixed realities that cross cultures.

These are summary points within the positivist paradigm. Theories and previous research are used to generate hypotheses or propositions in the form of research questions that can then be tested by further research. All knowledge is contingent and subsequent research will aim to confirm, modify or refute existing hypotheses through further study. Popper (1959) argued that scientists should aim to falsify their hypotheses rather than seek confirmation, as this is a more rigorous method for establishing new knowledge.

The key questions are those beginning with 'what' and 'why':

- What is going on? 'What' questions aim to obtain an accurate description and provide a foundation for research.
- Why is this happening? 'Why' questions aim to identify and explain causal relationships.

Positivist researchers go to some lengths to identify causal relationships (if X then Y): experiments have control groups to isolate the effects of a single change, as discussed in Chapters 12 and 13. However, it is important to bear in mind that the methods used by positivist researchers cover a wide range of designs. At one end of the spectrum is the RCT where, if bias is excluded and the study double-blinded and properly conducted, it can produce a clear outcome (Altman 2000). If this is replicated by other studies, then it is highly probable that X treatment will lead to Y outcome until it is shown that there are exceptions. However, with other positivist methods such as surveys, described in Chapter 10, causality is not so clear. Surveys using a questionnaire aim to establish correlations between independent and dependent variables in the analysis of results. This can infer cause by association, but does not establish a causal link as in an RCT. Positivist researchers claim that their research methodologies are based on scientific principles and quantitative methods that produce findings that are 'truthful'. The particular strengths in contributing to knowledge are outlined in Box 2.2 below.

Box 2.2   The advantages of quantitative methods

- *Measurement*: being able to demonstrate quantity is a powerful tool in producing reliable data on phenomena in the natural and social world. The measures themselves must be valid and should measure what they say they do.
- *Rigour*: the methods adopted by quantitative researchers are transparent. The methods followed are demonstrable, logical and mathematically and statistically sound.
- *Internal validity:* the methods are able to explain phenomena with independent and dependent variables explaining cause and effect, or through inference and association depending on the method.
- *Generalizability:* the findings of a study can be generalized to a large population – for example through sampling methods.
- *Replicability*: both natural and social scientists are concerned to make their methods transparent so research studies can be replicated by others and knowledge builds. Replication increases the reliability and validity of research findings. This is particularly important in biomedical research as interventions need to be shown to improve health and keep people well.

Critics of positivism base their arguments mainly on the inappropriateness of this approach to researching social life (see Glassner and Moreno 1989; Rubin and Rubin 2005; Silverman 2011; Bryman 2012). In general terms, they see positivism as assuming that the scientific method is the route to understanding human action. Unlike atoms and molecules, social life has a specific meaning for the beings living, acting and thinking within it (Schutz 1962). It is impossible to talk about, understand or communicate social phenomena without employing a particular language or conceptual scheme, as there is no such thing as a neutral stance. Moreover, it is claimed that all research instruments – such as the schedule for a survey, a clinical trial or a structured questionnaire – draw on social and cultural constructions. Researchers choose the questions and interpret the results. Ultimately, therefore, knowledge produced by positivist research methods has an element of subjectivity that may or may not be acknowledged. Some critics go so far as to argue that positivism represents an ideological and political position in the way it views the world (Rubin and Rubin 2005). As indicated in Chapter 18, feminist researchers claim that quantitative research is bound up with male values (Oakley 2000), while others have suggested that ethnic minority groups are side-lined in health research, as noted in Chapter 17. More specific criticisms of positivism are set out in Box 2.3.

Box 2.3   Specific criticisms of positivist methods

- The social world is different from the natural world and cannot be studied objectively in the same way as can objects in the natural world.
- The measures used by positivist researchers are artificial. They measure the constructs of the researcher and not life as it is lived by respondents. For example, surveys of patient satisfaction measure what health service managers think important, not patients' concerns.
- Cross-sectional studies (for instance, surveys) test for associations between variables through questionnaires, but make assumptions about how questions are interpreted – and we cannot be sure that questions have a consistent meaning for respondents.
- Surveys only measure responses at a single point in time, but people have the capacity for change and self-reflection. Their views may change. Questionnaires measure what people say, but this may be at variance with what they do.
- Positivist methods are less good at determining why people act as they do and how decision making is embedded in the complexity of individual social circumstance and relationships. For example, why do people delay in seeking a medical opinion for troubling symptoms when they know that an early diagnosis can prevent serious illness?
- In some situations, the more rigorous experimental methods such as RCTs cannot be used for ethical, practical or financial reasons. For instance, an RCT requires a control group of patients, but it may not be ethical to deny treatment to people who need it.
- Many of the measures used in quantitative studies are constructs or approximate measures. What does a one-off blood test actually measure, apart from a deviation from a predetermined scale? To be meaningful, it has to be interpreted in the context of the person's particular activities and taken over a period of time to establish a norm for that person. What does the concept of 'patient satisfaction' measure without a framework of meaning?

The Interpretivist Paradigm

Social scientists working within the interpretivist paradigm take a contrasting epistemological stance towards knowing about the world. Interpretivism developed due to a dissatisfaction with positivism and to new ways of undertaking social research that developed from the work of Weber (1947). Weber had argued that knowledge depended on *verstehen*, or 'an interpretive understanding of social action'. His view was that actions can only be understood in terms of their meaning for the people taking the action. In turn, a framework of meaning can only be understood in the context of the values, culture and mores of the time. In social life, there are no objective realities to be studied outside their social context. From this perspective, positivists with their claim to objectivity and to the existence of social laws are mistaken about the nature of social reality. The scientific method is not a route to understanding human action.

New methodologies and methods for researching the social world and social action had their origins in the 1920s and 1930s in the Chicago School (Silverman 2004). Sociologists and social psychologists based at the University of Chicago began to study social problems using ethnographic methods. They collected data about communities and groups through observation and developed theories and explanations from this base. In the late 1960s and 1970s, social scientists refocused their research on the ways in which meanings are constructed, negotiated and managed by different individuals and groups. For example, Schutz (1962) commented that in order to understand social action the social scientist had to understand the 'common-sense constructs' that people used to make sense of their world and that drove their actions. He argued that:

> The thought objects constructed by the social scientist, in order to grasp this social reality, have to be founded upon the thought objects constructed by the common sense thinking of people within the real world. (Schutz 1962: 59)

Various qualitative methodologies developed thereafter. Phenomenology was an approach that aimed to study how individuals themselves make sense of their own world. Symbolic interactionism was based on the assumption that the individual is constantly engaged in a process of interpretation through interaction with others. Authors such as Berger and Luckmann (1967), Geertz (1973), Lofland and Lofland (1984) and Rubin and Rubin (2005) held the view that social reality cannot be seen as external to social actors but is constructed through interaction and in response to events. Meaning and social action can only be understood in a specific context. Social researchers began to study health and illness behaviour, the careers of patients with particular illnesses, and how order is negotiated in health care settings through doctor–patient interaction and institutional rules and routines. Examples are the research by Bury (2001) on how people adapt to the onset of chronic illness; the meaning of the onset of symptoms; the process of coming to terms with the illness and the reconstruction of identity; and the study by Strong (1979) of encounters between patients and doctors in paediatric clinics.

Chapters 4–8 describe the methods of data collection commonly, though not exclusively, used by researchers within the interpretivist paradigm. Qualitative methodologies rely heavily on language, although visual images may also be used in research. The methods used to collect data include semi-structured or unstructured interviews, focus groups and observations by the researcher: covert or overt. Other methods include documentary research that draws on personal documents written by people themselves, such as diaries or through retrospective construction – or about them by others as, for example, in the case of hospital records. Qualitative data from focus groups can establish areas where there is a degree of consensus, conflicting views or a range of views. Action research is where the researcher and person or group collaborating on a project aim to bring about social change. These methods are often used where little is known about a research area and where there has been little conceptual or theoretical development. Another more specialist qualitative method is discourse analysis which analyses talk (Potter 1996; Becker et al. 2012). The aim is to show how social phenomena are constructed through language exchange and to identify the rules of talk that operate in different contexts.

All these methods seek to establish an understanding of people's lives and experiences through capturing the subjective meanings of social actors. Rather than seeking to measure attitudes, or predict behaviour through instruments constructed for the purpose, interpretivist researchers focus on understanding the world view of research respondents and how they negotiate meanings in interaction with others. It is identifying this complexity and subjectivity that characterizes qualitative research (Ezzy 2002).

Analysing qualitative data presents a challenge as the data collected must be linked to theoretical concepts and themes in order to reduce the quantity of data and to identify patterns that recur. These provide a basis for generalization. Glaser and Strauss (1967) proposed a systematic approach to the analysis of qualitative data through grounded theory. Here, the researcher aims to develop a theoretical framework for coding data from early on in the data collection process to identify themes. Coding means labelling or categorizing chunks of data. The coding framework is refined during the later stages through a process of 'analytical induction'. This strategy allows themes to be drawn from the data in a way that reflects the understanding of social actors and the way in which they act in the world. These general patterns or themes, it is argued, can be linked to an explanatory theory. Bryman (2012) suggests the term 'abduction' as shorthand for analytic induction. He comments:

> With abduction the researcher grounds a theoretical understanding of the contexts and people he or she is studying in the language, meanings and perspectives that form their world view. The crucial step in abduction is that, having described and understood the world from the perspective of participants, the researcher must come to a social scientific account of the world as seen from those perspectives. (Bryman 2012: 401)

Not all qualitative researchers are at ease with this method on the grounds that it fragments data. Another method is to use a narrative analysis to identify recurrent, or typical, patterns in the way that research participants account for an event or process. Here, the aim is to read interview data or documentary sources as accounts with a characteristic structure that develops in a temporal sequence of stages of adjustment or accommodation. At present, there is no agreement on which method of analysis is best (Silverman, 2011).

The key features of qualitative methods are outlined in Box 2.4.

Box 2.4   The features of qualitative methods

- The subjectivity of research practice is acknowledged. Knowledge is constructed by research subjects. It is not objective and neutral but partial and dependent on social position (class, gender, ethnicity, and so on). The methodologies and methods used seek to understand the subjective meaning of the phenomena to participants and how individual experiences are embedded in society and culture.
- Data are naturalistic: they are collected in the setting of everyday life.
- Data are complex: methods are concerned with the depth of analysis and with explaining the meaning of phenomena and interrelationships, rather than simply making inferences and pointing out associations between variables.
- There is no such thing as value neutrality. It is misleading to see research as something that can take place independently of social relations, including those between the researcher and researched.

It has been argued that there are a number of advantages in using qualitative methods. The main advantages are set out in Box 2.5.

Box 2.5   The advantages of qualitative methods

- *Flexibility in thinking:* researchers are less likely to become stuck in conventional ways of thinking. Rather than merely testing pre-existing ideas, they can make observations that demand the creation of new ideas and categories (Strauss and Corbin 1998; Ezzy 2002).
- *Flexibility in the research process:* researchers can adjust their approach in their interpretation of data. They may find themes or patterns in the data that contradict their initial assumptions.
- *Rich description:* qualitative methods present rich, subjective experience. Findings are based on an empathetic understanding of the views of research participants, whose experiences are embedded in specific social and historical contexts.
- *Compensation:* qualitative methods can be used to investigate areas where quantitative methods are inappropriate, where little is known. Examples are research in sensitive areas where behaviour can cause poor health with social consequences, such as drug taking, heavy drinking, sexual practices that increase risk and studies of informal decision making in organizational settings such as clinics or hospitals.
- *Validity:* such methods are high on internal validity as they draw on understandings of research subjects, but are not necessarily generalizable as they rely on the interpretation of the researcher.

Critics of interpretivist methodologies and methods argue that biological phenomena have a real existence that cannot be explained away. What can be more 'real' than cancer, diabetes or the pain from a broken leg? They are physiological conditions. It is all very well to use qualitative methods to understand society better, but this kind of research does not produce knowledge of use in treating patients and serve to diagnose and treat illness. Positivists' specific criticisms of qualitative methods are set out in Box 2.6.

Box 2.6   The specific criticisms of interpretivist methods

- *Observer bias*: researchers themselves construct categories. In semi-structured interviews, or focus groups, how can a distinction be made between what a participant actually thinks and what they have been prompted to say?
- *Lack of consensus*: qualitative researchers disagree among themselves over methods for data collection and analysis.
- *Lack of focus*: qualitative research is like a fishing expedition: the research question is loosely formulated and theoretical issues are not formulated prior to data collection. There can be data overload and analysis is time consuming.
- *Lack of generalizability*: interviews are often undertaken with a small number of participants. Methods of recruitment may depend on researcher or respondent self-selection through such procedures as snowballing, advertising or recruiting from a narrow base. There is no way of identifying bias or generalizing a larger group.
- *Poor replication:* studies are not replicable and data cannot be generalized so there is no cumulative addition to knowledge.
- *Lack of validity*: there may be internal validity if there is a plausible account, but external validity is absent. Data are interpreted by the researcher and methods of data are often poorly described. Without measurement, the strength of themes is impossible to assess. Anecdotes or snippets illustrate themes, but the question can be posed as to how representative they are.
- *Cost*: qualitative studies are costly in terms of time and therefore may not be cost-effective.

A Paradigm War?

Hammersley (1992) believes that there is a 'paradigm war' between positivism and interpretivism – an irreconcilable conflict between two methodologies that cannot be combined as they produce knowledge that is different in kind. Even if there are different arms to a project, the data from each arm will be not be commensurate. At an epistemological level, social reality cannot be an object for study and also a social construction. A researcher cannot both take an objective stance and at the same time allow for the subjectivity of social actors.

If a purist philosophical position is taken, the two approaches are logically inconsistent or mutually exclusive, and researchers wedded to a particular paradigm cannot accept that there is any alternative way of knowing.

The view in this volume is that one type of method is not superior to another. Rather, each serves a particular purpose, depending on the research question and the orientation of the researcher, but health researchers should be aware of the differences between the two paradigms in order to think critically about the kind of knowledge produced by the methods they use. It could also be argued that this overstates the differences between the positivist and interpretivist positions. The descriptions above present 'ideal types'. An ideal type, according to Weber (1947), is formed by the one-sided accentuation of one or more points of view.

It can also be argued that both positivists and interpretivists have much to contribute to health research practice. Both the biological and the social must be taken into account, from the lens of each of these paradigms. If there is hostility between researchers, there is little opportunity to find ways of working together. The dominance of the positivist paradigm carries a risk that the interests of researchers, health professionals and businesses that supply medical products will skew research priorities – and here there is a potential role for users of health care.

Health researchers have found various ways of working together and using the insights of each paradigm to enrich the research process, as illustrated by Chapter 20 on users of health care. Adjustments to research protocols have allowed patients to play a part in the research process without compromising results. For example, RCTs to evaluate the efficacy of cancer treatments have allowed patients to choose which arm of a trial they wish to enter in a situation where it is not known which of two treatments is likely to be the more effective. Another initiative is the James Lind Alliance where patients, carers and clinicians establish research priorities jointly. This provides an example of positivist researchers engaging with those who benefit from improved services to help determine priorities. One study showed that when patients with osteoarthritis of the knee or hip were asked for research priorities, they rated trials on the efficacy of surgery and physiotherapy above drug trials (Coulter 2011). For their part, some qualitative researchers, particularly those working with local communities, have used the issues identified by the group to shape the health research agenda (Culley et al. 2009). This sets up a situation where participants are partners rather than subjects, moving away from the positivist detached observer role.

Recent Developments: Refining Methods and Mixing Methods

Refining methods

Researchers in the health field have a professional interest in continuing to refine methodologies and methods of enquiry to produce results that can be trusted. As discussed in Chapter 23, a common reason for journal articles to be rejected is inadequate discussion of methods and data analysis (Hargens 1988). Competition for research funding has become more intense and so have procedures and criteria for evaluating research quality. Quantitative researchers carrying out surveys have now to take care to design questions that capture concepts and meaning. The analysis of patient narratives, or stories, has led to understanding the patient perspective and patient pathways through the health system that can contribute to service improvements (Greenhalgh and Hurwitz 1999).

Within both biomedical and social scientific research, patient narratives have been used to understand how a particular illness is understood or to examine patients' pathway through the health system. For example, Charmaz (1997) used semi-structured interviews with a small group of men suffering from a chronic illness to identify strategies to preserve their sense of self over time. Studies can also be made of organizational narratives within institutions such as hospitals, residential homes or clinics from the perspective of participants in different groupings.

Qualitative researchers have written extensively on ways to make data collection and analysis more systematic and produce accounts with greater external validity. Strauss and Corbin (1998) have refined the comparative method to identify and test dominant themes through seeking deviant cases and to test theory by seeking alternative explanations. Silverman (2011) suggests simple forms of counting as part of qualitative analysis to indicate quantity. Triangulation, that is checking data by using another method, has also been used as a strategy and is discussed further in Chapter 22. A further example is that of Bloor (1978), who undertook an observational study of a small number of ENT consultants' procedures in diagnosing the necessity (or not) for a tonsillectomy in their child patients. He checked his accounts with the consultants themselves to ensure they concurred with his analysis and found a high degree of agreement. These refinements in method utilize other methods from the same paradigm and therefore are philosophically congruent with either positivism or interpretivism.

Mixing methods

Since the 1980s, studies using mixed methods that cross the positivist/interpretivist divide have increased in number (Bryman 2012). This suggests a more flexible approach on the part of researchers. Bryman found out why and how a mix of methods was being used. Researchers said they used mixed methods to:

- Give greater validity to a research project by seeking corroborative findings.
- Offset the weaknesses of a single methodology.
- Develop research instruments.
- Deal with unexpected findings.

They used a mix of methods in different ways: as a qualitative element in a predominantly quantitative study; as a quantitative element in a predominantly qualitative study; or in a manner in which both were equally weighted. The methods were also used in different sequences. Qualitative methods have been used in quantitative studies where little is known about the context of the research. For example, focus groups, observations or a small number of unstructured interviews have been employed to provide information for sampling and designing a questionnaire. This helps to refine concepts, identify relevant theories and gain more information on the language, values and perspective of the group to be researched, as well as the likely range of views among participants. Alternatively, if an area has been well researched, and theories are well established, a study may begin with a questionnaire sent to the target population to collect basic descriptive data, with a qualitative study to follow to investigate the dynamics of interaction. Box 2.7 gives examples of two studies using both methods – further illustrations are given in Chapter 23.

Box 2.7 Case studies using quantitative and qualitative methods

This mixed methods design was used in a study by Baggott, Allsop and Jones (2004) to investigate how patient and carer groups represented their members in the policy process. For the first part of the study, a list of groups in five condition areas (arthritis, cancer, heart disease, maternity and mental health) was drawn up from existing databases. A questionnaire based on the positivist paradigm was designed to collect descriptive data on membership, finances and interaction between patient and carer groups and other stakeholders. Data from the questionnaire allowed a sample to be drawn for in-depth interviews with group leaders from an interpretivist perspective to identify the cultural practices that drove internal and external activities and how these differed between condition groups.

A similar sequence was adopted by Broom for his study of Australian men with prostate cancer and their use of the Internet. Broom (2005a, 2005b) began with a pilot survey of men diagnosed with the condition. This used a positivist paradigm in that it sought to establish and quantify patterns in men's experiences of online, as opposed to face-to-face, support groups. This showed positive and negative attitudes towards using an online service but no information on why men felt the way they did. In order to understand the cultural factors that shaped these men's perceptions of the Internet, an in-depth exploratory study was undertaken to investigate ways in which online support groups made an impact on the lives of respondents. The qualitative data showed how men with prostate cancer negotiated their masculinity and came to understand the nature of cyberspace.

In both these studies, two contrasting methods were used to show different aspects of group/individual activity. A mix of methods was used to provide a sample for a second qualitative study. The aim was not to triangulate, or corroborate, findings but to explain the dynamics of, and rationale for, behaviour. Potential users of mixed methods, though, should bear in mind that employing this approach adds to complexity and is therefore challenging.

Research Design and the Research Process

This section considers the more practical aspects of doing research by introducing the concept of research design, followed by a discussion of the early stages of the research process. Research design refers to the structure, or architecture, of a project: the analogy of a building has been used to express the concept of a research design. Buildings have a particular structure to suit their purpose. There will be guidelines and principles to be followed in their construction (methodology). Various methods (quantitative or qualitative) will be used to construct the building and certain materials (instruments) will be required. The purpose of the analogy is to make a distinction between a research design and research methods (De Vaus 2002). For each category of design, a range of quantitative or qualitative methods may be used. Prior to starting on a research project, three questions must be addressed:

- What is my research question?
- What research design am I using to address the question?
- What methods am I going to use and are they quantitative or qualitative?

Research design

The term research design may either refer to a typology of designs: experimental, cross-sectional, case study, longitudinal and comparative (De Vaus 2002), or be a term used more generally to describe a particular combination of methods used to investigate a research question. Some of the chapters in this volume use it in this way. Whichever concept is used, the overall design of a project should be mapped out before deciding on particular methods. As Figure 2.2 below shows, a range of methods may be used within any of these categories of design.

Experiments are set up to test a hypothesis within any of the natural or social science disciplines, although they are more common in the clinical sciences and psychological studies. However, there have been recent examples of experiments to change attitudes in public policy (John et al. 2011) referred to in Chapter 19, and in Chapters 12 and 13 to determine the effect of an intervention. In essence, experiments seek to introduce an independent variable and control for a range of other variables, in order to identify the

Design type	Experiment	Cross-sectional	Case study	Longitudinal	Comparative
Method of data collection	Questionnaire	Questionnaire	Questionnaire	Questionnaire	Questionnaire
Method of data collection	Interview	Interview	Interview	Interview	Interview
Method of data collection	Observation	Observation	Observation	Observation	Observation
Method of data collection	Document analysis	Document analysis	Document analysis	Document analysis	Document analysis

FIGURE 2.2   The range of methods on offer
Source: De Vaus (2002: 10)

effect of the independent variable by using one of two or more groups in a before-and-after study. If experiments involve human subjects, their informed consent is required. If there is a control group, this allows for a causal explanation of the effect of introducing the independent variable. An RCT that is double-blinded is the most highly developed form of experiment. It is known that not blinding a trial introduces bias (Schulz et al. 1995). Experiments are rare in sociology and social policy due to the difficulties in setting up a control group and manipulating the independent variable. For example, if we wished to test the effect of social class on health status, it would not be possible to do this through an experiment because social class is an attribution that cannot be changed. It is also ethically contentious to have a control group where treatment is denied – as in an experiment to test the efficacy of a walk-in psychotherapeutic service for people with mental illness. However, as highlighted by the experiments in public policy in Chapter 19, there may be opportunities for a researcher to study naturally occurring situations. This is illustrated by the case of a school vaccination session where, in error, one of two batches of ampoules contained one and a half times the standard measure. This could provide an opportunity to record which children had received the correct amount against the group who had not, and recall the children at defined intervals to check for a specified range of side-effects.

Cross-sectional designs refer to studies that require the collection of data from a number of subjects/objects over a specified time, with the aim of establishing an association between variables. Methods can be quantitative where questionnaires or structured interviewing are used to collect data from more than one, and often a very large number of, respondents. The aim is to capture variation by using the same tool to measure difference and draw inferences from associations between variables. If the methods are sound, the findings can be extrapolated to larger populations, as indicated in Chapters 10 and 11. Data can also be collected through qualitative methods based on either documentary evidence or covert or open observation, as discussed in Chapters 4 and 6. The characteristic of this form of research design is that data are collected at the same time or within a short period of time. The aim is to select particular criteria to establish similarity and difference across the units being analysed to make generalizations (De Vaus 2001).

Case study designs involve a single organization, place or person as the subject of research. The case is the unit of analysis, and the research methods focus on the circumstances, dynamics and complexity of a single or small number of cases. Yin (2009) defines five types of case: the critical, the unique, the typical, the revelatory and the longitudinal. An example of a case study is the research by Korman and Glennerster (1990) on the closure of a large mental handicap hospital. A number of methods were used to collect both quantitative and qualitative data. Bryman (2012) warns that the term 'case study' is often used loosely. Some so-called case studies are in fact cross-sectional studies.

Longitudinal designs study phenomena over time. They require a significant investment of resources and large teams so they are unlikely to be used by student researchers. An example of a longitudinal study is the National Child Development Study (www.esds.ac.uk/longitudinal/access/ncds). Data, including on health, illness and disability, were collected from a sample of children born in one week in 1958. Questionnaires and interviews were used to collect data for that year and at intervals subsequently. The design allows for a number of very interesting and profound questions about the influence of childhood events on, for example, health in adult life (Wadsworth 1991).

Comparative design is based on the value of studying similarity and difference between two or more contrasting cases. Typically, the same phenomenon is compared within two or more contrasting socio-cultural settings such as institutions, customs, traditions and cultures. Studies may be cross-national, cross-regional or cross-institutional. Studies use the same methods for data collection in each setting. For example, there can be a secondary analysis of national data followed by data collection through a questionnaire or observation. If the study is cross-national, particular problems can arise in identifying comparable concepts and data, and in dealing with institutional differences. These are discussed in Chapter 21.

The research process

This chapter concludes with some general guidelines on starting on a small-scale research study for an undergraduate course, or a dissertation for a postgraduate degree or doctorate.

These differ in the depth of theoretical sophistication and scope of empirical research between what is expected for, say, a 10,000-word project and an 80,000-word PhD, but the general principles apply to all forms of research. The activity of research is essentially a problem-solving exercise that requires project management skills as much as intellectual ability. Chapter 23 provides further details on how to proceed with your research after your initial proposal is accepted.

Task 1: What are the requirements for my project?

Institutions or courses will have information on producing a research project. There will be timescales for presentation of the finished study with instructions on length and other matters. These must be followed. You will have a tutor/supervisor to guide you through the process and you should see them at regular intervals. If things do not work out with them, ask to change.

End point: Obtain the required information.

Task 2: Decide on a topic for your research

A topic must be translated into a research question or a number of related questions. There are likely to be both What and Why questions. A question is likely to be answerable if it is explicit, focused and feasible. Your own life, experience and interests may provoke questions, or ideas may come from your immediate circle of friends and family. Almost everyone has experience of episodes of health and illness, has looked after others who have been ill or has used health services. You may have read something that identifies a puzzle or a gap in knowledge. Curiosity about why things are as they are, persistence in working through ideas and finding out what has already been written about the subject are important (see Denscombe 2010 on types of research question). Chapter 3 in this volume provides techniques for carrying out a literature review – finding out what data are available and what others have written. Chapters 4 to 14 provide a guide to methods in the health field and give examples of the type of research questions that can be investigated, while Chapters 15 to 21 give an indication of some interesting contemporary issues in the health field. Do not forget that it is possible to replicate an existing study or re-analyse existing data sets. Some survey agencies, such as IPSOS MORI, have data that they have not fully analysed. The University of Essex holds a data archive with a catalogue (www.data-archive.ac.uk) and so have many other institutions.

End point: Give yourself a time target for providing a short description of your project topic with questions and discussing it with others and your supervisor.

Task 3: Writing a proposal

Writing a proposal requires thinking through how to answer the research question(s). What is the purpose of the research in the context of related studies, theoretical explanations and key concepts? What is the research design: an experiment, a cross-sectional study, a case study or a comparative study? What methods will be used to gather data? How will the data be collected? How will access to research participants be achieved? How will the anonymity of participants be safeguarded? How will the confidentiality of data be maintained? How will data be analysed? What resources will be needed for data collection?

End point: provide a written proposal to be agreed with your supervisor.

A basic structure for a research plan is set out in Box 2.8.

Box 2.8   Elements of a research plan

- A short descriptive title
- The aims of the project: your research questions
- The objectives, or rationale for the project: the problem to be addressed, the existing literature, the key concepts and theory to be used
- The research design
- The method(s) for data collection and rationale
- Access to participants/institutions
- Data storage
- Method of analysis
- The resources needed
- The timetable for the research
- Ethical issues.

Conclusion

This chapter aimed to give health researchers a critical understanding of the positivist and interpretivist paradigms that inform quantitative and qualitative methodologies and methods. It has outlined the features, advantages and criticisms of each type of approach in terms of knowledge production. Until recently, positivist research methodologies have been seen by many stakeholders within the health care community as the only useful way of providing evidence to practitioners and patients. It is still the case that research funding is more likely to be awarded to researchers using quantitative methods. However, qualitative approaches have advantages in researching areas not amenable to quantitative methods. Researchers on either side of the quantitative/qualitative divide are concerned with the quality and rigour of their research and have become more flexible in their approach. A mix of methods from each paradigm can provide a greater depth of understanding. Ultimately, the appropriateness and usefulness of a particular paradigm is tied to the nature of the research question asked and the skills and inclinations of the researcher. This point is tested out in the exercise for the reader below on research into prostate cancer.

Exercise: Different methodological approaches to researching the use of the Internet in the case of men with prostate cancer

Based on what you have read in this chapter, what different sorts of information are yielded by the data sources set out in Boxes 2.9 and 2.10 centred on the work conducted by Broom (2004) in a study of Australian men with prostate cancer? Which do you think are the most important? Give reasons for your answer.

Box 2.9 An example of questions from a pilot survey (a quantitative method) with results

Selected Questions

Data

1 = strongly disagree; 2 = disagree; 3 = neutral; 4 = agree; 5 = strongly agree

| 1 | It would be easier to share my personal experiences in an anonymous environment like an online (Internet) support group. | 1 | 2 | 3 | 4 | 5 |
| 2 | In face-to-face support groups, the threat of embarrassment stops some men from sharing concerns about fears, emotional distress, symptoms or complications of treatments. | 1 | 2 | 3 | 4 | 5 |

Results

Of the 50 men surveyed, 46 per cent agreed that it would be easier to share their experiences online. Approximately 30 per cent of respondents agreed that face-to-face support groups can deter self-expression.

Box 2.10   A qualitative in-depth interview study and example of output

Selected interview themes:

The reasons patients gave for their decision of whether or not to use online support groups.

Patients' perceptions of the benefits and limitations of online support.

Examples of data:

Andrew: 'One of the things you find is an amazing openness and frankness about these sort of matters that I'm sure men if they were meeting face-to-face would not talk about ... we're doing it through this medium [the Internet] and we can be a lot more frank ... There's the anonymity, there's the disembodiment ... you're able to project in a way that isn't having any comeback on you.' (Six months' post-treatment, organ-confined disease, Internet user/online support, 40–50 years)

David: 'Some men don't want to be face-to-face. Maybe they're frightened of it; maybe they don't want to travel the distances. Maybe they're scared of being ridiculed or something ... all sorts of reasons like that. Maybe they're a bit anxious about having the problem [prostate cancer] and not wanting to share it with other people. I think that's men for you. Some will find it easier to talk online.' (Three years' post-treatment, organ-confined disease, Internet user/online support, 61–70 years)

Acknowledgement

This chapter has been developed from 'Competing Paradigms and Health Research' by Alex Broom and Evan Willis in the previous edition of this book. Their case study and exercise that appeared in the first edition have not been changed.

 ## Online Reading

Moore, S. (2010) 'Is the healthy body gendered? Toward a feminist critique of the new paradigm of health', *Body and Society*, 16: 95–118.
How different is the new paradigm of health to the old paradigm? How does feminism challenge the new and old paradigm? Does practice always change with new paradigms?

Atkins, M. And Frazier, S. (2011) 'Expanding the toolkit or changing the paradigm: Are we ready for a public health approach to mental health?', *Perspectives on Psychological Science*, 6: 483–87.

How do paradigm shifts challenge current practice? What are the biggest barriers to adopting new ways of thinking about health and illness? How can research help support the adoption of new practices?

Recommended Further Reading

Brown, B., Crawford, P. and Hicks, C. (2003) *Evidence-based Research: Dilemmas and Debates in Health Care*. Maidenhead: Open University Press.

This book focuses on charting the philosophical background and debates surrounding the use of health research methods, including the importance of paradigms.

Bryman, A. (2012*) Social Research Methods*, 4th edition. Oxford: Oxford University Press.

This is highly recommended as a comprehensive and up-to-date text on quantitative and qualitative methods that is written with research students in mind. It is well referenced so that readers can easily find answers to their questions.

De Vaus, D. (2002) *Research Design in Social Research*. London: Sage.

This book deals with the technical questions of research design.

Silverman, D. (2011) *Interpreting Qualitative Data: Methods for Analysing Talk, Text and Interaction*, 4th edition. London: Sage.

This is a useful book for researchers wishing to analyse and interpret qualitative data.

References

Altman, D. (2000) 'Blinding in clinical trials and other studies', *British Medical Journal*, 321: 504.

Aydon, C. (2002) *Charles Darwin: The Story of the Amateur Naturalist who Created a Scientific Revolution and Changed the World*. London: Constable.

Baggott, R., Allsop, J. and Jones, K. (2004) *Speaking for Patients and Carers: Health Consumer Groups and the National Policy Process*. London: Palgrave.

Becker, S., Bryman, A. and Ferguson, H. (eds) (2012) *Understanding Research: Methods and Approaches for Social Work and Social Policy*. Bristol: Policy Press.

Berger, P. and Luckmann, T. (1967) *The Social Construction of Reality: A Treatise in the Sociology of Knowledge*. London: Allen Lane.

Bloor, M. (1978) 'On the analysis of observational data: a discussion of the worth and uses of inductive techniques and respondent validation', *Sociology*, 12(3): 545–57.

Bowling, A. (2009) *Research Methods in Health*, 3rd edition. Maidenhead: Open University Press.

Broom, A. (2004) 'Virtually he@lthy: the impact of Internet use, by Australian men with prostate cancer, on patient/medical specialist interaction and disease experiences', PhD thesis, La Trobe University, Australia.

Broom, A. (2005a) 'The eMale: prostate cancer, masculinity and online support as a challenge to medical expertise', *Journal of Sociology*, 41(1): 87–104.

Broom, A. (2005b) 'Virtually he@lthy: a study into the impact of Internet use on disease experience and the doctor/patient relationship', *Qualitative Health Research*, 15(3): 325–45.

Brown, B., Crawford, P. and Hicks, C. (2003) *Evidence-based Research: Dilemmas and Debates in Health Care*. Maidenhead: Open University Press.

Bryman, A. (2012) *Social Research Methods*, 4th edition. Oxford: Oxford University Press.

Bury, M. (2001) 'Illness narratives: fact or fiction?', *Sociology of Health and Illness*, 23: 263–85.

Charmaz, C. (1997) *Good Days, Bad Days: The Self in Chronic Illness and Time*. New Brunswick, NJ: Rutgers University Press.

Cochrane, A. (1972) *Effectiveness and Efficiency: Random Reflections on Health Services*. London: Nuffield Provincial Hospitals Trust.

Coulter, A. (2011) *Engaging Patients in Healthcare*. Buckingham: Open University Press.

Culley, L., Hudson, N. and Rooij, F. (2009) *Marginalised Reproduction: Ethnicity, Reproduction and Reproductive Technology*. London: Earthspan.

Denscombe M. (2010) *Ground Rules for Good Research: Guidelines for Good Practice*, 2nd edition. Maidenhead: Open University Press.

De Vaus, D. (2001) *Surveys in Social Research*, 5th edition. London: Routledge.

De Vaus, D. (2002) *Research Design in Social Research*. London: Sage.

Ezzy, D. (2002) *Qualitative Analysis: Practice and Innovation*. Crows Nest, Australia: Allen & Unwin.

Geertz, C. (1973) *The Interpretation of Cultures: Selected Essays*. New York: Basic Books.

Giddens, A. (1987) *Positivism and Sociology*. London: Heinemann.

Glaser, B. and Strauss, A. (1967) *The Discovery of Grounded Theory: Strategies for Qualitative Research*. Chicago, IL: Aldine.

Glassner, B. and Moreno, J. (1989) 'Introduction: quantification and enlightenment', in B. Glassner and J. Moreno (eds), *The Qualitative–Quantitative Distinction in the Social Sciences*. Boston, MA: Kluwer Academic.

Greenhalgh, T. (2010) *How to Read a Paper: The Basics of Evidence-based Medicine*. Chichester: Wiley & Sons.

Greenhalgh, T. and Hurwitz, B. (1999) 'Why study narrative?', *British Medical Journal*, 318: 48–50.

Hammersley, M. (1992) 'The paradigm wars: reports from the front', *British Journal of the Sociology of Education*, 13: 131–43.

Hargens, L.L. (1988) 'Scholarly consensus and rejection rates', *American Sociological Review,* 53: 139–51.

Hughes, S. (2002) *Consciousness and Society.* Piscataway: Transaction Publishers.

John, P., Cotterill, S., Moseley, A., Richardson, L., Smith, G., Stoker, G. and Wales, C. (2011) *Nudge, Nudge, Think, Think. Experimenting with Ways to Change Civic Behaviour.* London: Bloomsbury Academic Publishing.

Korman, N. and Glennerster, H. (1990) *Hospital Closure.* Milton Keynes: Open University Press.

Kuhn, T. (1970) *The Structure of Scientific Revolutions.* Chicago, IL: University of Chicago Press.

Lofland, J. and Lofland, L. (1984) *Analysing Social Settings: A Guide to Qualitative Observation and Analysis,* 2nd edition. Belmont, CA: Wadsworth.

Oakley, A. (2000) *Some Experiments in Knowing: Gender and Method in the Social Sciences.* Cambridge: Polity Press.

Popper, K. (1959) *The Logic of Scientific Discovery.* London: Hutchinson.

Porter, R. (1997) *The Greatest Benefit to Mankind: A History of Medicine.* London: Harper Collins.

Potter, J. (1996) *Representing Reality: Representing Discourse, Rhetoric and Social Construction.* London: Sage.

Rubin, H. and Rubin, I. (2005) *Qualitative Interviewing: The Art of Hearing Data,* 2nd edition. London: Sage.

Schulz, F., Chalmers, I., Hayes, R. and Airman, D. (1995) 'Empirical evidence of bias: dimension of methodological quality associated with estimates of treatment effects in controlled trials', *Journal of the American Medical Association,* 273: 408–12.

Schutz, A. (1962) *Collected Papers I: The Problem of Social Reality.* The Hague: Martinus Nijhof.

Silverman, D. (2004) *Qualitative Research: Theory, Method and Practice,* 2nd edition. London: Sage.

Silverman, D. (2011) *Interpreting Qualitative Data: Methods for Analysing Talk, Text and Interaction,* 4th edition. London: Sage.

Strauss, A. and Corbin, J. (1998) *Basics of Qualitative Research,* 2nd edition. London: Sage.

Strong, P.M. (1979) *The Ceremonial Order of the Clinic.* London: Routledge.

Wadsworth, M. (1991) *The Imprint of Time: Childhood and Adult Life.* Oxford: Clarendon Press.

Weber, M. (1947) *The Theory of Social and Economic Organisation.* New York: Free Press.

Williams, M. and May, T. (1996) *Introduction to the Philosophy of Social Research.* London: UCL Press.

Yin, R.K. (2009) *Case Study Research: Design and Methods,* 4th edition. Los Angeles, CA: Sage.

3

Doing a Literature Review in Health

KATHRYN JONES

Introduction

- The literature review aims to identify, analyse, assess and interpret a body of knowledge related to a particular topic and is normally required as part of a dissertation or thesis. In this case, it sets a context for a research study and provides a rationale for addressing a particular research question in the light of an existing body of literature. Research proposals to funding bodies also typically include a literature review. Here the purpose is to justify the proposal in terms of a gap in existing knowledge. Some literature reviews are substantive, stand-alone studies in their own right that serve to assess what is known and what is not known in an area of study. The aim is to show how a particular topic has been approached by other scholars. Within the health field, the literature review can also aim to assess existing knowledge on the efficacy of an intervention, such as the evidence base for the preferred treatment of a particular disease, or the response to a social problem.

- This chapter describes how to undertake a rigorous and thorough review of the literature and is divided into three sections. The first section examines the two main types of review: the narrative and the systematic review. The second section describes techniques for undertaking a comprehensive search, while the third gives guidance on how an analysis of the literature can be presented. It is assumed in the chapter that those undertaking a review will have access to college or university library resources and to the Internet. The majority of sources can now be accessed electronically. Those who have not previously searched using an online catalogue or database are advised to seek assistance prior to starting out. Most college and university libraries offer courses, publish guidelines or make help available online. Throughout the chapter, examples are drawn from recent studies undertaken by the author and others.

Types of Literature Review

All reviews aim to provide an overview of what is known about a particular phenomenon and what the gaps in knowledge are (see, for example, Aveyard 2010). However, narrative reviews, which are used widely in social scientific research, place an emphasis on identifying the key concepts or specific terms used in the literature and the particular theoretical approaches adopted by different authors to understand a phenomenon. Concepts and theories may be employed implicitly or explicitly in the investigation of a topic. A review of the literature will identify the range of approaches and offer a critique of their contribution to knowledge (on approaches relating to grounded theory, see Dunn 2011).

A systematic review of the literature in health and social care has a different focus. It aims to contribute to practice through an assessment of the efficacy of a particular health care intervention and underpins much evidence-based practice. Initially developed as a means for synthesizing quantitative research, in recent years the value of systematic reviews on qualitative research has been acknowledged (Suri 2011). A basic overview is given here but the researcher should seek advice from a trained information specialist prior to undertaking a systematic review.

The narrative review

The narrative review is the most common form of literature review. It aims to show how concepts, theories and methods have developed within particular subject areas. The key differences between concepts, theories and methods are:

- Concepts: terms and ideas used to describe a particular phenomenon.
- Theories: ideas that have been developed to explain a specific phenomenon.
- Empirical research: research that has already been undertaken to observe the phenomena.
- Methodology: the philosophical approach adopted by a researcher to study a particular phenomenon and not to be confused with methods.
- Methods: techniques such as questionnaires, observation or interviewing used to collect data.

In a narrative review, the reviewer offers a critique in order to assess, analyse and synthesize previous research, and place it in its current context. The review can take a number of forms: a chapter within a dissertation showing the context of the research; a section of a proposal justifying the work; or a stand-alone summation of thinking about a particular subject area. In each, the reviewer draws on and critiques the conceptual and theoretical approach of different authors and offers an assessment and interpretation.

When reading the item concerned, the reviewer seeks to identify the particular conceptual and theoretical approach taken by the author. This is likely to be influenced by the author's background and discipline. So, for example, a political scientist interested in public involvement in health policy making is likely to draw on theories related to interest groups in the policy process, participation and representation. A sociologist of health and illness writing on the same topic might place their work in the context of people's experience of illness and how this may affect their wish to participate in decisions and policy making. Identifying the conceptual and theoretical approaches taken by different authors is the first step to understanding the literature and, in the writing up stage, will influence the structure of the report, another vital component of the narrative review, as will be seen below.

The systematic review

Over the past few decades, evidence-based practice has achieved growing recognition as a means of increasing the efficacy of health care interventions. Initiatives such as the international Cochrane Collaboration (see Chapter 20 for a fuller description) and organizations such as the National Institute for Health and Clinical Excellence in England assess available evidence to inform guidelines, policy and practice. A systematic review enables the reader to appraise critically the most robust evidence available in an attempt to synthesize what is known, and not known, about the efficacy of a particular intervention. According to Petticrew (2001), systematic reviews can be characterized by the following criteria:

- They aim to answer a particular question or test a hypothesis – usually in relation to a specific health care intervention on a particular population group.
- They attempt to be as exhaustive as possible, identifying all known references.
- Studies included in the review are chosen as a result of explicit inclusion and exclusion criteria. They assess the evidence and provide a synthesis of results based on the thoroughness of a study's research method.

Systematic reviews place an emphasis on judging the quality of evidence. Here, the priority is to utilize studies where the research design minimizes bias – as highlighted by the list below showing the traditional hierarchy of evidence for reviews that assess the effectiveness of a particular intervention. Street (2001) notes that the quality levels of evidence in systematic reviews of health care interventions can be categorized as follows:

- Level I: evidence obtained from a systematic review of all relevant randomized controlled trials.
- Level II: evidence obtained from at least one properly designed randomly controlled trial.
- Level III.1 : evidence obtained from a well-designed controlled trial without randomization.
- Level III.2: evidence obtained from a well-designed cohort or case-control analytic study, preferably from more than one centre or research group.

- Level III.3: evidence obtained from multiple time series with or without the intervention, or dramatic results in an uncontrolled experiment.
- Level IV: the opinion of respected authorities based on clinical experience, descriptive studies or a report from an expert committee.

Clearly, this hierarchy is biased towards quantitative research, but across health care and the social sciences there is a strong history of qualitative research that explores the experience and perspectives of people living with a particular medical condition or welfare intervention. If a review is attempting to understand why a particular intervention works, rather than what interventions work, then other research methods, including qualitative studies, are likely to provide more relevant data (Dixon-Woods et al. 2001; Graham and McDermott 2006). Guidelines for approaching a qualitative synthesis in systematic reviews have been developed and a growing body of research is pointing to their value in building evidence-based policy (Petticrew and Roberts 2006). For example, Graham and McDermott (2006) used a synthesis of qualitative studies on teenage mothers in the UK to offer additional insights and provide further understanding of how teenage mothers experience social exclusion. They argued that the use of such evidence was necessary, given policy makers' increasing emphasis on public engagement in service development. The authors adopted the approach by Noblit and Hare (1988) to meta-ethnography. Here, findings from disparate studies were cross-checked in a matrix, and used to identify 'second-order inferences' or new interpretations of existing data. In a similar way to quantitative synthesis, a key aspect of qualitative reviews is the establishment of an audit trail of search parameters and explicit criteria for article selection. However, a qualitative synthesis does allow more flexibility in selecting studies with different research designs, and the approach to synthesis gives greater acknowledgement of the interpretivist paradigm which underpins much social science research (Suri 2011).

A specialized technique in quantitative systematic reviews is the use of a meta-analysis where the results from studies identified in a literature search are reanalysed and reinterpreted. The use of statistical techniques can account for differences in quantitative methods and enables the researcher to pull together the findings of numerous studies to offer a more substantive assessment of the available evidence. This is particularly useful when studies are based on a small sample. However, meta-analysis is a highly sophisticated tool and should only be undertaken by researchers with statistical skills. The NHS Centre for Reviews and Dissemination at York (www.york.ac.uk/inst/crd) provides useful guidelines that explain the various statistical techniques available.

The key source for identifying systematic reviews is the Cochrane Collaboration, an international network of those working on systematic reviews (www.cochrane.co.uk). Its website includes a searchable database. The TRIP (Turning Research into Practice) database of evidence-based articles covering medical science may also be searched (www.tripdatabase.com), alongside the Bandolier website (www.medicine.ox.ac.uk/bandolier).

In addition, it may be useful to search the EPPI-Centre database (Evidence for Policy and Practice) for systematic reviews in the social sciences and public policy (www.eppi. ioe.ac.uk).

Carrying Out a Literature Search

This section outlines good practice in how to undertake a literature search: that is, how to set search parameters; identify appropriate databases; write a search strategy; and record results (for further guidance, see Gash 2000). In a sense, literature searching is like detective work – the aim is to identify the most appropriate sources to answer a question within a field of study. The key sources used by information specialists are listed below:

- Bibliography: a bibliography is a list of publications relating to a particular subject area.
  - o *General bibliographies*: the *British National Bibliography* published online by the British Library, provides a searchable list of all new books published in the UK (http:// bnb.bl.uk).
  - o *Specialist subject bibliographies*: produced by research centres, scholars or specialist information services, such as the US National Library of Medicine or the King's Fund library.
  - o *Publications*: journal articles note the works the author has quoted in a list of references at the end. Research monographs and textbooks will also provide a list of sources but will often include all items read by the author rather than just those quoted in the text.
- Catalogues: most academic libraries and specialist institutions maintain a catalogue that shows the details and location of all items in stock. This is the most obvious place to start any search. COPAC (www.copac.ac.uk) is the merged catalogue of a number of university libraries and the British Library and national libraries of Scotland and Wales. Most academic libraries have reciprocal access arrangements for students via the SCONUL scheme (www.sconul.ac.uk).
- Abstracting and indexing journals: an abstract is a short summary of an academic journal article. This is an aid to assessing relevance without reading the full article:
  - o *Abstracting journals* provide details of articles drawn from a range of journals within a particular subject area. They tend to be arranged alphabetically by author, with a subject index to locate relevant papers.
  - o *Indexing journals* are usually arranged in subject order and provide basic bibliographic details of articles (title, author, journal, date, volume, page numbers).

Most abstracting and indexing journals are now available electronically on specialist databases. The Internet and electronic sources have made the search process quicker and broadened the range of sources that can be accessed. This can be a problem as an overwhelming number of potentially useful articles may be retrieved. It is imperative, therefore, to plan a search effectively, and to review the strategy as the search progresses.

Library catalogues typically allow searches based on author, title, subject classification and keyword. Subject codes are assigned to books and other publications using classification schemes such as the Dewey Decimal System. The majority of classification systems are based on numeric codes. For example, in the Dewey System, books on the medical sciences are located at 610. In addition, most cataloguers apply keywords to publications. The classification of articles in electronic databases is more sophisticated and has a higher degree of specificity than items in library catalogues. In other words, database searching can be more precise and retrieve more items of relevance as they are coded in more depth. A number of subject headings are assigned to summarize the coverage of each article. An example is the US National Library of Medicine, which uses MeSH (Medical Subject Headings) in the Medline database. In addition, databases assign keywords to each item drawn from the abstract or provided by the author. Some databases also make abstracts searchable. A keyword or abstract search can be a useful way to narrow down the focus of a search.

The reviewer may use various sources to identify the best database to search. Most academic libraries produce guides to the subject areas they cover and list the databases they subscribe to. It is usually possible to check where journals are abstracted and indexed on publishers' websites, although no one database will cover all journals within a subject area. Databases are generally free at the point of use for students. If a library does not subscribe to a particular database, it may be possible to gain access on a pay-as-you-go basis. Table 3.1 summarizes some of the main subject databases covering health care. In addition, there are numerous specialist databases such as AgeInfo, or PsycINFO that focus on particular sub-specialities in the health care field.

How to set the search profile

While it might be tempting to start immediately entering search terms into library catalogues, Internet sites and databases, an effective literature search requires careful planning. The reviewer should begin by setting down on paper a brief title for the review and a summary of the areas of interest, including the type of evidence and publications required and any parameters for the search, such as the date or language of publication. A search profile serves two key purposes. First, it requires the researcher to clarify the scope and parameters of the study and, second, it acts as an *aide-mémoire* throughout the search process. In this way, the searcher is encouraged to remain focused and not be side-tracked down interesting but irrelevant byways. Narrative reviews offer more temptations to the unwary researcher. Systematic reviews usually set explicit inclusion and exclusion criteria. The search profile shown in Box 3.1 below for a study on the effects of overcrowding on health and education (Brown et al. 2004), funded by the Office of the Deputy Prime Minister in the UK, was adapted from guidelines provided by Gash (2000). The profile was also used as a structure for describing the literature search process in the final report of this project.

TABLE 3.1 Key databases in health care

Database	Scope	Content	Years
General:			
Applied Social Sciences Index and Abstracts	Health, social services, psychology, sociology, economics, politics, race relations and education. International in scope	Indexes and abstracts 500+ journals	1987–
International Bibliography of Social Sciences	Anthropology, economics, health, politics and sociology. International in scope	Bibliographic references to journal articles. Abstracts and some full-text access are provided. Includes research notes, responses and short essays, book reviews and book chapters	1951–
ScienceDirect	Science, technology and medicine full text. International in scope	Bibliographic details and abstracts from around 2,500 journals. Currently retrospectively digitizing pre-1995 journals including *The Lancet*	1995–
Health:			
Cumulative Index to Nursing and Allied Health Literature	Nursing, allied health, biomedicine, alternative/ complementary medicine, consumer health and health sciences librarianship. International in scope	Bibliographic references to nearly 3,000 journals. Abstracts are also provided for about 1,000 journals. Includes a citation index from 1994. Some access to full text	1982–
Health Management Information Consortium	Clinical medicine, health policy, occupational and environmental health, health systems and services, public health, health administration and management. International in scope	Bibliographic references and abstracts from three institutions: the UK Department of Health and Nuffield Institute for Health (Leeds University Library) and King's Fund Library	1983–
Medline	Biomedicine and health. International in scope	Bibliographic references and abstracts. Some links to full text	1950s–

Box 3.1   Search profile for the effects of overcrowded housing on health and education

Scope:

Health impacts: for example, mental health and infectious disease.
Educational consequences: for example, attainment and child development.
Empirical and conceptual studies: the academic literature, excluding publications that merely report on levels of overcrowding in particular areas.
Adopt a snowball technique: read reference lists in articles and books for follow-up. Citation search of key articles to identify other potential sources of data.

Date

1970s onwards –

Language

English

Type

Academic literature – excluding newspaper articles and policy reports.

Sources

Academic and policy databases, websites of key research organizations, charities and government departments.

Country

OECD countries.

Keywords

'academic achievement', 'child development', 'crowding', 'deprivation', 'educational attainment', 'health', 'houses in multiple occupation', 'mental health', 'overcrowding', 'physical health'.

Known references

Thomson, H. et al. (2001) 'Health effects of housing improvement', *British Medical Journal,* 323: 187–90.
Marsh, A. et al. (1999) *Home Sweet Home.* Bristol: Policy Press.

Source: Adapted from Gash (2000)

While the search profile provides an overview of the scope and parameters of the search, it is the search strategy that is actually used to retrieve journal articles and books from databases. The strategy requires the identification of terms that best describe the area of interest. These can be found in the definitions provided in subject-specific dictionaries and encyclopaedias. This list should include synonyms, abbreviations and related terms. As most databases have an international scope, researchers should allow for possible variations in language. For example, while UK authors use the word 'overcrowding' in relation to overcrowded housing, North American authors tend to use 'crowding' to describe the same phenomenon. Browsing the subject index of the database can ensure that the most appropriate words are searched for. It may also be worth checking how a key reference has been indexed in the database to see what subject terms and keywords were used to catalogue the article.

Once a list of search terms is identified, a search strategy must be written and decisions made on how these terms should be entered into the computer. It is rare that a search can be completed by inputting one or two words. Often, the search strategy is built using Boolean operators: 'and', 'or', 'not', which can be used to combine search terms to retrieve the most relevant articles. These three simple words can be used to broaden or narrow the search. For example, using the 'or' operator ensures that synonyms for the chosen term can be searched. The 'and' operator provides a narrower focus. The 'not' operator ensures that records with this term are not retrieved. Prior to entering the strategy in the database, it is important to check how the Boolean operators must be entered. Some databases use symbols rather than words. Table 3.2 provides working examples of how Boolean operators were used in the overcrowding and health review.

Refining the literature search

Always be prepared to rethink the search strategy in the light of results. The search may retrieve too many results. A useful technique is to download or print out the complete references (or a sample of them) – together with the abstract and subject classifications – and use these to identify the relevant articles. The enquirer should look to see how these have been catalogued and then refine the search strategy. If this does nothing to reduce the numbers, then limits such as date, language or place of publication should be applied. Most, if not all, databases offer on-screen help or prompts for this. More recent articles are likely to give a summary of previous research, and from these it should be possible to judge how far back the search needs to be taken. With luck, the search may identify an earlier review article that can be updated. If there are still too many references, then the focus of study will need rethinking in order to narrow the search further.

Conversely, searches may end with no results, or very few. This could be because little has been written on the subject, or it may be due to inconsistencies in cataloguing and indexing on different databases. Each database will have its own house style so differences may occur in subject and keyword classification or in the logging of bibliographic details such as author name. For example, in any database the name of the author could be indexed as *Jones, K; Jones, K. L.; Jones, Kathryn* or *Jones, Kathryn L.* So an author search for *Jones, K. L.* in one database may come back as having no hits, because papers are listed in the author index under *Jones, K.* Most databases offer the possibility of browsing the author index or searching for the surname alone. In the case of a common name such as Jones, this should be combined with a subject term to narrow the search focus.

Keyword searching may not retrieve results because different authors may assign different words for the same phenomena. For example, some academics may use 'patient group', 'self-help group', 'health consumer group' or 'health care user group' to describe similar types of organization. Or cataloguers could use the same word to describe different phenomena. For instance, 'complaint' may mean an illness or an allegation that something has gone wrong. In addition, different cataloguers may code the same article under different subject headings. Most databases give the option of truncating search terms, by using a particular symbol (usually * or $) to retrieve more references. For example, a search on 'consum$' would retrieve articles on consumers, consumerism and consumption. It is essential to browse both subject and keyword indexes in databases. Recognizing that

TABLE 3.2 The use of 'and', 'or', 'not' in a search strategy

	Search	Outcomes	Uses
	Using the **AND** operator:		
#1	Overcrowding		
#2	Asthma		
#3	#1 and #2	Records that contain both 'overcrowding' and 'asthma'	Narrowing the focus of the search by including particular terms
	Using the **OR** operator:		
#1	Overcrowding		
#2	Crowding		
#3	#1 or #2	Records that contain either 'overcrowding' or 'crowding' or both terms	Ensuring synonyms are included in search strategy
	Using the **NOT** operator:		
#1	Overcrowding		
#2	Trains		
#3	#1 not #2	Records that contain 'overcrowding', but not 'overcrowding' in 'trains'	Narrowing focus of search by excluding particular variables

inconsistencies can occur ensures a healthy scepticism of retrieved results. A quick way of testing the results is to look at the reference list of a relevant journal article to see if at least some of the same articles are cited.

Another technique is to search for authors who have quoted an important journal article as this can help to snowball the search to ensure a comprehensive coverage. The *Science* or *Social Science Citation Index* allows a researcher to identify articles, and, increasingly, also books and book chapters that have cited a particular reference. This provides access to further work on the subject, and gives an indication of how others view this work. In addition, many databases now include a 'cited by' function to find out who cited the article, or a 'reference' function which lists the references cited by the author.

The literature within a particular subject area is never static, so it is essential to build in a mechanism for keeping a search up to date. Some databases will save searches that can be rerun later. Many libraries and institutions produce a 'current awareness service' of publications. For example, the King's Fund Information and Library Service (www.kingsfund.org.uk) specializes in health policy and economics and publishes a bimonthly 'current awareness service'. The latest versions of journal content pages are produced by zetoc Alert email service (http://zetoc.mimas.ac.uk).

Searching for grey literature

Grey literature refers to literature published independently by, for example, specialist research units rather than mainstream publishers. The *Aslib Directory of Information Sources in the UK* is a useful starting point for identifying specialist collections. Grey literature may be difficult to obtain, but can be extremely valuable as it can include cutting-edge research. Some research bodies such as the King's Fund or the Institute of Health Services Management Research in the UK have websites that list, and increasingly provide, their publications online. It is also worth looking at the websites of research-funding bodies such as the Economic and Social Research Council (www.esrc.ac.uk), the Medical Research Council (www.mrc.ac.uk) and the Department of Health (www.dh.gov.uk). Some research reports are available electronically. There are also various specialist indexes that cover particular types of publication such as conference papers, dissertations and official documents. These may provide access to information that has not been formally published. In the overcrowding study, grey literature was identified through hand searching specialist journals, specialist indexes and the websites of key research units and housing charities.

Although it is tempting to rely on Internet search engines to locate information in relation to grey literature and other material, it is important to remember that this does not substitute for properly constructed search strategies using specialist databases. First, a search engine will not search with the same degree of rigour as an online database. Second, some literature found on the Internet may look official but it may be inaccurate and unverified by external experts.

Recording the search

The type and extent of information provided in the results of the database search will vary according to the database publisher. Most databases provide options for how results can be viewed online. At a minimum, the bibliographic details (such as author, date, title, journal, volume/issue number and page number[s]) will be provided for each item. The majority of databases will also provide the abstract and subject classification. An increasing number now offer access to the full article. It is worth downloading or saving the bibliographic and abstract details of the search into an email account or some form of specialist software such as EndNote, RefWorks or Mendeley, so they can be looked at more comprehensively at a later stage. The database will generally offer prompts to achieve this. It is vital to keep track by noting the databases searched, the years covered, the number of retrieved articles and the search strategy used, to ensure that the search is undertaken as systematically as possible. This record will also be useful if the search strategy needs to be revised.

The bibliographic details and abstract of each item retrieved should provide a good indication of whether the full article is worth reading. If a journal or book is not available locally, it can be obtained via an interlibrary loan. For each item read, the reviewer should complete a data extraction form, which can then be used to summarize key details from the item, as set out in Box 3.2.

Box 3.2   A data extraction form

Article no:		Review date:	
Title:			
Author(s):		Publication date:	
Publisher:		Place of publication:	
Journal:		Volume: number: page no:	
Keywords/definitions:			
Conceptual framework:			
Findings/argument:			
Author conclusions:			
Own notes:			
Rating: quality of research		Rating: relevance to study	
A	High quality	1	Extremely relevant
B	Medium quality	2	Quite relevant
C	Low quality	3	Marginally relevant

The type of information logged will depend on the purpose of the review, but keeping a record is essential. In the example given at the end of the chapter, the bibliographic details necessary for referencing are noted as well as information on definitions of keywords; the concepts that make up the conceptual framework; the findings or results of the study; the argument put forward; and the conclusions drawn. The form also provides space for personal comment, and a prompt for a rating of the quality and relevance of the paper.

For the literature review on overcrowding, a more complex form was devised that recorded details about the type of study and the methods used. It also included stricter guidelines for judging the quality of the papers (see Brown et al. 2004). Completing a form for each item may seem cumbersome, but it is essential. A number of sources are likely to be identified and it will be impossible to remember everything that has been read. In addition, most reference-managing software now enables you to log this information electronically and support searches and sorting by these criteria. Some software such as Mendeley allow you to store and add 'e-notes' on pdf versions of articles. Recent improvements in the user-friendliness of reference-managing software mean it is worth taking time to learn how to use them, especially if you are writing a dissertation at Masters or PhD level. Figure 3.1 below shows a screen print from a Mendeley library created by the author as part of a recent literature review to scope the role of argument and persuasion in policy documents on community in health, housing and local government (Hamalainen and Jones 2011). The study was funded by the Arts and Humanities Research Council.

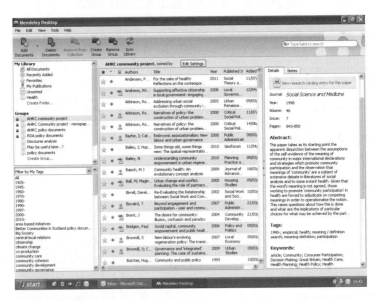

FIGURE 3.1   Screen dump from Mendeley Reference Managing Software for AHRC Scoping (Hamalainen and Jones 2011)

Assessing relevance and quality in a literature review

A major part of the literature review will involve making a judgement on the relevance of what is being read. The significance of the findings to a project should be assessed, as well as the effect of the research design and methods on the outcome of the study. Once a number of studies have been read, it should be possible to make an accurate assessment of the importance of each item extracted.

Even within a narrative review, an attempt must be made to judge the relative merits of the methods employed in each study. For example, a study rated as highly relevant may be based on only a small sample. A researcher may use this to make a case for a larger study. Alternatively, a search may identify issues that were explored using quantitative methods, but there may be a benefit in further investigation using qualitative methods and vice versa. The reviewer should comment on the reliability and validity of the methods used, and the extent to which they can be generalized to a larger population. It is also important to note whether findings support or contradict previous research.

A number of guides are available which describe approaches to evaluating different types of research in the clinical and social sciences. These have been developed for researchers wishing to undertake a systematic review. However, they raise questions pertinent for any review (see, for example, NHS CRD 2001; Greenhalgh 2010). The key questions for assessing the quality of studies in a literature review are summarized in Box 3.3 below.

Box 3.3 Questions for assessing the quality of studies in a literature review

- Conceptual framework:
  - Are the aims clearly stated and research questions clearly identified?
  - Does the author link the work to an existing body of knowledge?
- Study design and methods:
  - Are the methods appropriate and clearly described?
  - Is the context of the study well set out? Did the research design account for possible bias?
  - Are the limitations of research explicitly identified?
- Research analysis:
  - Are the results clearly described, valid and reliable?
  - Is the analysis clearly described?
- Conclusions:
  - Are all possible influences on the observed outcomes considered?
  - Are conclusions linked to the aims of the study?
  - Are conclusions linked to the analysis and interpretation of data?

Writing the Literature Review

A literature review is not simply a regurgitation of who said what on a particular subject. A successful review is an interpretive piece of work that offers an assessment of the quality and scope of existing studies in a particular subject area. It brings together what is known in order to state what further research or analysis is required. In essence, a review acknowledges what has come before and how this can be built upon and expanded.

The review should define the key concepts to be used in the research and how these will be used within the reviewer's own work. It is good practice to draw attention to different definitions of key terms and why the researcher has decided to follow one definition rather than another. For example, the term 'consumer' is contested; different authors attach different meanings. In a study undertaken by the author and others of health consumer groups, attention was paid to explaining why this term was used rather than 'patients' group' or 'patients' association' or 'health user group' by discussing debates in the literature (Baggott et al. 2005).

In discussing the theoretical framework for a study, the researcher must justify why a certain theory has been adopted and spell out what research questions are raised by this approach. Some studies use a number of theories, a strategy termed by Sabatier (1999) as a 'multiple-lens' approach. For example, in the health consumer group study, the research team drew on a number of different theoretical perspectives that raised different questions to assess the influence and impact of health consumer groups on the policy process. These included theories about the configuration, and relative power, of various structural interests in health care; explanations of the power and influence of particular pressure groups; and theories about issue networks and policy communities within the policy process. Theories of representative and participative democracy were also reviewed in the context of questions about how health consumer groups represented their members, and how representatives were seen by health care stakeholders. These theories informed the questionnaire design and the semi-structured interviews with health consumer group leaders, and contributed to developing a theoretical framework for the subsequent analysis of qualitative data.

A literature review should also report on previous empirical work undertaken, what methods have been adopted and relevant findings. In the study of health consumer groups, previous work on patient groups and patient and public involvement in policy making at local and national level provided the basis for identifying gaps in the research. In addition, factors that limited the validity or generalizability of previous research findings were noted.

Deciding on a structure for the literature review

One challenge for the researcher is to select the most relevant articles for inclusion from a large quantity of material. The basis for inclusion in the narrative review is the relevance of the conceptual, theoretical and methodological approach taken by different authors to the study in question. A second challenge is to find a logical structure in writing the review. This will depend on its purpose. A review that seeks to assess the evidence base for a particular health care intervention will be structured differently from a review for a dissertation, thesis or project. Thus, for example, the overcrowding review took a themed approach. In the introduction, issues relating to definitions and methods were discussed. Subsequent chapters reported evidence on the impact of overcrowding on various aspects of health (such as the higher incidence of respiratory illness) and education (like the effect of overcrowding on educational attainment).

It would be unusual to follow a simple chronological arrangement in the literature review by, for instance, starting a discussion with the earliest work on the subject and ending with the latest. A review is more likely to be arranged according to themes drawn from the literature or framed around certain research questions. Within a narrative review, the reviewer should take care to ensure that the structure follows the logic of their argument. In effect, the reviewer aims to establish that a gap in knowledge exists and suggests a way forward, through further research (see Hart 1998).

Effective planning is essential in order to identify the most logical structure. Before writing, an outline or plan for the review should be put together. This will involve jotting down key themes identified from the reading and making links between them to establish an appropriate order. It is helpful to identify headings and subheadings. These may not be used in the final review, but can help to ensure a logical flow to the argument.

Style and referencing in a literature review

The writing style adopted in a review will depend on what is being reviewed. One benefit from reading widely around a subject area is to gain a feel for scholarly writing. Sentences commonly used to develop an argument are summarized below:

- Where there is agreement and disagreement on particular issues: 'While there is general agreement that this has occurred (references), there has been some debate about whether this is due to x (references) or y (references).'
- On the criticisms levelled at particular studies: 'Jones' work has been criticized because of a, b, c (references), but it is of relevance to this study because it suggests x, y, z.'
- Offering suggestions of what can be surmised or understood from the literature: 'In summary, it is possible to suggest that x is related to y; however, what is still not known is how z fits into this, which is the purpose of the study.'

A review will go through several drafts. Early drafts are likely to be more descriptive than analytical as the reviewer must first decide how the literature fits together before they can present a coherent argument. As the argument develops, the literature can be revisited. The extraction forms will be invaluable at this point to identify key findings. Articles that contradict findings, or question theoretical or conceptual frameworks, are also important. A good review offers a balanced perspective.

It is not necessary to cite or quote every reference retrieved, only those that are relevant to the question. The primary aim is to construct a clear narrative and to distinguish the author's argument from the works referenced. In deciding what to include, the researcher should bear in mind the intended audience. For example, a supervisor or external examiner will already have a general background in the subject area. The literature should be analysed with reference to the research aims or questions. A common mistake is simply to describe the literature – the approach must be analytical and critical.

Correct attribution is also important. Failure to acknowledge a source can lead to an allegation of plagiarism. For dissertation or research students, a preferred citation style may be recommended. One common style is the Harvard system – as used in this volume – based on an author and date (year) system, with fuller details listed in alphabetical order at the end of the work. Another style is the Oxford system where numbers for each source are used in the text and then full bibliographic details are given in a footnote or endnote. Legal or historical texts tend to favour page footnoting as readers may wish to see precise amplification as they read. If guidelines are provided by a book publisher or editors of a journal, they should be followed to the letter and consistently applied. Moreover, if a source is quoted directly, it should always be cited and the page number given. If particular ideas or arguments are summarized, this should also be acknowledged. Chapter 23 discusses writing style further.

CASE STUDY

The Black Report

In 1977, the Secretary of State for Health and Social Security requested a review of existing knowledge on the differences in health status between social classes, their causes and implications for policy and future research. The review was chaired by Sir Douglas Black (then Chief Scientist at the Department of Health and Social Security, and later President of the Royal College of Physicians). This hard-hitting report on the evidence of inequalities in health (Department of Health and Social Security 1980) was finally made more widely available by Townsend and Davidson (1988) and subsequently has been updated in the light of further evidence. The aim was to provide evidence of the extent of inequality in health and offer an assessment of its implications. The report reviewed the following:

- *Concepts of health*: How are health, ill health and inequality defined?
- *Concepts of health and inequality*: definitions of health, indicators of health and illness, including disablement, and inequality indicators based on occupational group, income and expenditure.
- *Theoretical debates*: Which theoretical approaches explain why health inequalities occur?
- *Empirical evidence*: sources of evidence on health inequalities, for example the statistical returns from the General Household Survey, birth cohort studies and published reviews of data.
- *The pattern of present inequalities*: mortality by gender, race, region, occupational class, incidence of common illnesses.
- *Trends in inequality of health*: inequality in the availability and use of the health service: a review of published studies and critique of methods.
- *International comparisons*: comparison with other developed countries, particularly in Europe.
- *Towards an explanation of health inequalities*: theoretical approaches to understanding health inequalities assessed against the human life cycle.
- *Recommendations*: these outlined (a) the need for further primary and secondary research on particular issues and in policy terms; and (b) the need for a comprehensive anti-poverty strategy covering a range of social services and based on a broader concept of inequalities in health.

Carrying out a literature review for a short paper: Health consumer networks and alliances

This review was undertaken for a chapter in a book by Baggott et al. (2005), entitled *Speaking for Patients and Carers,* on health consumer groups in the national policy process, and was funded by the Economic and Social Research Council (R000237888). The chapter formed a link between the early part of the book, which had set out research into the general conceptual, theoretical and policy context and explored the characteristics and social and political resources of health consumer groups, and the later chapters which dealt with the relationships between such groups and other actors/institutions in the policy process. The aim of the chapter was to explore how and why contacts and links between health consumer groups were formed; how these alliances supported the groups' role in policy; and the factors that encouraged collaboration rather than competition. The issues were identified as:

(Continued)

CASE STUDY

(Continued)

- *Conceptual issues*: How are networks and alliances defined?
- *Theoretical debates*: How can an alliance working in the policy process be understood and explained?
- *Empirical evidence*: What evidence exists on current patterns of alliances and networking within the health consumer group and the voluntary health sector?

Conclusion

This chapter has emphasized the importance of the literature review in identifying concepts, theories and existing empirical studies of a particular phenomenon in the early stages of developing a research proposal or project. This enables a researcher to build on the basis of existing knowledge and on what other scholars have achieved, but also to identify gaps in the literature and to identify interesting new questions. While systematic reviews are a specialized form of study, narrative reviews are fundamental to any project.

The Internet has brought access to a vast range of electronic sources for the researcher. A well-written review will provide enough background to bring readers up to speed in the subject area and give them a framework within which to assess the evidence. In order to navigate a way through the quantity of sources available, two strategies may be employed. First, it is important to plan a search strategy carefully and to record sources and their content meticulously. The chapter outlines ways in which this can be done, so that with practice the researcher can be quick and efficient at finding the sources most likely to be relevant to their research question. Second, the expansion of the Internet has led to an increase in information specialists who are employed by many organizations, and not only higher education institutions, to assist people in gaining access to information and what they need to know. This is particularly the case in the health field where a wide range of people, both professionals and the lay public, now wish to inform themselves better using both national and international sources. An exercise now follows for readers to help develop further their understanding of this chapter.

Exercise: A literature search on New Labour's expert patients' agenda from a consumer/citizen perspective

The following exercise provides an opportunity to think through the process of developing a search strategy and a structure for a literature review. While the subject area may not be one you are familiar with, the process described in this chapter should give you a framework to plan a successful search.

Think about the type of literature review that you would undertake for a dissertation entitled 'A critical analysis of New Labour's expert patients' agenda in the UK from a consumer/citizen perspective'.

1 What conceptual and theoretical issues will you need to consider?

- Consider what definitional issues you will need to address.
- How will perspectives on consumerism/citizenship influence the analysis of the literature?

2 Which electronic databases will you need to search?

- Consider the scope and coverage of the database. How important is it that it is international in scope?
- Are you going to attempt to identify primary research studies, secondary policy analysis or both?

3 What search strategy will you build?

- Consider what keywords and phrases you will need to use.
- Consider what the most appropriate limits might be for your search – for example, language and date of publication.
- Are there any terms that can be truncated to broaden the search?

4 What will be the most relevant sources of grey literature?

- Which key research organizations may have an interest in the Expert Patients' Programme?
- What information will you need to obtain from the Department of Health website?

5 What key data will you need to log from the literature?

- Consider how these may change according to the type of information – for example, policy documents, policy critiques and policy analyses that draw on field research.

6 How will you structure the review?

- What information will the reader require on the Expert Patients' Programme?
- What information will the reader require on the theoretical and conceptual issues underpinning your review?
- Will you tackle the advantages/disadvantages of the Expert Patients' Programme separately or by theme?
- Will you discuss primary and secondary research together or separately?

Acknowledgement

The author would like to thank the following for permission to draw on projects undertaken while part of a larger research team: Judith Allsop; Rob Baggott, Health Policy Research Unit, De Montfort University; and Tim Brown and Ros Hunt, Centre for Comparative Housing Research, De Montfort University.

Recommended Further Reading

Gash, S. (2000) *Effective Literature Searching for Research*. Aldershot: Gower.
This is an excellent, easy-to-understand guide for students and other researchers on the process of planning, executing and recording a literature search, covering both print and electronic sources.

Hart, C. (1998) *Doing a Literature Review: Releasing the Social Science Research Imagination*. London: Sage.
This book provides a comprehensive guide to the process of accessing, analysing and understanding the arguments presented in academic texts, giving useful advice on how the literature review fits into undergraduate and postgraduate dissertations.

Petticrew, M. and Roberts, H. (2006) *Systematic Reviews in the Social Sciences*. Malden, MA: Blackwell.
This highlights how systematic reviews of research evidence are becoming increasingly important in the social sciences, much of which is also relevant to narrative reviews as well.

Online Readings

Morris, S., Wilmot, A., Hill, M., Ockenden, N. and Payne, S. (2012) 'A narrative literature review of the contribution of volunteers in end-of-life care services', *Palliative Medicine*, 26.
What are the similarities and differences between systematic and narrative reviews? Should narrative reviews follow same process as systematic review? What are the advantage/disadvantages of different approaches?

Kavanagh, J., Oakley, A., Harden, A., Trouton, A. and Powell, C. (2011) 'Are incentive schemes effective in changing young people's behaviour? A systematic review', *Health Education Journal*, 70: 192–205.
Compare and contrast narrative and systematic reviews. What is the value of systematic reviews as form of evidence-based health care? What are the barriers to undertaking systematic reviews?

References

Aveyard, H. (2010) *Doing a Literature Review in Health and Social Care*, 2nd edition. Maidenhead: Open University Press.
Baggott, R., Allsop, J. and Jones, K. (2005) *Speaking for Patients and Carers: Health Consumer Groups and the National Policy Process*. Basingstoke: Palgrave.

Brown, T., Baggott, R., Jones, K. and Hunt, R. (2004) *The Impact of Overcrowding on Health and Education: A Review of the Research Evidence and Literature*. London: The Office of the Deputy Prime Minister.

Department of Health and Social Security (DHSS) (1980) *Inequalities in Health: A Report of a Research Working Group* (Chair: Sir Douglas Black). London: DHSS.

Dixon-Woods, M., Fitzpatrick, R. and Roberts, K. (2001) 'Including qualitative research in systematic reviews: problems and opportunities', *Journal of Evaluative Clinical Practice*, 7: 125–33.

Dunn, C. (2011) 'The place of the literature review in grounded theory research', *International Journal of Social Science Research Methodology*, 14: 111–24.

Gash, S. (2000) *Effective Literature Searching for Research*. Aldershot: Gower.

Graham, H. and McDermott, E. (2006) 'Qualitative research and the evidence base of policy: insights from studies of teenage mothers in the UK', *Journal of Social Policy*, 35: 21–37.

Greenhalgh, T. (2010) *How to Read a Paper: The Basics of Evidence Based Medicine*. Chichester: Wiley-Blackwell.

Hamalainen, L. and Jones, K. (2011) Conceptualising community as a social fix, argument and persuasion in health, housing and local governance [online]. Available at: www.ahrc.ac.uk/FundingOpportunities/Documents/CC%20scoping%20studies/Hamalainen.pdf

Hart, C. (1998) *Doing a Literature Review: Releasing the Social Science Research Imagination*. London: Sage.

NHS CRD (2001) *Undertaking Systematic Reviews of Research on Effectiveness: CRDs Guidelines for Those Carrying Out or Commissioning Reviews*. York: CRD.

Noblit, G.W. and Hare, R.D. (1988) *Meta-ethnography: Synthesizing Qualitative Studies*. Newbury Park, CA: Sage.

Petticrew, M. (2001) 'Systematic reviews from astronomy to zoology: myths and misconceptions', *British Medical Journal*, 322: 98–101.

Petticrew, M. and Roberts, H. (2006) *Systematic Reviews in the Social Sciences*. Malden, MA: Blackwell.

Sabatier, P.A. (1999) 'The need for better theories', in P.A. Sabatier (ed.), *Theories of the Policy Process*. Boulder, CO: Westview Press.

Street, A. (2001) 'How can we argue for evidence in nursing?', *Contemporary Nurse*, 11(1): 5–9.

Suri, H. (2011) 'Purposeful sampling in qualitative research synthesis', *Qualitative Research Journal*, 11(2): 63–75.

Townsend, P. and Davidson, N. (1988) *Inequalities in Health*. London: Penguin.

PART II
Qualitative Methods and Health

4

Using Documents in Health Research

ANDY ALASZEWSKI

Introduction

- Documents, especially personal documents such as diaries and letters, provide a relatively neglected resource for health service researchers. They can be used to access data that are difficult to obtain in other ways. For example, such documents can tell us about individuals who died several centuries ago; people from marginalized and stigmatized groups who are often reluctant to participate in research; or activities, such as gay sex, that are otherwise concealed. In this respect, the overall aim of this chapter is to examine the ways in which documents have been and can be used for health research. This includes describing documentary research, identifying the type of resources it requires, and examining the research issues for which it is appropriate. The chapter will also, among other things, outline the strengths and weaknesses of documentary research and consider how documentary data can be coded, analysed and presented.

Defining Documentary Research

A document can be defined as a human artefact that contains information. This artefact can take different forms. In Europe, a document is usually one or more pieces of paper (a file if loose and book if bound) containing written symbols, usually words, often numbers and sometimes diagrams, drawings or illustrations. With the development of computer technology, documents increasingly take the form of computer files. Thus, *The Chambers Dictionary* defines a document as: 'a paper, *esp* of an official character, affording information, proof or evidence of anything, a file of text produced and held on a computer' (2008: 454). It is possible to argue that any human artefact is in fact a document as it was created for a purpose, and deciphering that purpose provides insight into human activity. For example, Prior (2003: 2) in the introduction to his textbook on documentary research argued that 'paintings, tapestries, monuments, diaries, shopping lists, stage plays, adverts, rail tickets, film, photographs, videos, engineering drawings, the content of human tissue archives and World Wide Web (WWW) pages' could all be thought of, and treated as, documents. However, in this chapter I will restrict my discussion to a more conventional definition of documents, focusing on how and in what ways the knowledge encoded in documents can be deciphered and used.

Both the nature of technology underpinning the creation of documents and access to that technology have changed. The first documents created nearly 5,500 years ago were records made by specialist scribes for political and religious elites. Examples are the clay tablets inscribed with cuneiform writing in Mesopotamia and hieroglyphs on papyruses in Egypt. Initially, documents were accounts of transactions, but they developed into more literary representations and mathematical texts (see MacGregor 2010: 91–110 for an analysis of three early documents). As I noted in my textbook on one type of document, the diary, in the last 400 years the development of paper, simple writing tools and printing, as well as more open access to education, has resulted in a reduction in the cost of creating documents and wider access to the skills needed to create them (Alaszewski 2006). In contemporary society, most people can create a personal document such as a diary, letter or blog.

Although there has been a democratization of document creation, the systematic creation of documents remains an organizational activity. As Weber (1978: 957) pointed out, modern society is characterized by the development of bureaucratic organizations in which management is 'based upon written documents ("the files") that are preserved'. In the area of health, such bureaucracies include agencies that fund and provide health care, and which, during the course of their routine activities, build up records. In the context of health, documentary research involves the use of any 'records relating to individuals or groups of individuals that have been generated in the course of their daily life' (Clarkson 2003: 80). Such records may be created by individuals working in and for organizations. For example, a hospital will over time build up a store of records, including patients' notes, letters of complaint and minutes of meetings.

While such official documents can provide evidence on the activities of official agencies and about the nature of health issues, they are more limited in providing insight into individuals' experience of health and illness. The best source of such evidence is 'documents of life' (Plummer 2001). These are personal and family records such as letters or diaries that can be used as the basis for biographical case studies or life stories (Clarkson 2003). Not only can health researchers access and make use of official and personal documents, they can also access more ad hoc sources. For example, in the course of legal actions in the USA, courts have forced tobacco companies to make public documents relating to their activities. As a result, the University of California San Francisco Legacy Tobacco Documents Library has built up a 60-million-page archive of documents that can be used to examine how tobacco companies have marketed and tested their products (Wertz et al. 2011).

As I have already noted, documents can take a variety of forms. The traditional – and the one that tends to predominate and is the easiest to use for research – is written text, such as hospital records, letters and diaries. These may be stored in archives or published in collected works or as memoirs, autobiographies and institutional histories. However, with the development of other media, written text can be supplemented, or even replaced, by photographs, film, and audio and video recordings, and some archives include both types of material. For example, at the University of Cambridge, MacFarlane and his colleagues have created an ethnographic archive of written texts, photographs and audio-visual material relating to the Naga, an indigenous people who live in North East India (MacFarlane and Turin 2008).

Documents in archives and published locations are unsolicited; the researcher is therefore reusing material that others have created, used and stored. Researchers can also solicit the creation of documents specifically for the purposes of research (Alaszewski 2006). In particular, diaries – which can be seen as the 'document of life' par excellence (Plummer 2001) – can be used in a range of health-related research. These have been used to keep a record of the symptoms experienced by individuals who have relapsing-remitting multiple sclerosis (Parkin et al. 2004), the sexual activities of men who have sex with men (Coxon 1996) and illness behaviour and decisions to seek expert advice (Robinson 1971).

The defining characteristic of documentary research is that the researcher uses documents created by others. This is self-evident when the researcher is accessing unsolicited documents that are stored in archives and created by individuals who died long before the research started. However, when researchers solicit documents for the purposes of a research project, they can then influence the way in which the document is created. This influence should fall short of control. The key feature of documentary research is that the person creating the document has ultimate control and ownership of it. They can choose to destroy it or give others access to it. For example, Elliott (1997) undertook a study of the help-seeking behaviour of eight people who were aware of having musculo-skeletal problems, and invited them to keep a health diary. Diarists were asked to record their personal details and the time period covered by the diary on the first page, and on subsequent pages to keep a daily record. To help them structure their records, they were invited to respond to a set of questions about their health. Elliott argued that the documents created by these diaries and follow-up interviews were texts mainly authored by informants and used informants' own words and ideas, rather than those of the researcher.

Why Use Documentary Research?

Documents are readily available, albeit as I will discuss further with increased concern about ethical issues, there are restrictions on access to contemporary documents in organizations such as the NHS in the UK. In some cases, documents provide the only available source of information. For example, when a researcher is interested in how social processes and relationships have changed over a long period of time, documents are often the sole source of evidence. Pollock (1983) wanted to examine the commonly held view that parenting and childrearing have become less strict and violent over time. Using the timeframe 1500–1900, she used a variety of bibliographic sources to identify 496 relevant documents, most of which contained information on child rearing practices: 36 were autobiographies and 350 were American or British diaries, including 98 diaries written by children or at least started during childhood. Pollock was able to use these sources to challenge the received wisdom that childcare had become more liberal and less violent over time.

Even when researchers can access other sources of data, documentary sources are important where a researcher needs to minimize memory or recall problems. Documents are often based on records that were made shortly after the actual events. Stone et al. (2003: 182), in a review of medical research diaries, noted the value of diaries in 'capturing experience close to the time of its occurrence', especially medical symptoms which are 'subjective and/or variable'. They estimated that these types of documents feature prominently in drug trials and have been used in nearly 25 per cent of clinical trials.

Documentary sources also provide a way of collecting data that minimizes the intrusiveness associated with much social research. This is self-evident when the researcher uses unsolicited documents. Solicited documents may also minimize intrusion. The researcher specifies what sort of information is wanted. Participants are then free to decide when, and how, they record this information. Minimizing intrusion is important when a researcher wants to address sensitive issues or work where groups or individuals want to avoid scrutiny of their activities. In a Hong Kong study of men who have sex with men, Jones and his colleagues recruited 16 men to keep a daily record of their activities, relationships and feelings. The researchers asked participants to submit their records weekly and offered a variety of media for doing so, including mail, fax, anonymous email, tape recording and face-to-face interviews (Jones et al. 2000; Jones and Candlin 2003).

Resources Needed for Documentary Research

The resources required for documentary research depend on the type of documents the researcher wants to use. Researchers who wish to use unsolicited documents need to locate and access relevant documents and sources, while researchers who use solicited documents must invest resources in creating, collecting and analysing these documents.

Unsolicited documents

Researchers using unsolicited documents need to identify where such documents are held. Historic documents are likely to be stored in archives and the researcher will need to ensure resources are available to identify and access appropriate archives. Until relatively recently, this involved using published bibliographies and other sources to identify possible archives and then physically visiting each place to access suitable documents (see Jordanova 2000; Corti 2003). This required resources to cover travel costs as well as photocopying, where that was permitted, and the costs of subsequent analysis. The development of electronic and Internet resources has increased access to, and reduced the costs of using, archives. Bibliographies and other resources can increasingly be accessed through the Internet. For example, Penn Library (2004) has specifically produced a research guide to finding diaries. Some archives are also available on the Internet. In the UK, the DIPEx website (www.primary-care.ox.ac.uk/research.dipex) is an online archive of personal experiences of health and illness. The Mass Observation archive maintains a website that provides information both on the diaries archived and on publications based on the diaries. Mass Observation recruited 500 men and women to develop an 'anthropology of [them]selves' (Sheridan 1991: 1). Most recruits kept a diary from 1939 until 1945 and some continued until 1965.

Researchers dealing with recent documents may need to identify who is holding the documents and who can provide access to them. Searching for such individuals can be a difficult and time-consuming activity and generally researchers use intermediaries. Miller (1985), in his study of Irish migrants in the USA, followed the approach pioneered by Thomas and Znaniecki (1958) in their classic study of Polish migration that drew on unsolicited personal documents, such as letters and diaries. Miller used institutions and individuals with contacts in the Irish migrant community to access documents. Researchers can also advertise through media such as newspapers and the Internet. For example, the British Broadcasting Corporation used public interest in the Second World War, stimulated by 60th anniversary events, to promote an Internet archive of personal stories. Individuals were encouraged to contribute to a rapidly growing archive of personal documents by sending their stories and associated photographs electronically (WW2 People's War Team 2004). While setting up and promoting a website is expensive, it may be possible for researchers to use established websites. For example, there is a range of websites for users of health services, such as the Different Strokes website for stroke survivors (www.differentstrokes.co.uk), which could be used to contact document holders.

Solicited documents

The resources needed by researchers who are using solicited documents specifically created for a research project will be determined by the purposes of the study and its design. The study may be based on experimental, survey or other methods. The major resource implications are those normally associated with using such designs. For a survey design, resources are needed to:

- Identify the Population.
- Select and recruit a sample.
- Collect data from the subjects or units in the sample.
- Code and enter the data into a database.
- Analyse the data statistically.
- Write a report.

The additional resources needed for a survey of documents are those associated with the creation of suitable documents. For example, when monitoring the impact of different treatment regimes on chronic illnesses such as diabetes or multiple sclerosis, the researcher may need the research subject to record not only compliance with the prescribed treatment regime, but also relevant clinical data such as blood sugar levels or level of pain. In this context, the researcher will wish to recruit subjects who can be trusted to follow the instructions and keep an honest and accurate record. The researcher will also need to provide appropriate recording equipment. Traditional record keeping requires basic competence in literacy (Corti 2003), although subjects can now use audio and video recorders as well. The chances of creating documents suitable for research purposes increase when adequate resources are provided for:

- The initial recruitment process.
- Training and support for diarists.
- Checking the reliability of entries and providing feedback.

The use of incentives, such as the payment of modest sums of money, is controversial but not uncommon in research soliciting documents from subjects (Coxon 1996; Jones et al. 2000).

Strengths and Weaknesses of Documentary Sources

Authenticity

Documents offer an authenticity which is difficult to gain through other methods. Documents such as diaries capture the richness of everyday life as it happens. Plummer (2001: 48) noted that 'each diary entry – unlike life histories – is sedimented into a particular moment in time'. Bolger et al. (2003: 580) have argued that such documents facilitate 'the examination of reported events and experiences in their natural, spontaneous context'.

The authenticity of unsolicited documents makes them a particularly valuable resource for social or ethnographic histories. For example, MacFarlane (1970: 11) used Ralph Josselin's diary to 'step back 300 years and to look out through the eyes of an Essex vicar of the mid seventeenth century'. He used the diary to examine demographic and social issues, such as Josselin's relationship with his kin, godparents, servants and neighbours. He was interested in the cultural dimensions of these relationships and other aspects of Josselin's life. MacFarlane (1970: 3) noted that such a document 'enables us to probe a long-vanished mental world, as well as to describe the social characteristics of a previous civilization'.

If the researcher is careful not to impose an over-rigid structure, then solicited documents can also be used as a means of obtaining authentic accounts of contemporary social events and experiences. Coxon (1996), in discussion of the use of diaries in Project SIGMA which studied gay men, noted that the diary method arose out of the researchers' experience as sexually active gay men. This use of solicited documents was 'natural' as it was not imposed on, or alien to, individuals who participated in the research. Diary keeping was common among gay men, and several of the researchers had kept sexual diaries for a number of years before the research. Thus, the researchers drew on their own experience in developing the method and encouraged the diarists to describe their experiences in their own words.

Nonetheless, the authenticity of such documents is problematic. Documents such as letters and diaries are created to perform a particular function and achieve this using specific structures and forms. As Thomas and Znaniecki (1958) commented in their study of Polish migration in the early part of the twentieth century, the existence of extensive family correspondence is fairly remarkable, as in the peasant community literacy skills were not highly developed. The letters were the product of a social duty and written by, or to, an absent family member, including those who had migrated to the USA. They tended to follow certain well-established conventions. As Clarkson (2003: 82) has noted, documents need to be treated with caution as they 'are tricky; they tell us what the author wants us to know, which is not necessarily what the researcher is really interested in'.

Flexibility

Data from letters or diaries can be used in combination with other sources of data in a range of research designs. In historical research, different types of documents can be used to triangulate findings, since convergent views from multiple sources can help to overcome potential weaknesses arising from a single source. Sahlins (1995) in his analysis of how Hawaiian Islanders made sense of an unprecedented event – their first encounter with Europeans – used a variety of diaries and other documents kept by Captain Cook and his crew, and compared them with oral traditions and histories from the Islands. Sahlins argued that the comparison of these interpretations helped better explain Cook's death.

Various methods can also be combined in research on contemporary issues. For example, Zimmerman and Wieder (1977) have developed a diary-interview approach that has three components:

- An initial interview.
- The research diary.
- A debriefing interview.

The initial interview is to provide participants with a briefing about how they should use their diaries and answer their questions. The participants maintain their diary for a specified period and at an agreed time they return their diaries. Zimmerman and Wieder developed their approach as an alternative to participant observation to access settings and activities that they could not directly observe. Elliott (1997) also used this approach in her diary study of illness and help-seeking behaviours. She maintained close contact with participants in the research, visiting them at least three times: once to brief them and give them their diary; a second time to give them another diary and to have an initial 'conversation' about the diary; and a third and final time to conduct an in-depth interview. She used both the conversations and interviews to explore themes identified in the diaries. For example, in the interviews, participants discussed not only actions which they had recorded in their diaries, but also actions they had considered but did not take, as well as actions they intended to take at some time in the future.

So why don't health researchers make more use of documents?

Documents are relatively easy to access and contain interesting useable data, albeit data protection regulations restrict access to some contemporary records. However, researchers using unsolicited documents contained in archives can, as I discuss below (see also Chapter 15), avoid engaging with much of the governance and ethics bureaucracy that now consumes so much health researcher time and energy. So it is puzzling that health and other researchers do not make more use of documents, as Prior (2003: 4) has noted: 'In most social science work[,] documents … are placed at the margins of consideration.'

Prior (2003) offers an explanation for this. He argues that social scientists and other researchers tend to value the spoken word, accessed through interviews and other methods, more highly than the written word, the key component of most documents. However, there is a more fundamental problem. An interviewer is in direct contact with those providing the information and can directly influence the interview process. In contrast, the researcher using documents, especially unsolicited ones, can exert no influence. They have to accept and work with what is available. One response to such limitations is to focus on the ways in which documents are created and used rather than on the intrinsic information they contain. Thus,

Prior et al. (2002) showed that documents played a key role in a cancer genetics clinic where clinicians used them to identify and communicate individuals' cancer risk. For example, Prior et al. noted that clinicians used a computer program, Cyrillic, 'that draws a family tree and provides a numerical estimate for an individual' (2002: 248) as a means of explaining and making visible risk estimates.

Those researchers who want to make use of the information contained within documents have to deal with the issue of 'second-hand' data as they are reusing material that was not specially created for the purposes of research. Thus, they have to consider how the documents were created and used and how this might affect the purpose for which they wish to reuse them. Garfinkel (1967: 191) tried to use routine clinical records to identify the criteria used by a psychiatric outpatient clinic to select patients and allocate treatments. He found that in most of the 661 files accessed, key data were missing. Garfinkel argued that while the records were 'bad' from a research perspective, they were 'good' from the organization's perspective, as they fitted within organizational routines and were fit for organizational purposes. The main purpose of the records was not to collect accurate research data and they did not work as an actuarial record such as a bank account. Case files recorded and justified the decisions made by the clinic staff about the person who was the subject of the file. It was both a record and an account of the treatment the clinic agreed to provide. It was a form of therapeutic contract designed to provide a basis for the relationship between the patient and the clinic. Garfinkel (1967) argued that such documents did not have fixed meanings, but were used and interpreted in the context of interactions with patients, and professionals used them to 'make a case' and justify a course of action. Thus, researchers seeking to use documents need to reflect on the nature and purpose of those documents and the ways in which this fits with the nature and purpose of their research.

Analysing Documentary Material

Statistical analysis

Researchers using experimental or survey methods will see the entries in such documents as recording specific forms of social reality that are reflected in recurring themes in the data. These can be coded within each case and organized into categories or variables. The data relevant to each variable for each case can then be expressed as a number (Moser and Kalton 1971). Such coding creates a data set which can be analysed using statistical techniques. The aim of the analysis is to identify relationships between variables and demonstrate that they are unlikely to be a product of chance. Parkin et al. (2004) used a statistical analysis of their diary data to examine the ways in which the symptoms of individuals with relapsing-remitting multiple sclerosis varied over time. The cross-sectional time series data enabled them to analyse the stability and variability of their main measuring instrument, the EuroQol Visual Analogue Scale.

Content analysis

Documents that have not been created within a closely defined structure tend to produce qualitative data, which in written documents take the form of written text. Data may take other forms, such as audio or video recordings, which are usually transcribed to form written text. One approach to such text is to analyse it to identify and isolate the information that it contains. This approach to analysing text usually involves some form of content analysis (Brewer 2003). While the term 'content analysis' may be used to refer to all forms of textual analysis, it can also refer more narrowly to the identification of specific information.

The starting point for such analysis is the identification of constituent units in the text. If the researcher does not start with a clear idea of the specific characteristics that they are interested in, then the categories and overall scheme will develop following further investigation and comparison. Such an approach has been formalized as part of grounded theory, following a set of analytical strategies that can be applied to a variety of data collection techniques (Charmaz 2003). In this approach, which is considered further in Chapter 5, researchers develop their coding categories through a process of constant comparison. As they collect data, so they identify emerging themes and issues – and, as new themes emerge, they reconsider previously analysed texts in the light of the developing categories.

Griffiths and Jordan (1998) used this approach in their exploratory diary/interview study of patients' experiences during recovery from a lower-limb fracture. The study was based on a convenience sample of nine patients who were recovering from emergency surgery following a lower-limb trauma. The researchers developed a grounded theory by reading the texts and identifying categories. From their analysis, they found three major themes which were consistent with a theoretical model evident in the literature. The patients went through three stages during their recovery: first, feeling stressed and uncertain, then seeking control and finally returning to normal.

Structural analysis

An alternative approach to analysing texts is to treat each text as an entity in its own right as a form of social reality which is the product of, and provides information on, the social processes that shaped its creation and are evident in the form and structure of the narrative. This method involves identifying the structure of each text; the similarities and differences between the structures of each text; an explanation of why a particular structure exists; and how this is used to create a form of social reality.

Conversational analysis provides a way of examining the structure that underlies social interactions (Bryman 2012). Jones and his colleagues (Jones et al. 2000; Jones and Candlin 2003) used diaries to explore the ways in which men who have sex with other men accounted for their actions. They recruited 18 gay men who kept diaries in which they recorded their sexual activities and their reflections on sex and AIDS. In these diaries, they identified 49 'sexual narratives', which they defined as 'accounts of specific sexual encounters with specific partners in specific settings which contained three or more clauses arranged in chronological order' (Jones and Candlin 2003: 203). They found that most of these narratives had a distinctive form, as they took the form of 'paired actions'. This structure was used to present the reported behaviours, even when these were 'risky', such as having unprotected sex, as reasonable and rational within the specific context.

Narrative analysis provides a further approach that explores the structure of the text. Rather than examining the structures of interactions which underpin the text, it addresses the ways in which the narrator structures and uses the narrative. It examines the role of the author in telling the story in a convincing way. Thus, in a narrative analysis the focus is on the production of the text; the identity and intention of its author; the extent to which the author appears in the text; and the devices used in the text. In the case of documents such as letters, the identities and relationships of the person writing the letter and the person receiving it may be important in interpreting the narrative. For example, Honkasalo (2006) has contrasted the suicide notes of men and women in Finland, noting that women write mostly to family or loved ones while men tend to write for, and justify themselves to, a wider audience.

Crossley (2003) used a narrative approach to analyse John Diamond's account of living with oral cancer, which was originally published as a regular column in *The Times* and then reprinted in a posthumous collection of writings (Diamond 2001). Crossley treated Diamond's account as a text in which the author tried to make sense of challenges to his very existence. Crossley suggested that Diamond uses four main devices to structure and communicate his experience of cancer. The first related to the early pre-cancer stage in which Diamond raised the possibility of cancer, but distanced himself from the experience. The second and main device of the narrative involved detailed descriptions of treatment or therapeutic employment when Diamond was engrossed in the treatment process. This alternated with periods of remission when the third device, relative silence about the cancer, was used – before culminating in the final unspoken narrative of dying.

How Documentary Material Can be Used When Presenting Findings

Using numbers

If a researcher uses numbers and statistical analysis, it is important to present these in an interesting way, for example by using visual presentations. Generally, the simpler the analysis, the easier it is to present visually. For example, the products of univariate analyses can be presented as bar charts, pie charts or histograms. Bivariate analyses can be presented as scatter diagrams, though it may be more difficult to present the results of multivariate analyses visually.

Coxon, in his analysis of the Project SIGMA diaries, started his analysis and discussion of sexual sessions with a simple description of the number of sexual acts per session: 'The average (mean) is quite low (1.75 for most data-sets), but there is a very long tail: some sessions are quite long, and a few very long' (1996: 109).

He then moved on to more complex analysis to explore the structure of acts – that is the relationship between different sex acts. He used multidimensional scaling to produce a table of the co-occurrence of sex acts and a map in which each act was positioned to indicate its association with other acts. Using this analysis, Coxon was able to explore the relationship between sex acts showing that some acts such as oral sex tended to be reciprocal, while others such as penetrative sex tended to be asymmetric or 'gendered'.

Developing themes in qualitative data

Content analysis of documents involves taking a number of written texts, breaking them into their constituent parts and reassembling these parts into a new scientific text. The most effective way of presenting such ideas is to describe how they developed out of the analysis of the text, and then to provide illustrative sections of that text. Griffiths and Jordan (1998) used this approach in their study of patients' experiences during recovery from lower-limb fracture, and identified ways in which individuals reconstruct their lives. They use quotes from their texts to illustrate key themes such as loss of control:

> The last few months I really lost control over my life, and I feel I am just existing at the minute. That is how I feel. I feel I am on pause, as if someone has turned on a pause button on my life ... I know it is not going to last. (Griffiths and Jordan 1998: 1281)

Identifying structures

Structural analysis relies on identifying the ways in which documents are created and how they achieve their effect. This involves a comparison of key features of different texts, and therefore the findings are often presented in the form of broad comparisons. Geertz (1988) showed how ethnographers created accounts of other cultures that their readers could understand. He compared, inter alia, two journal-like ethnographies – the diary of Malinowski (1989), with its account of fieldwork in the Melanesian Islands, and the account by Read (1965) of life in Highland New Guinea:

> Instead of the Dostoevskian darkness and Conradian blur [of Malinowski's text], the Readian 'I' is filled with confidence, rectitude, tolerance, patience, good nature, energy, enthusiasm, optimism – with an almost palpable determination to do what is right and think what is proper. If the Diary presents the image of the womanizing cafe intellectual cast among savages, The High Valley presents one of an indefinite country vicar. (Geertz 1988: 85)

Using documents to examine the ways in which nurses learn to manage risk in everyday practice

This example draws on a project that ran from 1996 to 1998, funded by the English National Board for Nursing, Midwifery and Health Visiting. The project was designed to evaluate whether current nurse education adequately prepared nurses to identify and manage the risks associated with supporting vulnerable people in the community (Alaszewski et al. 1998, 2000). In one part of the project, we examined the types of risk nurses identified in their practice and the ways they addressed these. In the other part, we examined current nurse education and the ways in which it prepared nurses to manage risk. In both parts, we used documents alongside other sources of data. To examine risk in nursing practice, we invited a number of nurses to record their everyday practice in diaries and to examine current education we accessed course documentation.

For the study of current practice, we used an interview/diary approach. We felt that using interviews alone would introduce recollection bias – for example, a tendency to remember dramatic events and forget more mundane activities – and was likely to result in generalized and idealized accounts. Observation was an alternative but it would have intruded into the potentially sensitive relationship between the nurses and their clients and might have distorted the very processes that we were seeking to capture. We therefore decided to use a less intrusive approach and invited nurses to act as self-observers and to record their observations in diaries (Alaszewski et al. 2000). We recruited 26 diarists, 10 student nurses, 8 new practitioners and 8 experienced nurses. To examine educational preparation, we sampled 24 current nurse education programmes. We interviewed lecturers, practice teachers and students engaged with each programme and examined course documentation – especially programme validation documents. We found that the latter were especially useful as they were very detailed.

In our analysis of the diaries, we started by identifying decisions – choices which the diarist made between different courses of action. Some decisions could be identified relatively straightforwardly, for example one diarist wrote: 'Decision 1: to allow client to make her own choice where she slept.' Other decisions were embedded in a general discussion of interactions and activities and we needed to examine whether the diarist had implicitly identified a choice, but chosen not to make it. For example, 'Next chap regular. Contriving to support wife regarding catheter care although I end up doing work; wife prefers to watch.' Although the diarist was reporting an activity, she had chosen not to confront the issue of handing over responsibility to the carer and she noted: 'I am allowing the wife to accept her responsibilities slowly.' Having identified the decisions, we then examined them to consider their nature, especially the ways in which nurses identified and managed the risk and uncertainty intrinsic to each decision. From each diary, we selected two contrasting decisions to discuss with the diarist in more detail in a follow-up interview.

(Continued)

(Continued)

Our research team also analysed the content of all the documentation from the 24 selected courses. Each set of documents was read by at least one member of the team and a sample read by two to check for the accuracy of coding. In some documents, risk was explicitly identified within the documentation. But usually risk-related teaching was identified using other categories such as 'safety', 'empowerment', 'advocacy' or 'challenging' behaviour. Using these categories, we were able to identify how, and in what ways, risk was identified and treated within each teaching programme. We could then compare this with lecturers', practice teachers' and students' discussions of risk in a teaching situation.

The documentary material in our study made an important contribution to our published findings. It added both interest and authenticity. For instance, entries in the diaries help to establish the seriousness and urgency of some decisions:

> *Message on answer phone from Client M. She needs to talk to me. When I phone back she says she doesn't need me she is going to [famous landmark on English coast] … My decision is to cancel my first client and go round to M. I find her staring from the window, refusing to let me in. Eventually I persuade her to open the door. She then indicated to me that she is going to drive off [famous landmark on English coast] to join her sister. I arrange for ward to take her and she is admitted.*

The diary material also enabled us to explore the content, complexity and difficulty of many of the risk assessments and of risk management. In focus group interviews, nurses tended to emphasize the importance of identifying and managing hazards. In the diaries and follow-up interviews, a richer and more complex picture emerged. Nurses were often managing dilemmas and conflicts of interest rather than obvious hazards. For example, one set of diary and follow-up interviews allowed us to explore the ways in which a district nurse dealt with pressure from the family of a terminally ill patient to move beyond pain management, to an acceleration of the dying process.

The material from the course documentation provided an insight into the ways in which nurse education prepared nurses for the risks of everyday practice. Overall coverage of risk management was patchy. In only 13 of the 24 sets of documents could we identify risk-related issues and, in most of these, risk did not form a prominent theme in the curriculum. For example, in one registration course on adult nursing, risk was only identified as a theme within a health promotion unit. However, we did identify courses that highlighted risk. In one learning disability course, risk management formed one of the 12 units of competence that successful students were expected to develop. Furthermore, a clear and coherent rationale was given for risk teaching within the documentation that included a well-developed statement of the importance of risk management within professional practice.

Ethical Issues

All health research must not only be ethical, it must also be seen to be ethical. When researchers solicit documents, they need to be aware of their responsibility to protect those who participate in their research. The creation of a personal document such as a diary involves an investment of time and energy and in some cases a personal risk if the subject matter of the document challenges social norms. The researcher needs to be aware of the commitment and ensure that such investment is properly recognized and undue pressure is not placed on individuals to participate. The researcher should provide a written description of the research project and what is expected of the participant and gain their consent. They should also provide a 'document creator' so that the participant knows what is expected and how to contact the researcher if they need further support.

When the researcher uses unsolicited documents contained in public archives, then much of the bureaucracy of governance and ethics is redundant. As the documents are in the public domain, they are freely available. However, it is prudent to consider how, and in what ways, the researcher has a responsibility to those who created the documents and, if they are dead, their descendants. In this context, it may be appropriate for the ethical issues involved in the research to be reviewed by a university or college-based ethical committee.

Researchers who want to use contemporary records relating to current patients cannot follow the precedent set by Garfinkel (1967), namely just to obtain the consent of the doctors responsible for particular patients. The development of the electronic record system has brought about regulations in most developed countries, designed to protect the interests of individuals who are the subject of electronic records. While the scope of such regulation is often restricted to electronic records only, some health care agencies, such as the NHS, have decided to treat traditional paper records in the same way as electronic records. Thus, the researcher who wishes to use contemporary health records not only has to gain the approval of relevant keepers of these records, but also must find a way of gaining access to records that have been anonymized. Otherwise, they must obtain the consent of each and every person whose records they want to use.

Reading Health Research Based on Documents

In reading health research based on documents, as with all research publications you should start by considering the author's description of how and why they used documents. In particular, you should reflect on the following issues:

- The design of the project: was it fit for purpose and was the use of documents necessary and appropriate?
- Which documents were selected, and how, and in what ways, could the selection process introduce bias?
- What was the nature of these documents, who constructed them and for what purpose? How and in what ways was the original purpose aligned with the aims and objectives of the researcher?

Having considered the appropriateness of the documents in terms of the aims and objectives of the research, you should also consider how the documents are used in the publication. In particular, you should consider whether the research is focused on the ways in which the documents are constructed and used, or whether data is being accessed by analysing the content of the documents. If it is the former, then questions should be asked as to what sort of additional information is being used to provide insight into the purpose of the document and its process of construction. If the researchers are employing the documents as a source of information, it is important to ask how relevant information is being extracted and how the analysis of the data is structured.

Conclusion

The case study of nursing illustrates the practical use of documentary analysis in health research, the relevance and applicability of which have been clarified in this chapter – as well as the resources that it requires, its strengths and weaknesses, and the way that data so derived can be coded, analysed and presented. As this chapter shows, the value of this comparatively neglected qualitative method in health research cannot be overstated, particularly given the insights it provides into areas that are otherwise often difficult or impossible to access directly through the use of other research techniques. While further qualitative and quantitative methods are examined in detail in subsequent chapters of this book, its distinctive value is further underlined by the exercise set out for the reader below on the experience of stroke over the past three centuries in the UK.

Exercise: The use of documents in research into the experience of stroke

The following exercise is designed to make you think about the ways in which documents can be used in health research. While the material contained in this chapter may help you consider many of the issues, you may wish to access additional material from a library or the Internet. If you would like to prepare a formal answer, then write a research proposal or protocol.

You want to apply to a charity for funding to undertake a study of the ways in which the experience of stroke has changed over the last 300 years in the UK.

1 What sort of documents could you use?

- Consider the range of possible documents, including personal documents such as diaries and letters, literature, newspapers and pamphlets, medical textbooks, records of care and treatment.
- Consider where such documents might be held for different time periods.
- How could you access appropriate documents?

2 How will you select the documents for your study?

- Consider what sort of design you want to use.
- Consider whether you wish to concentrate on one type of document or compare and contrast.
- How will you judge how 'typical' documents are?

3 How will you analyse documents?

- Will you need to transcribe them?
- Will the analysis be primarily qualitative, quantitative or both? Do you have access to appropriate support such as statistical advice or support for qualitative software packages?
- Will you want to use a software package to help with the analysis?

4 What sort of resources will you need?

- Can you calculate an approximate time budget and identify travel and equipment costs?

5 How will you present your findings?

- Who do you see as the main users of your findings and what are their needs?
- How will you structure publications, such as reports, articles and presentations?
- How will you present the evidence supporting your findings?

Recommended Further Reading

Alaszewski, A. (2006) *Using Diaries for Social Research*. London: Sage.
This book provides a comprehensive overview of the different ways in which diaries can be used for social and health research, describing their development and examining how the method can be most effectively used in all stages of the research process.

Plummer, K. (2001) *Documents of Life 2: An Invitation to Critical Humanism*. London: Sage.
This is a key text that explores the ways in which personal or documents of life can and should be used in social and health research. Plummer argues that such documents can restore the humanism to research.

Prior, L.F. (2003) *Using Documents in Social Research*. London: Sage.
This is an overview of the strategies and debates surrounding the diverse range of documents that can be employed in research, giving examples of their use. Prior adopts a very broad definition of documents and is interested in how they are created and used, as well as in the insights that this provides into social construction. He draws many of his examples from studies of health and illness.

Valles, M.S., Corti, L., Tamboukou, M. and Baer, A. (2011) Qualitative archives and bio-graphical research methods: an introduction to the *FQS* Special Issue. *Forum Qualitative Sozialforschung/Forum: Qualitative Social Research*, 12(3), Art. 8. Available at: http://nbn-resolving.de/urn:nbn:de:0114-fqs110381

FQS is an open-access electronic journal. Although the articles in this special issue do not explicitly focus on health services research, they explore the nature of qualitative research archives and the ways in which they can be used for social research. This introductory article provides an overview plus links to the other articles in the issue.

 ## Online Readings

Barnes, E. (2007) 'Between remission and cure: Patients, practitioners and the transformation of leukaemia in the late twentieth century', *Chronic Illness*, 3: 253–64.

What are the challenges of identifying documents for research? To what extent should documentary analysis be supported by the use of other research methods such as interviews?

Sargeant, S. and Gross, H. (2011) 'Young people learning to live with inflammatory bowel disease: Working with an "unclosed" diary', *Qualitative Health Research,* 21: 1360–70.

What are the challenges of using audio diaries as a research method? What benefits does this type of research tool bring to the research subjects?

References

Alaszewski, A. (2006) *Using Diaries for Social Research.* London: Sage.

Alaszewski, A., Alaszewski, H., Ayer, S. and Manthorpe, J. (2000) *Managing Risk in Community Practice: Nursing, Risk and Decision Making.* Edinburgh: Ballière Tindall.

Alaszewski, A., Alaszewski, H., Manthorpe, J. and Ayer, S. (1998) *Assessing and Managing Risk in Nursing Education and Practice: Supporting Vulnerable People in the Community.* London: ENB.

Bolger, N., Davis, A. and Rafaeli, E. (2003) 'Diary methods: capturing life as it is lived', *Annual Review of Psychology*, 54: 579–616.

Brewer, J. (2003) 'Content analysis', in R.L. Miller and J.D. Brewer (eds), *The A–Z of Social Research.* London: Sage.

Bryman, A. (2012) *Social Research Methods,* 4th edition. Oxford: Oxford University Press.

Charmaz, K. (2003) 'Grounded theory: objectivist and constructivist methods', in N.K. Denzin and Y.S. Lincoln (eds), *Strategies of Qualitative Inquiry.* Thousand Oaks, CA: Sage.

The Chambers Dictionary (2008), 11th edition. Edinburgh: Chambers Harrap Publishers.

Clarkson, L. (2003) 'Documentary sources', in R.L. Miller and J.D. Brewer (eds), *The A–Z of Social Research*. London: Sage.

Corti, L. (2003) 'Documentary sources', in R.L. Miller and J.D. Brewer (eds), *The A–Z of Social Research*. London: Sage.

Coxon, A.P.M. (1996) *Between the Sheets: Sexual Diaries and Gay Men's Sex in the Era of AIDS*. London: Cassell.

Crossley, M.L. (2003) '"Let me explain": narrative employment and one patient's experience of oral cancer', *Social Science and Medicine*, 56: 439–48.

Diamond, J. (2001) *Snake Oil and Other Preoccupations*. London: Vintage.

Elliott, H. (1997) 'The use of diaries in sociological research on health experience', *Sociological Research Online*, 2(2). Available at: www.socresonline.org.uk/socresonline/2/2/7.html

Garfinkel, H. (1967) '"Good" organizational reasons for "bad" clinical records', in H. Garfinkel, *Studies in Ethnomethodology*. Englewoods Cliffs, NJ: Prenctice-Hall, pp. 187–207.

Geertz, C. (1988) *Works and Lives: The Anthropologist as Author*. Cambridge: Polity Press.

Griffiths, H. and Jordan, S. (1998) 'Thinking of the future and walking back to normal: an exploratory study of patients' experiences during recovery from lower limb fracture', *Journal of Advanced Nursing*, 28: 1276–88.

Honkasalo, M.-J. (2006) 'Fragilities in life and death', *Health, Risk and Society*, 8(1): 27–41.

Jones, R.H. and Candlin, C.N. (2003) 'Constructing risk across timescales and trajectories: gay men's stories of sexual encounters', *Health, Risk and Society*, 5: 199–213.

Jones, R.H., Kwan, Y.K. and Candlin, C.N. (2000) *A Preliminary Investigation of HIV Vulnerability and Risk Behavior among Men who have Sex with Men in Hong Kong*. Hong Kong: City University of Hong Kong.

Jordanova, L. (2000) *History in Practice*. London: Arnold.

MacFarlane, A. (1970) *The Family Life of Ralph Josselin: A Seventeenth-Century Clergyman: An Essay in Historical Anthropology*. Cambridge: Cambridge University Press.

MacFarlane, A. and Turin, A. (2008) 'The digitization of Naga collections in the West and the "return of culture"', in M. Oppitz, T. Kaiser, A. von Stockhausen and M. Wettstein (eds), *Naga Identities: Changing Local Cultures in the Northeast of India*. Ghent: Snoeck, pp. 367–78.

MacGregor, N. (2010) *A History of the World in 100 Objects*. London: Allen Lane.

Malinowski, B. (1989) *A Diary in the Strict Sense of the Word*. London: Athlone.

Miller, K.A. (1985) *Emigrants and Exiles: Ireland and the Irish Exodus to North America*. New York: Oxford University Press.

Moser, C.A. and Kalton, C. (1971) *Survey Methods in Social Investigation*. London: Heinemann.

Parkin, D., Rice, N., Jacoby, A. and Doughty, J. (2004) 'Use of a visual analogue scale in a daily patient diary: modelling cross-sectional time-series data on health-related quality of life', *Social Science and Medicine*, 59: 351–60.

Penn Library (2004) *Finding Diaries – Research Guide.* Available at: http://gethelp.library.upenn.edu/guides/general/diaries.html

Plummer, K. (2001) *Documents of Life 2: An Invitation to Critical Humanism.* London: Sage.

Pollock, L.A. (1983) *Forgotten Children: Parent-child Relations from 1500 to 1900.* Cambridge: Cambridge University Press.

Prior, L.F. (2003) *Using Documents in Social Research.* London: Sage

Prior, L., Wood, F., Gray, J., Pill, R. and Hughes, D. (2002) 'Making risk visible: the role of images in the assessment of (cancer) genetic risk'. *Health, Risk and Society*, 4(3): 241–58.

Read, K.E. (1965) *The High Valley.* New York: Scribner.

Robinson, D. (1971) *The Process of Becoming Ill.* London: Routledge and Kegan Paul.

Sahlins, M. (1995) *How 'Natives' Think: About Captain Cook, For Example.* Chicago, IL: University of Chicago Press.

Sheridan, D. (ed.) (1991) *The Mass-Observation Diaries: An Introduction.* The Mass-Observation Archive (University of Sussex Library) and the Centre for Continuing Education, Falmer: University of Sussex. Available at: www.sussex.ac.uk/library/massobs/diaries

Stone, A.A., Shiffman, S., Schwartz, J.E., Broderick, J.E. and Hufford, M.R. (2003) 'Patient compliance with paper and electronic diaries', *Controlled Clinical Trials*, 24: 182–99.

Thomas, W.I. and Znaniecki, F. (1958) *The Polish Peasant in Europe and America*, Volume 1. New York: Dover.

Weber, M. (1978) *Economy and Society.* Berkeley and Los Angeles, CA: University of California Press.

Wertz, M.S., Kyriss, T., Paranjape, S. and Glantz, S.A. (2011) 'The toxic effects of cigarette additives. Philip Morris' project mix reconsidered: an analysis of documents released through litigation', *PLoS Med* 8(12): e1001145. doi:10.1371/journal.pmed.1001145

WW2 People's War Team (2004) *About WW2 People's War.* Available at: www.bbc.co.uk/dna/ww2/About

Zimmerman, D.H. and Wieder, D.L. (1977) 'The diary-interview method', *Urban Life*, 5: 479–98.

5

Unstructured and Semi-structured Interviews in Health Research

JACQUELINE LOW

Introduction

- The unstructured interview, also referred to as the in-depth, the open-ended, the narrative or the long interview, has become a favoured method in qualitative research, in research generally (Riessman 2008; Silverman 2010, 2011) and in research into health and health care in particular (Silverman 1998; Miczo 2003). This is the case not only in the social sciences, but also in the field of nursing (Sorrell and Redmond 1995) and evidence-based medical and other clinical research (Boulton et al. 1996) where 'lay knowledge' has been deemed essential to the development of health policy and practice. Semi-structured interviews in qualitative research are no less useful in these contexts and are of particular relevance where researchers have more narrow and specific research questions. Almost all of the methodological techniques employed in both the unstructured and semi-structured interview are standard, irrespective of substantive context (Booth and Booth 1996). However, in health research, especially where there are sensitive issues or vulnerable informants, the researcher faces particular challenges (Corbin and Morse 2003).
- In this chapter, the advantages of unstructured and semi-structured interview as central techniques in qualitative research are explored, which is followed by an account of the stages of a project using these methods. Issues of data collection and techniques for data analysis are considered. The validity, reliability and generalizability of these forms of data collection are discussed and a checklist for ways of demonstrating rigour is provided. Finally, an indication is given of how to present research findings in such a way that enhances their credibility and how to read research in this area. This is complemented by a case study.

The Advantages of Using Unstructured and Semi-structured Interviews

Unstructured and semi-structured interviews have certain advantages over survey research and the structured questionnaire. As discussed in Chapter 2, quantitative methods set out with particular questions in mind to test a particular hypothesis. In contrast, interpretivist or constructivist theoretical perspectives using qualitative methods take an inductive approach that provides access to the subjective perceptions of individuals, as well as the means by which they give meaning to their experiences. For example, survey data can provide an invaluable context for qualitative data (Silverman 1998) by furnishing data concerning the number and demographic characteristics of people with a chronic illness. However, it can tell us less about the experience of living with chronic illness. The latter is better achieved through the use of the unstructured and semi-structured interview. Many argue that these methods of data collection are the best way to gain access to experiences of health and illness where people already feel disempowered by their illness. They are essential tools too in gathering data from people who, due to illness and/or disability, may be physically unable to participate in other types of research. For instance, Higgins and Daly (1999) used unstructured interviews successfully with people on mechanical ventilation.

Corbin and Morse (2003) and others have discussed with clarity the advantages of the unstructured interview, which also apply to the semi-structured interview. These can be summarized in Box 5.1 as follows:

Box 5.1 The advantages of unstructured interviews

- They are a cost-effective way of collecting a great deal of data in a relatively short time frame.
- They are useful when exploring research areas that are complex or about which little is known.
- They can address how and why questions from the perspective of subjective experience – that is, they allow researchers to explore the perceptions of individuals and how they give meaning to, or interpret, their experiences.
- They are flexible, allowing the researcher to pursue emergent themes and follow the lead of the interviewee as to how they construct particular phenomena, thus gaining new insights.
- The pace of unstructured and semi-structured interviews can be adjusted throughout. This is particularly useful in dealing with people on matters of health and illness. For example, people who are ill may tire easily or begin to feel pain during the interview.

Source: Corbin and Morse (2003)

Other qualitative researchers have noted that unstructured and semi-structured interviews:

- Allow the researcher the opportunity to seek ongoing informed consent. This is important when dealing with sensitive issues in research in health and illness (Miczo 2003).
- Give informants more power and control over what gets discussed in the interview and how it gets discussed (Johnson 2002).
- Allow researchers the opportunity to reflect on, and distance themselves from, their tacit knowledge of the topic under study (McCracken 1988).

Stages of Research Using Unstructured or Semi-structured Interview Techniques

The first step in carrying out research is to decide on your research question and then carry out a literature review. Having decided that questions you wish to address, which dictate the use of unstructured or semi-structured methods of data collection, you must plan your research. The next initial task is to recruit informants.

Recruiting research participants

Most commonly, 'purposeful' sampling is used where informants are selected who have specific knowledge about the research question (Curtis et al. 2000). This is made easier if informants are members of a pre-existing group or if they congregate at one locale (Johnson 2002). Alternatively, organizations such as physicians' professional associations or health consumer groups like the Multiple Sclerosis Society, can be approached in order to make contact with potential informants. Hospital administrators can also be asked for help in recruiting health personnel to participate in health service research. This is known as the 'health services' model of recruitment where health service providers or agencies provide contact information and/or client or patient lists to the researchers, or do the recruiting on behalf of the research team (UyBico et al. 2007). In many cases, this means that the service provider undertakes to send a recruitment letter from the researchers to clients or patients who are invited to contact the researchers directly if they are willing to participate in the project. In other situations, a two-stage process is followed. Here, the service provider or other third party with privileged access to people's names and addresses approaches potential research participants with an outline of the project and what it would involve, to ask if they would be prepared to take part. Only when permission has been received should details be given to a researcher. Chapter 15 discusses this and other ethical issues in research further.

However, in many cases, there simply is no specific setting in which to recruit people to take part in interviews, whether unstructured or semi-structured. For example, when I first began researching the lay use of alternative therapies in Canada, there were few holistic health centres and, as I did not want to limit my analysis to the clients of any one alternative practitioner, there was no one setting in which to recruit informants (Low 2004a). I therefore had to use a combination of snowball sampling (that is, asking one informant to suggest another) and convenience sampling (that is, contacting known, rather than randomly selected, informants) in making contact. Using 'insider awareness', where the researcher has personal experience of the substantive topic or social world under study, I began convenience sampling by approaching an acquaintance who had used alternative health care (Douglas 1976). Snowball sampling occurred at the end of each interview when I asked informants if they knew of anyone else who would be interested in taking part in the study. Researchers should keep track in field notes of how they have made contact with informants, as well as noting the nature of any relationships between informants. They can then differentiate in their analysis between patterns that reflect friendship or other related networks from more general patterns in the data (Low 2004a). The technique of sampling is discussed further in Chapter 9.

Decisions must also be made about how many informants to recruit, as well as how many interviews to conduct. For instance, in grounded theory research it is the concept or basic item being counted or studied, not the informant, which is the unit of analysis (Corbin and Strauss 1990). Theoretically, therefore, one interview is sufficient provided it is adequate in terms of conceptual richness. In reality, however, one interview is seldom enough. A commonly used guideline is that at least 20–30 informants should be interviewed and re-interviewed. In narrative analysis, and some types of linguistic or discourse analyses, the number of interviews is typically very small. Nonetheless, enough data must be collected to enable the researcher to reach 'theoretic saturation' (Glaser and Strauss 1967). Theoretic saturation is satisfied when no new information is generated by subsequent interviews, and when the data reflect a conceptual richness that both accounts for 'variations' in the data, and allows for a detailed description of the 'processes' informants experience. This also enables the researcher exhaustively to analyse relationships between concepts and the categories identified (Strauss and Corbin 1990).

The unstructured and semi-structured technique

It would be a mistake to conclude that the central difference between the unstructured and semi-structured interview is the absence or presence of structure as, in practice, there is no interview technique that is totally devoid of structure. At the very least, the unstructured interview must be informed by a research question or questions and researchers should have some idea of how they will begin the interview. As the name suggests, unstructured interviews do not follow a set path and may vary in length and/or richness. The questions employed in the unstructured interview should be open-ended and as non-directive as possible. McCracken

(1988) likens this type of interview to a conversation where the researcher says as little as possible, allowing informants to tell their stories in their own fashion. The unstructured interview is a dynamic event that 'often takes unexpected turns or digressions that follow the informant's interest or knowledge' (Johnson 2002: 111). Both the informant and the researcher are deeply involved in the emergent narrative. The unstructured interview typically opens with a 'grand tour' question (McCracken 1988). These are questions that encourage informants to begin speaking without directing the content or substance of their discourse. For instance, a researcher might begin by saying something like: 'Tell me about your experiences in communicating with your physician.' In contrast, when using the semi-structured interview, several questions will be asked of all informants. These should be prepared in advance and attention must be paid to crafting questions that are not leading. However, unlike a survey questionnaire, which features consistently worded, close-ended and strictly ordered questions, there is no epistemological imperative to ask questions in exactly the same way or in the same order in each unstructured or semi-structured interview. Indeed, questions may need to be modified to fit the biographical and socio-cultural contexts that shape informants' lives.

In cases of both the unstructured and the structured interview, subsequent questions are based on what the informant says, and prompts are used to support informants in telling their story, and to solicit further information, clarification or explanation. According to McCracken (1988), 'floating prompts' like features of everyday speech – such as eyebrow raises or the repetition of a keyword – maintain the flow of responses without undue interruption of the informant's narrative. In contrast, planned prompts, or probes, are used when further explanation is required, or when the researcher wishes to delve deeper (Crabtree and Miller 1991). Recapitulation probes are also used where informants are asked to 'retell parts of stories'. In so doing, they may add new details (Sorrell and Redmond 1995). When to prompt is a matter of researcher judgement. Some researchers choose to wait until the interview is complete before probing, as they believe that any type of interruption of the informant's speech will affect the meaning of the findings. Others choose to prompt as the interview progresses, which is often a better strategy as themes can be pursued in the context in which they emerge. Any potentially sensitive question, including those related to age, gender, class, income and ethnic background, should be asked at the conclusion of the interview after trust and rapport between the researcher and informant have been established.

Researchers must also be aware of the implications of silence in unstructured and semi-structured interviews (Sorrell and Redmond 1995). As Charmaz (2002: 303) points out:

> Not all experiences are storied, nor are all experiences stored for ready recall. Silences have meaning too. Silences signify an absence – of words and/or perceivable emotions ... [and] may ... reflect active signals – of meaning, boundaries, and rules.

Periods of silence may also indicate that the informant is becoming tired, that illness and/or disability is compromising their ability to speak, or that they are in pain. Silence may also indicate a breach of communication norms. For example, something the researcher says may literally 'silence' the informant. Finally, informants may silence the researcher as well when they decline to answer a question (Charmaz 2002). The researcher therefore must listen carefully and prompt judiciously in response to what informants say, or do not say. Silence should be noted and accounted for in the analysis. As important, for researchers using an unstructured or structured interview technique, is reflexivity. The interviewer must be aware of their 'tacit' or assumed knowledge about the topic they are researching, and they should be able to distance themselves so they do not make unwarranted assumptions about their informants' views. They must remember to ask informants to explain what they mean (McCracken 1988).

Resourcing the unstructured and semi-structured interview

In addition to technical skills, unstructured and semi-structured interviews require significant interpersonal skills, as well as access to resources. One such resource is willing and informed research participants. Not all potential informants are sufficiently motivated to participate in an unstructured interview as a greater commitment in terms of time and emotional energy is required (Johnson 2002). Furthermore, not all informants are articulate and not all interviews result in an equally high degree of conceptual richness (Charmaz 2002). However, it would be a mistake for the researcher to equate succinct responses with a lack of richness of the data, especially in cases where illness or disability constrain the informant's speech. As Booth and Booth (1996: 66) argue, '… it is possible for people to communicate a story in one word answers. Even single words can leave a big wash.'

If unstructured and semi-structured qualitative interviews require more of informants, they also require more from the researcher. Glaser and Strauss (1967) argue that researchers must develop 'theoretic sensitivity' so that they can judge when theoretic saturation and conceptual richness have been reached. Furthermore, locating and contacting informants, especially in medical settings, can be difficult and requires reserves of energy and ingenuity. Unstructured and semi-structured interviews also mean that researchers need to invest much of themselves and their emotions in the interview process (Charmaz 2002). Corbin and Morse (2003: 344) argue that interviewers can 'become involved in the story and reach out with empathy to participants'. Consequently, the unstructured and semi-structured interview method is always demanding and can often be exhausting for the researcher.

Collecting and Analysing Unstructured and Semi-structured Interview Data

Recording data

It is important to record unstructured and semi-structured interviews as an informant's words must be presented verbatim in the analysis to preserve meaning (Johnson 2002).

Silverman (1998) advocates the use of video recording to better record the interactive aspects of the structured or unstructured interview. However, this may be felt to be too intrusive and to jeopardize confidentiality. Digital audio-recorders are currently the best means of audio-recording interviews. They are typically very small and even the least expensive have sharp sound and little if any interference in playback. This is a huge improvement over analogue audio-tape recording. Digital recorders also have the added advantage of enabling interviews to be shared via digital audio files, thus facilitating team research. In addition, such audio files can be imported into qualitative analysis software and synchronized with the corresponding transcript. NVivo 9 also has a function that allows direct coding of audio files. Nonetheless, there are situations where audio-recording is difficult. An informant may refuse to give permission for the interview to be recorded or the interview might take place in noisy or crowded locations that are not the best setting for unstructured or semi-structured interviews. In cases where audio or video recording is impossible, researchers must use their note-taking skills during, and after, the interview to preserve as much of the informant's actual words as possible. Even when able to audio or video record the interview, field notes should be taken that include non-verbal aspects of the interview, such as facial expressions, body language, the setting and informant/researcher interaction, as these may affect interpretation (Miczo 2003).

The setting chosen for the interview should be one in which the informant feels comfortable and affords a degree of privacy. For instance, if the researcher was interested in interviewing domiciliary care workers about their relationships with their clients, interviewing them in their place of work would not be appropriate. Likewise, if the interviews are with hospital nurses and focus on workplace stress, interviewing them in the hospital where they work would not engender trust and thus their workplace would not be a suitable setting for the interview. In all cases, the researcher should ask the informant where he or she would like the interview to take place and efforts must be made to accommodate the informant's wishes.

Allowing time

A fundamental resource required using unstructured and semi-structured interview techniques is time. Setting up and conducting interviews, and particularly transcribing and analysing data, are time-greedy activities. Time is required to recruit informants, schedule interviews and allow for re-interviews. In health research, more time may be required as, for example, informants with a chronic illness may tire easily and several short interviews may be necessary. Analysis of the vast amount of data that results from unstructured and semi-structured interviews is also time-consuming. Unstructured and semi-structured interviews are typically long, and transcription of one audio-taped interview can take 'several hours ... generat[ing] 20–40 pages of single-spaced text' (Pope et al. 2000: 114). Crabtree and Miller (1991: 148–9) report that it took them up to six hours 'to highlight and make notations on a twenty-four page transcript' when using a fairly simple coding scheme. More complex methods of coding, such as thematic or comparative coding where transcripts are read and re-read several times throughout the analysis, can take much longer.

Methods for data analysis

Discussions about how to analyse, like making decisions about how to collect, semi-structured or unstructured interview data are informed by the theoretical assumptions held by the researcher (Kvale 1996). For instance, if the researcher is aiming to develop a grounded theory, analytic induction is a technique for deriving theory from empirical research, in contrast to a deductive approach, where data are collected to support or refute an existing theory (see also Chapter 2). In the case of grounded theory, theoretic sampling and comparative coding are the forms of analysis mode employed. According to Glaser and Strauss (1967: 45), theoretic sampling is a method by which 'the analyst jointly collects, codes, and analyses data and decides what data to collect next and where to find them, in order to develop theory as it emerges'. Open coding is 'the process of breaking down, examining, comparing, conceptualizing, and categorizing data' (Corbin and Strauss 1990: 61) – an area also covered in Chapter 6 of this book.

Other theoretical approaches dictate different types of coding. For instance, Baker (2002: 778) asserts that within ethnomethodology, informants' stories are understood 'as accounts rather than reports'. Such analysis therefore involves coding individuals' explanations for their beliefs and behaviour. Depending on the mode of analysis followed, the style of transcription will also vary. Thus, in the case of narrative analysis transcription, this will include recording pauses, hesitations, the timing of responses and other linguistic devices, in addition to the words spoken by the informant. The analyst will then be able to discern how a text is structured and organized in order to bring out its meaning (Kvale 1996).

Data coding

Regardless of the particular mode of analysis chosen, coding of unstructured interviews takes the form of a thematic analysis (Ryan and Bernard 2003). More specifically, it is the rigorous and systematic analysis of data that results in the development of concepts and categories that emerge from the words of informants, culminating in the development of conceptual and explanatory models – what Glaser and Strauss (1967) would call 'formal theory' (Silverman 1998). This kind of content analysis means more than merely counting occurrences of key terms. Rather, the researcher analysing unstructured or semi-structured interview data more often codes for similarity of meaning rather than for words or phrases, as informants hardly ever express themselves in exactly the same way. This does not indicate that they are inconsistent in terms of the conceptual meaning intended. For example, in my analysis of the lay model of alternative health and healing, one informant used the words 'inner self' while another spoke about her 'higher self', but what they were both talking about was the importance of drawing on their own spiritual power to heal themselves (Low 2004a).

How the researcher goes about the practical task of coding and categorizing is a matter of preference. Some highlight transcripts; others use word-processing search, copy and paste functions; and still others photocopy and physically cut up the transcripts to categorize data. Increasingly, qualitative researchers make use of qualitative analysis software as a tool to aid in categorizing data from unstructured and semi-structured interviews. It is important to be aware that qualitative analysis software does not do the conceptual or analytic work for the researcher. They must still discern themes and develop concepts and categories by reading and re-reading the transcripts as well as making analytic notes. Software merely helps in storing, moving and collating large amounts of text-based data – to paraphrase Silverman (1998): 'garbage in, garbage out.' However, the current generation of qualitative analysis software does have some very useful functions (Bringer et al. 2006).

What is most valuable about using qualitative analysis software is the time that it can save in analysing interview transcripts. For example, in an interview project with 30 informants, it would not be uncommon to have almost one thousand pages of single-spaced interview transcript. If one wished to see if there was a relationship between gender and a particular emergent theme, qualitative analysis software can search for, and collate, all the places in those thousand pages of transcript where such a relationship exists in a matter of minutes. This is a task that would take hours if it was attempted by reading through the transcripts and manually noting instances of the relationship. In addition, qualitative analysis software like NVivo 9 can facilitate inter-rater reliability, as more than one researcher can code the same transcript and the program keeps track of, and displays, the coding of different researchers.

Further, such qualitative analysis software allows researchers to code audio and video files, photographs or other images in the same way as they would code text and with equal ease. For the most part, qualitative analysis software makes what one would do manually easier and faster. There is at least one task in qualitative analysis that is accomplished better by qualitative analysis software than could be done manually and that is analytic modelling, or what Ryan and Bernard (2003) call meta-coding. This is where concepts and categories are linked conceptually and in this case NVivo 9's automated modelling feature is invaluable. Once data is coded into concepts and categories, it can be loaded onto a modelling screen where the concepts and categories appear as labelled shapes. These can be easily highlighted and dragged to different positions on the screen as the researcher makes decisions about the hierarchical arrangements within their emergent conceptual model. This kind of diagramming can be done by hand but it cannot be modified as quickly as is possible using the software. The critical point here is that thinking conceptually often happens very quickly and the software can keep up with the researcher's thought processes in a way that drawing by hand could never do.

Regardless of the type of analysis or the practical method of coding employed, attention must be paid in the analysis to divergent themes: what some researchers call 'deviant cases'

(Silverman 1998). This is essential for capturing conceptual richness and enhancing the validity of unstructured and semi-structured interview findings. For instance, only one participant in my research on the users of alternative health care said that a desire for control over the healing process motivated her use of these therapies. This was significant as it allowed me to critically address assumptions in the literature about what motivates people to seek out alternative health care (Low 2004a). It is also important to pay attention to discordant elements or seeming contradictions within the discourse of informants as they can give insight into its deeper meaning (Corbin and Morse 2003). Divergent cases can also illuminate the way in which an informant's story has been influenced by the researcher (Miczo 2003).

Enhancing Rigour: Validity, Reliability and Generalizability

Validity

The validity of unstructured and semi-structured interview findings centres on the richness of the data that are generated by this method. The information disclosed by informants is so detailed that it guards against

> … bias by making it difficult for [informants] to produce data that uniformly support a mistaken conclusion, just as [it makes] it difficult for observers to restrict [their] observations so that [they] see only what supports [their] prejudices and expectations. (Becker 1970a: 52)

This richness derives, in part, from the fact that the researcher allows the informant to direct the flow of conversation, saying as little as possible. This bolsters the validity of the finding as statements volunteered by informants are 'likely to reflect the observer's preoc-cupations and possible biases less than [those] made in response to questions posed by the researcher' (Becker 1970b: 193). Furthermore, the non-directive nature of open-ended questions enhances validity as informants are able to articulate their experiences, rather than having to conform to predetermined answer categories imposed by the researcher (Cicourel 1982). Informants can be asked to review the analysis and provide feedback on whether or not concepts and categories reflect their understanding of their experience. This also enhances the validity of findings from unstructured and semi-structured interviews. It has been said by advocates of these methods that unstructured or semi-structured inter-view data is not valid or is invalid in relation to an 'objective' truth. Instead, the unstruc-tured interview is seen as a 'social occasion' (Johnson 2002) and is therefore governed by power relations and rules of communication (Miczo 2003). The narrative or story which emerges from the unstructured interview is one that is jointly constructed between the researcher and the informant and this makes it both 'process and product' of that interac-tion (Charmaz 2002).

Reliability

The quantitative notion of reliability, that research instruments 'continually yield an unvarying measurement', is not only inappropriate to research employing the unstructured or semi-structured interview, but also impossible to achieve using this method of data collection (Kirk and Miller 1986: 42). This is because the social world is dynamic, not static. Consequently, two researchers who interview the same informant at different times using the same questions will invariably collect different data (Becker 1970a). However, this should not be taken as an indication that the unstructured or semi-structured interview method is unreliable. Rather, it is that the social context and the informant's perspective have changed over time. The unstructured or semi-structured interview, though, must satisfy the standards of synchronic reliability, that is, achieve a 'similarity of observations within the same time period'. They must also achieve consistent observations with regard to the researcher's conceptual concerns (Kirk and Miller 1986: 42). More simply, the words that informants use will rarely be the same, yet they can still be conceptually consistent.

Techniques to enhance validity and reliability so that the reader can assess the overall credibility of the findings include those as set out in Box 5.2.

Box 5.2   Techniques to enhance validity and reliability

- Audio-taping interviews and taking comprehensive field notes
- Systematic transcription and analysis, allowing others to assess how researchers have analysed their data and developed theoretic constructs
- Using a combination of methods or sources of data, such as observation or documentary analysis (see Chapter 6 and Chapter 22 for discussions of triangulation)
- Employing inter-judge or inter-rater techniques – here, more than one researcher codes the transcripts. Comparing coding can increase consistency, reliability and validity in both coding and the subsequent analysis
- Using a 'member test' or informant validation – here, analysis and early findings are assessed through the informant's confirmation that these reflect accurately their perspectives and experiences.

Generalizability

However valid and reliable the findings from unstructured interview research are, the analyst must also pay attention to the nature of the generalizations that can be made from the findings. For instance, what Williams (2000) refers to as moderatum generalization or 'generalizations about everyday life' are important for research where the intention is theoretic or conceptual generalization, rather than statistical generalization. This is where an informant's individual perceptions, beliefs and experiences can be seen as indicators of larger socio-cultural features or generic social processes (Blumer 1969). Williams (2000: 215) illustrates what he means by moderatum generalization by invoking Geertz's classic ethnographic analysis of the cockfight, in writing:

> Geertz's claim ... 'that every people loves its own form of violence' is an example of such a general feature, which is then reworked and enriched through the specific inferences about the [particular] 'cockfight'.

Silverman (1998) argues that attention to the historical, cultural, political and contextual grounding of informant discourse is necessary to enhance generalizability of the findings from unstructured or semi-structured interview research. Analyses must be situated in the historical context, and the political factors behind informants' experiences must be addressed. Attention must also be paid to how cultural constructs and discourses are both reflected in, and shape, informants' beliefs and action. For example, Lupton and Chapman (1995) ground their analysis of media coverage of the role played by cholesterol in heart disease in the socio-cultural context of contemporary discourses about food as being healthy or unhealthy. Contextual grounding refers to the fact that social phenomena take on a variety of meanings in different contexts and that individuals construct contexts for their actions. Thus, analyses of unstructured interview data must also take account of how salient aspects of informants' personal biographies shape their experience and behaviour (Lupton 1997). For instance, health status, such as living with chronic illness, may be one biographical factor that shapes experience, perception and action (Low 2004b).

Presenting Unstructured and Semi-structured Interview Findings

Demonstrating credibility in presentations

How findings from unstructured and semi-structured interview analysis are presented impacts directly on the credibility of the research. For example, informants' speech should be used verbatim in presentation of the findings as rewording or summarizing inevitably reduces validity by changing the meaning of words. It also detracts from the reliability of the findings as readers cannot assess the validity of the data for themselves. Ideally, research questions and informant responses should be presented together as answers are inextricably linked to the questions to which they are a response. Furthermore, in order to allow the reader to assess validity, the researcher needs to indicate whether or not the labels applied to concepts and categories presented in the findings emerge from the actual words of the informants or are researcher constructs (Silverman 1998).

Sufficient informant quotations must also be included so that readers are able to evaluate the findings for themselves (Boulton et al. 1996). Here, it is important for researchers to indicate whether the quotations selected are representative of some, many or all of the participants in the research. Researchers must also make plain how contradictory cases have been accounted for. To this end, Silverman (1998) argues that counting events and therefore 'quasi statistics' should be included in presentations. However, others caution that presenting findings in the form of percentages or relative frequencies may be misleading when the findings are derived from a small number of interviews (Pope et al. 2000). In contrast, presenting precise counts can sometimes be important. For instance, the finding that only one out of 21 informants in my study of the lay use of alternative therapies said that they had a desire for control over health and healing, was essential to the credibility of my conclusions. I argued that the generic social process of problem solving and not individual motivating factors, better explained informants' health-seeking behaviour. Demonstrating credibility in presentations also involves setting out the theoretical perspective taken in the study. This can be done by giving detailed descriptions of how reliability and validity have been ensured, and including excerpts from field notes that describe how the data were collected, transcribed and analysed to provide a paper trail. The drawback is that if all of the aspects of the unstructured and semi-structured interview method described above are included, this can fill several pages of the article or report. Researchers should be aware that many journals, especially those in medicine and nursing, typically publish only very short articles. Editors of such journals may object to lengthy methodology sections or to the inclusion of the large amount of data necessary to present the findings adequately. This may inhibit the publication of qualitative studies (Boulton et al. 1996). It may therefore be wise for health researchers using this method to include, in the covering letter accompanying their submission, the argument that such information is essential so that both referees and readers can assess the reliability and validity of their study.

Weaknesses of the Unstructured and Semi-structured Interview Method

While conducting unstructured and semi-structured interviewing can be more cost-effective than survey research, a corresponding weakness of the method is the greater amount of time invested in the analysis of unstructured interview data compared with statistical analysis. In addition, Silverman (1998) concludes that the unstructured interview should never be used as a substitute for observation. He thus calls into question its usefulness as a stand-alone method. He asserts that while unstructured interviews are an effective method of gathering data about what people say, they are less useful as a means of capturing what they do. However, what people say about what they do provides valid and useful information. It is an account of their experience of what they do. As Trow (1970) convincingly argues, observation and interview are different methods that measure different things. One is not inherently better than the other. However, it is also the case that when more than one method of data collection is used, the findings can be triangulated and based on more robust evidence.

Silverman (1998) also asserts that a weakness of the unstructured interview method is that the data collected are retrospective. It is an informant's description of event(s) that happened in the past, and therefore cannot be an accurate account of their experience at the actual time the event(s) occurred. However, the moment we experience something, it becomes part of our past, thus we always make sense of our lives retrospectively. In the end, all methods have strengths and weaknesses. Good researchers are aware of them and use their informed judgement in selecting the method appropriate to the research question at hand. This applies no less to the use of unstructured or semi-structured interviews in health research than for other methods.

CASE STUDY

Case study: The use of semi-structured interviews in alternative and complementary health care

The research I conducted on how lay people assess the efficacy of the alternative and complementary therapies they use is illustrative of many of the methodological issues already discussed in this chapter. In this study, I used semi-structured interviewing to collect data from people with Parkinson's disease who used alternative and/or complementary health care. In addition to the symptoms of Parkinson's disease and the adverse reactions caused by Parkinson's medication, some of the people I spoke to also experienced difficulty with verbal and non-verbal communication. Thus, having Parkinson's disease is a salient aspect of these informants' personal biographies that needed to be taken account of in recruitment, data collection and analysis.

Contacting informants

I was able to make contact with informants through the pre-existing groups of the Parkinson's Disease Society (1999) and Young, Alert, Parkinson's Partners and Relatives. In the end, 14 people were eligible to participate in the interviews, a relatively small number of informants. However, this did not present a problem concerning the generalizability of my findings as the data collected were conceptually rich and my intent was to develop a theoretical explanation of how these people determined efficacy, not to make statistical generalizations about how people assess efficacy.

Conducting interviews

This research demonstrated the flexibility of the semi-structured interview approach to data collection which allowed me to start and stop interviews in response to informants when they became tired, were experiencing pain, and when the effectiveness of their medication began to wear off. Moreover, the method also proved invaluable in coping with the communication difficulties that occurred during some of these interviews. This flexibility meant that there was more scope for probing for clarification; repeating questions or keywords; and checking and rechecking that we had understood each other.

Some communication difficulties resulted in several virtually unintelligible portions of the audio-recorded interviews, reinforcing the need to take systematic field notes in addition to audio-recording. Transcription and analysis of the interviews took much longer than anticipated as it was necessary to verify with informants that I had interpreted their voices correctly. This also meant noting the length of informant pauses, the types of questions that generated problems in communication, and informant requests for repetition. The symptoms of Parkinson's disease also impacted on the nature of the data collected. Some interviews were quite short and, due to speech difficulties, some informant responses were very brief. However, it was possible to probe in order to expand upon brief responses (Low 2006).

Selecting deviant cases

Finally, the importance of accounting for contradictory cases, and attention to contextual grounding, in the analysis of unstructured interview data were highlighted by this research. Through the process of comparative coding, for instance, I noted that some informants believed that a therapy is effective if it works for one person – arguing that, even if it did not work for them, it might for someone else. In seeming contradiction, they also believed that therapies need to work for most people to be considered efficacious. However, what appeared to be a contradiction was actually a reflection of these informants' internalization of both an alternative healing ideology, which posits an individual notion of efficacy, as well as the view that state-subsidized health services lack the funds to provide services that do not work for all (Low 2003).

Reading Health Research Based on Unstructured/ Semi-structured Interviews

As will be apparent from the foregoing, in reading health research based on unstructured and semi-structured interviews, it is important, among other things, to consider how far:

- The form of the interviews is appropriate in addressing the research question(s).
- The relevant data is being gathered, with suitable richness.
- Interviews are appropriately recorded and coded, in relevant settings.
- Explicit consent has been obtained from the participants.
- There are sufficient, well-selected participants to make the interviews credible.
- The interviews are appropriately contextualized.
- The analysis links back to the theoretical approach of the researcher.
- Due attention is paid to validity, reliability and generalizability.
- Sufficient quotations are given to enable evaluation of the findings.
- Suitable consideration is given to triangulation of the results.

The complexities of using this method are thrown further into relief by recent efforts to innovate by gathering material using cell phones (Zuwallack 2009) and Internet forums

(Seale et al. 2010) rather than through face-to-face interaction. The reader should reflect on the implications for conducting research in this manner – not least in appraising articles in the health field underpinned by the use of new technologies.

Conclusion

The strengths and weaknesses of unstructured and semi-structured interviews in health research have been covered in this chapter – along with the issues that they raise in practice in the various stages of research, from recruiting research participants and resourcing interviews, to analysing data and presenting research findings. These highlight that unstructured and semi-structured interviews can be extremely helpful as a qualitative research method, but are not as straightforward to carry out as first meets the eye. A contrast with structured questionnaires can be made by referring to Chapter 10 in this book, which covers quantitative survey methods in health research. It is hoped, though, that this chapter will help the reader to negotiate some of the potential challenges of unstructured and semi-structured interviews, as discussed in the brief case study above. Questions now follow in a practical exercise which should further highlight the benefits and limitations of the method and the issues that it raises in the context of research into the experience of burns.

> ### Exercise: The use of unstructured interviews to conduct research into the experience of burns
>
> Using unstructured or semi-structured interviews, you intend to conduct research focused on how individuals who have suffered serious burns experience and cope with pain. The burns have left those concerned with severe scarring over large portions of their bodies. Address the following questions:
>
> 1 How would you go about purposeful sampling in this research?
>
> 2 What problems would you anticipate in recruiting informants for your study?
>
> 3 How many informants would you need to participate in the interviews?
>
> 4 What kind of probing questions do you anticipate would be useful in interviews with these informants?
>
> 5 What aspects of informant biographies would you have to be aware of?
>
> 6 What particular socio-cultural, historical and political contexts would you have to ground your analysis in?
>
> 7 How might class, gender, stigma and cultural notions of beauty, among other contextual factors, shape the experiences of your informants?
>
> 8 In addition to unstructured or semi-structured interviews, are there other sources of data you could draw on in increasing the validity, reliability and generalizability of your analysis?

Recommended Further Reading

Corbin, J. and Morse, J.M. (2003) 'The unstructured interactive interview: issues of reciprocity and risks when dealing with sensitive topics', *Qualitative Inquiry*, 9(3): 335–54.
This is a very focused article that highlights the issues that make aspects of unstructured interviewing unique in the context of health research.

Gubrium, J.F. and Holstein, J.A. (eds) (2002) *Handbook of Interview Research: Context and Method*. Thousand Oaks, CA: Sage.
This is an accessible and comprehensive text covering the unstructured interview method in general.

McCracken, G. (1988) *The Long Interview*. Newbury Park, CA: Sage.
This is a classic book on the unstructured interview, in which unstructured interview techniques such as probing are very nicely described and explained.

Silverman, D. (2011) *Interpreting Qualitative Data*, 3rd edition. London: Sage.
This is a comprehensive text that can be recommended on qualitative data analysis.

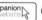 ## Online Readings

Freidin, B. and Timmermans, S. (2008) 'Complementary and alternative medicine for children's asthma: Satisfaction, care provider responsiveness, and networks of care', *Qualitative Health Research*, 18: 43–55.
Why are unstructured interviews useful in this research context? What are the advantages and disadvantages of such an approach?

Johnson, N. and Dickson-Swift, V. (2008) '"It usually happens in older women": Young women's perceptions about breast cancer', *Health Education Journal*, 67: 243–57.
Could this research data have been collected using different tools? What are the advantages of using semi-structured interviews? What are the challenges?

References

Baker, C.D. (2002) 'Ethnomethodological analyses of interviews', in J.F. Gubrium and J.A. Holstein (eds), *Handbook of Interview Research: Context and Method*. Thousand Oaks, CA: Sage.
Becker, H.S. (1970a) *Sociological Work: Method and Substance*. Chicago, IL: Aldine.
Becker, H.S. (1970b) 'Problems of inference and proof in participant observation', in W.J. Filstead (ed.), *Qualitative Methodology: Firsthand Involvement with the Social World*. Chicago, IL: Markham.
Blumer, H. (1969) *Symbolic Interactionism: Perspective and Method*. Englewood Cliffs, NJ: Prentice Hall.

Booth, T. and Booth, W. (1996) 'Sounds of silence: narrative research with inarticulate subjects', *Disability and Society*, 11: 55–69.

Boulton, M., Fitzpatrick, R. and Swinburn, C. (1996) 'Qualitative research in health care: II. A structured review and evaluation of studies', *Journal of Evaluation in Clinical Practice*, 2(3): 171–9.

Bringer, J.D., Johnston, L.H. and Brackenridge, C.H. (2006) 'Using computer-assisted qualitative data analysis software to develop a grounded theory project', *Field Methods*, 18(3): 245–66.

Charmaz, K. (2002) 'Stories and silences: disclosures and self in chronic illness', *Qualitative Inquiry*, 8(3): 302–28.

Cicourel, A.V. (1982) 'Interviews, surveys, and the problem of ecological validity', *American Sociologist*, 17: 11–20.

Corbin, J. and Morse, J.M. (2003) 'The unstructured interactive interview: issues of reciprocity and risks when dealing with sensitive topics', *Qualitative Inquiry*, 9(3): 335–54.

Corbin, J.M. and Strauss, A.L. (1990) 'Grounded theory research: procedures, canons, and evaluative criteria', *Qualitative Sociology*, 13(1): 3–21.

Crabtree, B. and Miller, W.L. (1991) 'A qualitative approach to primary care research: the long interview', *Family Medicine*, 23(2): 145–51.

Curtis, S., Gesler, W., Smith, S. and Wasburn, S. (2000) 'Approaches to sampling and case selection in qualitative research: examples in the geography of health', *Social Science and Medicine*, 50: 1001–14.

Douglas, J.D. (1976) *Investigative Social Research: Individual and Team Research*. Beverley Hills, CA: Sage.

Glaser, B.G. and Strauss, A.L. (1967) *The Discovery of Grounded Theory: Strategies for Qualitative Research*. Chicago, IL: Aldine.

Higgins, P.A. and Daly, B.J. (1999) 'Research methodology issues related to interviewing the mechanically ventilated patient', *Western Journal of Nursing Research*, 21: 773–84.

Johnson, J.M. (2002) 'In-depth interviewing', in J.F. Gubrium and J.A. Holstein (eds), *Handbook of Interview Research: Context and Method*. Thousand Oaks, CA: Sage.

Kirk, J. and Miller, M.L. (1986) *Reliability and Validity in Qualitative Research*. Newbury Park, CA: Sage.

Kvale, S. (1996) *Interviewing: An Introduction to Qualitative Research Interviewing*. Thousand Oaks, CA: Sage.

Low, J. (2003) 'Lay assessments of the efficacy of alternative/complementary therapies: a challenge to medical and expert dominance?', *Journal of Evidence-based Integrative Medicine*, 1(1): 65–76.

Low, J. (2004a) *Using Alternative Therapies: A Qualitative Analysis*. Toronto: Canadian Scholar's Press.

Low, J. (2004b) 'Managing safety and risk: the experiences of people with Parkinson's disease who use alternative and complementary therapies', *Health: An Interdisciplinary Journal for the Study of Health, Illness and Medicine*, 8(4): 445–63.

Low, J. (2006) 'Communication problems between researchers and informants with speech difficulties: methodological and analytical issues', *Field Methods*, 18(2): 153–71.

Lupton, D. (1997) 'Consumerism, reflexivity and the medical encounter', *Social Science and Medicine*, 45(3): 373–81.

Lupton, D. and Chapman, S. (1995) '"A healthy lifestyle might be the death of you": discourses on diet, cholesterol control and heart disease in the press and among the lay public', *Sociology of Health and Illness*, 17(4): 477–94.

McCracken, G. (1988) *The Long Interview.* Newbury Park, CA: Sage.

Miczo, N. (2003) 'Beyond the fetishism of words: considerations on the use of the interview to gather chronic illness narratives', *Qualitative Health Research*, 13(4): 469–90.

Parkinson's Disease Society (1999) *The Drug Treatment of Parkinson's Disease: For People with Parkinson's and their Families.* London: Parkinson's Disease Society.

Pope, C., Ziebland, S. and Mays, N. (2000) 'Qualitative research in health care: analysing qualitative data', *British Medical Journal*, 320: 114–16.

Riessman, C.K. (2008) *Narrative Methods for the Human Sciences.* Thousand Oaks, CA: Sage.

Ryan, G.W. and Bernard, H.R. (2003) 'Techniques to identify themes', *Field Methods*, 15(1): 85–109.

Seale, C., Charteris-Black, J., MacFarlane, A. and McPherson, A. (2010) 'Interviews and internet forums: a comparison of two sources of qualitative data', *Qualitative Health Research*, 20: 783–91.

Silverman, D. (1998) 'The quality of qualitative health research: the open-ended interview and its alternative', *Social Sciences in Health*, 4(2): 104–18.

Silverman, D. (2010) *Doing Qualitative Research: A Practical Handbook*, 3rd edition. London: Sage.

Silverman, D. (2011) *Interpreting Qualitative Data*, 3rd edition. London: Sage.

Sorrell, M.J. and Redmond, G.M. (1995) 'Interview in qualitative nursing research: differing approaches for ethnographic and phenomenological studies', *Journal of Advanced Nursing*, 21: 1117–22.

Strauss, A.L. and Corbin, J. (1990) *Basics of Qualitative Research: Grounded Theory Procedures and Techniques.* Newbury Park, CA: Sage.

Trow, M. (1970) 'Comment on participant observation and interviewing: a comparison', in W.J. Filstead (ed.), *Qualitative Methodology: Firsthand Involvement with the Social World.* Chicago, IL: Markham.

UyBico, S.J., Pavel, S. and Gross, C.P. (2007) 'Recruiting vulnerable populations into research: a systematic review of recruitment interventions', *Journal of General Internal Medicine*, March 21: 852–63.

Williams, M. (2000) 'Interpretivism and generalisation', *Sociology*, 34(2): 209–24.

Zuwallack, R. (2009) 'Piloting data collection via cell phones: results, experiences, and lessons learned', *Field Methods*, 21: 388–406.

6

Participant Observation in Health Research

DAVID HUGHES

Introduction

This chapter discusses the method of participant observation (PO) in health research. The term PO is sometimes used interchangeably with 'sociological ethnography', but traditionally ethnography is a broader category that includes methods such as the ethnographic interview and the analysis of cultural arte-facts, as well as observation. PO is one of the oldest and least 'high tech' research methods, emphasizing as it does the importance of gathering data through observing, interacting with, and listening to, the human subjects under study. The participant observer typically spends an extended period of time in a natural setting, such as a hospital ward or an intensive care unit, following the activities of staff members, observing particular classes of activities, or generally 'hanging out' with a view to understanding what is going on. It is this requirement for the researcher to participate in social interaction as part of the research process that separates PO from the systematic observational methods used in psychology and organizational studies where the observer looks on and records, but does not interact (Emerson 1981; McCall 1984). In consequence, there is an extensive literature on field relations and the participant observer role. Although natural-istic observation takes many forms and involves varying degrees of participation, all PO methods share the need to manage social interaction with subjects in the field (Gold 1958).

This chapter examines the characteristics of PO and the types of study that have been carried out in health care settings. It looks at the problems of access and ethics raised by PO studies, the strengths and weaknesses of the approach, the methods and techniques for collecting, coding and analysing data, and identifying and writing up findings. Finally, it presents a case study to illustrate how the method is used in practice.

The Characteristics of Participant Observation

Almost all recent PO research takes the form of a case study where there is intense observation in a specific setting. PO would not, for example, undertake an investigation of the ecology of a city, nor would it be the method of choice to examine the characteristics of a geographically dispersed social group. In the health field, most PO studies examine a patient or staff group or particular social processes associated with selected settings, such as the emergency ambulance service, the accident and emergency department, the outpatient clinic, a hospital ward, hospice or nursing home. A typical study might last between six months and two years, with the researcher completing several observation periods per week. Usually, a period of relatively unfocused fieldwork, where the researcher 'feels out' the setting and attempts to develop an appropriate field role, will be followed by a strategy to spread observations between different categories of subjects and aspects of activity that need to be covered.

Typically, access will be negotiated first with senior staff who act as formal gatekeepers to the setting, and then with the various levels of actors who will be the subjects of study. Usually, access will need to be maintained or renewed on an ongoing basis, so that it will remain a preoccupation throughout the period of fieldwork. A handful of studies in settings such as mental hospitals or acute wards (Caudill et al. 1952; Porter 1995) have been carried out covertly, without the knowledge of people in the setting, but most studies now for ethical reasons depend on explicit access agreements, with researchers operating in an open researcher role.

The origins of PO are often traced back to anthropology (Hume and Mulcock 2004) and the Chicago School of Sociology, with the method as we know it today deriving more directly from the work of later 'neo-Chicagoan' sociologists, particularly in the sociology of deviance and medical sociology (Fine 1995). Initial classic health studies focused on the process aspects of health care, such as:

- Professional socialization in medical school (Becker et al. 1961).
- The temporal experience of polio (Davis 1963) and TB care (Roth 1963).
- The management of death in hospital (Sudnow 1968) and the organization of terminal care (Glaser and Strauss 1965).
- The professional socialization of nurses (Olesen and Whittaker 1968).

All involved long periods of fieldwork spent observing and talking with research subjects in natural settings, charting the various stages, transitions or attitudinal shifts associated with professional education, patient 'careers' or illness trajectories.

There is some evidence that changes in the nature of health care systems have resulted in a change in the focus of research. Zussman (1993) has pointed out that the once flourishing tradition of studies of hospitalized patients' social worlds has all but disappeared, as patient throughput speeds up and specialized units replace traditional wards. He contends that the focus of research has shifted from ward culture and felt experience to detailed studies of specialized locales. More exacting ethical requirements for informed consent by patient research subjects may have accentuated this trend (Edgerton et al. 1984). (See also Chapter 15 on this subject.) Most recent American studies focus on staff rather than patient perspectives in settings, such as:

- The intensive care unit (Zussman 1992).
- The neonatal unit (Anspach 1993).
- The surgical training programme (Bosk 1979).
- Paramedic ambulances and emergency rooms (Timmermans 1999).
- How medical examiners explain suspicious deaths through postmortems (Timmermans 2006).

A similar trend is discernable in British work, for example:

- The study by Atkinson (1995) on haematologists.
- Research by Fox (1992) on surgeons.
- The study by Allen (2001) of the division of labour in acute wards.
- Research on the health service as an organization by Strong and Robinson (1990), Bennett and Ferlie (1994) and Flynn et al. (1996).
- The work by Allen (2010) on care pathway development.

The Rationale for Employing Participant Observation as a Research Method

The rationale for using the PO method is bound up with its instrumental effectiveness in answering certain kinds of research question. Qualitative methods have traditionally been concerned with questions of explanation and understanding, rather than with questions about frequency or quantity. Such methods may be used at the exploratory stage of research to map out variables in a field and generate hypotheses for testing in later quantitative studies. They can also have a role in making sense of observed correlations or patterns in quantitative data by elucidating the social processes that produce these patterns.

Qualitative studies can provide a snapshot of the behaviour or perspectives of a hard-to-reach or stigmatized group inaccessible via other methods (Lambert et al. 1995). They have shed light on seemingly illogical aspects of illness behaviour, poor compliance with drug prescribing, unsafe sex practices and teenage smoking behaviour, and have demonstrated some of the reasons for the limited effectiveness of programmes such as the controversial World Health Organization 'Directly Observed Therapy, Short Course' (DOTS) strategy for TB control. In any situation where the context of a health care intervention or programme or policy is likely to affect outcomes, qualitative studies can help identify real-world factors that may slip below the gaze of experimental or survey research.

In an early and influential paper, Becker and Geer (1957) suggested that PO has clear advantages over interview studies where special in-group languages (such as medical argot) are used; in situations where informants are unwilling to talk or find it difficult to describe an unfolding or complex social process; or where group myths and stereotypes feature centrally in accounts. Other writers have emphasized the importance of obtaining accounts that give an authentic representation of the social world by 'being there' and 'telling it as it is' with respect to the group being studied (Melia 1982). However, while PO undoubtedly provides data that could not be obtained via other methods (Mays and Pope 1996), it is important to avoid a naive realism that overlooks the role of the observer in 'interpreting' or making sense of observational data. It is tempting to assume that direct experience of a setting provides greater validity for research findings (Hammersley 1992). However, as discussed further below, PO raises issues of differential focus and selective perceptions on the part of the researcher that rule out any simple equation between direct observation and the one true account of events.

The Resources Required for Participant Observation

PO is resource-intensive in terms of human resources rather than technology. It makes heavy time demands, but usually involves individuals or small teams rather than the large teams characteristic of survey research. The need to build up field relationships over time militates against the kind of 'hired-hand' research common in quantitative projects (Roth 1999). In recent times, many researchers have supplemented the classic tool of the research notebook with the audio recorder to collect and record data and the computer to analyse data using qualitative data analysis applications (discussed below).

Audio recording permits more rigorous recording of organizational discourse and is particularly useful when focused interactions, such as patient consultations, case conferences, ward rounds or management meetings occur at key junctures of organizational processes. Several contemporary ethnographies combine elements of field note-based data collection with recording conversation or discourse so that a general description of organizational processes may be illustrated through a series of detailed exemplars. However, the decision to audio-record has significant implications for costs and the nature of data analysis.

Transcribing and analysing recordings is an expensive and time-consuming process – a much slower process than the reading of conventional field notes – and will probably be beyond the capabilities of a lone researcher who cannot afford secretarial support. Making sense of data collected typically involves forms of sequential or discourse analysis which are very different from traditional forms of content analysis of documents that were described in Chapter 4, and will represent a steep learning curve for many qualitative researchers.

A number of qualitative data analysis (QDA) packages, such as *Ethnograph, ATLAS™, HyperRESEARCH, MAXQDA* and *QSR NVivo,* have been developed to assist with the management of field note and interview data (Lee and Esterhuizen 2000; Banner and Albarrran 2009). Most of these applications are essentially 'chunkers and coders', which attach electronic labels to passages of text and allow the retrieval of extracts coded under a chosen index term. Most packages permit more complex operations such as Boolean searches using the three logical operators 'or', 'and' and 'not' for search terms (see Chapter 3); searches for co-occurring categories; and the merging of codes. However, they are no substitute for the sophisticated processes of interpretation, synthesis and theory generation that researchers have traditionally performed on field data (see below). Such programmes are useful as a support tool for conventional thematic content, but can create problems with forms of process analysis where change over a series of sequential data entries or the narrative structure of a text are important.

More recent versions of these packages use embedded links to preserve the overall structure of field notes and may reduce the risk of fragmentation or de-contextualization of data but, in this researcher's view, the technology remains an imperfect one. My informal questioning of a small number of well-known qualitative health researchers revealed very mixed views on this subject, with many preferring to stick to the traditional manual approach to data analysis.

Ethics and Participant Observation

Although participant observation studies raise much the same ethical concerns that come up in other research (see Chapter 15), some issues arise in accentuated or changed form. Among the features of PO that give rise to special problems are:

- The close relationships between researchers and subjects developed during fieldwork.
- The 'emergent' nature of most research designs.
- The fact that PO characteristically involves 'thick description' of natural settings and subjects.

PO traditionally emphasizes the need to build empathy and rapport with subjects so as to gain full access to research settings and sustain relationships over time. The inductive logic of investigation means that the choice of subjects and topics is difficult to specify fully at the time of designing the study and agreeing research access, so that the focus of observations often changes in the light of early findings. PO studies typically contain detailed descriptions of research subjects, their attitudes and feelings, and even verbatim extracts of spoken interactions, which may make it difficult to hide the location of the research site and actors' identities. These characteristics of PO affect the way researchers think about the notions of informed consent, anonymity and confidentiality.

Informed consent implies that a participant freely agrees to participate, and fully understands the consequences of this agreement. The difficulty is that formal agreement in advance is more difficult to arrange in a PO study than, for example, in a social survey. There is rarely a single, initial stage where subjects are given full information about the research and the demands to be made on them, so they can agree or decline to take part. The research design at the time of the initial access approach may not be the same as the design three months later. Often, access will involve multiple gatekeepers, and it may be obtained step by step as the research moves through different sites and encounters new actors, or as research plans change. Moreover, the classic PO studies generally negotiated access in relation to settings rather than specific individuals, partly because the settings were populated by individuals who were not regular participants, and could not be approached in advance.

The period of agreeing access thus overlaps with the period during which the researcher seeks to cultivate the good relations needed to stay in the field. Research relationships may be embedded in social relationships with associated emotions, likes and dislikes, and so on. Consequently, informed consent may be sought against the background of personal pressures arising from the etiquette of social relationships. Where lower participants are asked for consent after superiors have agreed access, there are also issues of power and hierarchy.

These are difficult problems where issues of ethics and practicality are often intertwined. Any requirement that a PO study can only go ahead when all subjects within the field of observation have given informed consent in advance would limit the types of research that could be done, and the extent to which an initial research design could be varied at a later stage. Some researchers draw a distinction between focused interactions, such as closed meetings or restricted settings that will be attended and perhaps audio-recorded, and observation of more 'open' settings such as Accident and Emergency Departments, where the researcher cannot know which individuals will attend on a given day. They conclude that while it is viable to obtain advance consent (perhaps on prepared consent forms) in respect of focused interactions, they will not seek formal consent from occasional actors in open settings. In consequence, they may opt not to describe such individuals and their actions in great detail in research field notes and research reports. This is a controversial matter in qualitative research circles because the approach to access adopted in many of the classic PO studies would clearly not meet the requirements of today's research ethics committees. In January 2004, there was a fascinating discussion in the American Sociological Association MedSoc Section's online discussion group, when researchers such as Virginia Olesen and Robert Dingwall debated the rights and wrongs of informed consent without any exceptions, versus the argument that important knowledge gains could come from PO studies of the classic kind. The latter could be undertaken for altruistic motives and researchers could take additional care not to harm subjects. As yet, however, there is no consensus among PO researchers on this subject, which is discussed further in Chapter 15.

Researchers usually seek to manage any problems arising from thick description by promising to take special measures to safeguard anonymity and confidentiality. With regard to anonymity, they undertake to ensure that no uniquely identifying information is attached to the data, so that readers of research reports cannot trace the data back to the individual subject. Confidentiality is addressed by promising that the data will be handled and managed in such a way as to secure storage, use password-protected data files and remove real names from files, so that individuals are protected from the consequences of information leaks to third parties. But how far subjects can rely on such assurances may be open to doubt. If sites are identifiable, this may lead to the identification of certain office holders. If this were to happen, readers could associate detailed accounts of events and verbatim quotations with those individuals. In some circumstances, merely changing minor details to hide identities may not provide sufficient safeguards, and it may be necessary to agree a time embargo on the research (as sometimes happens with doctoral theses). One advantage of the long gestation and writing-up time of some PO studies is that partici- pants may have moved to other posts by the time later papers are published, thus reducing the risk of adverse consequences.

One contemporary problem that may seem remote, but affected the author recently, is that confidential research data may be requested when participants become involved in legal proceedings. The author was involved in a study of individual patient commissioning panels (Hughes and Doheny 2011) when a patient initiated judicial review proceedings against a health board that had declined to fund a high-cost drug. The health board requested copies of audio recordings of meetings involving that patient so that these were available if demanded by the court. This posed complicated issues beyond the scope of this chapter, which thankfully were resolved when the case did not proceed beyond an initial hearing. The relevant point for our discussion is that such requests are extremely difficult to resist, and may not have been covered by the original terms of consent – in this case on written consent forms which made no mention of the arrangements that would apply if the courts became involved. The possibility of legal proceedings should therefore be considered when deciding on the content of consent forms.

Strengths of Participant Observation

The strengths of PO studies lie in their ability to shed light on issues that other methods are less effective in investigating. Becker and Geer (1957) spell out the advantages of PO as a tool for exploring local cultures and the unfolding of social processes over time. However, in practice there are different sets of arguments about the strength of PO in illuminating culture and subjective experience and its strength in examining social organization and organizational practices.

The argument that PO is a naturalistic method concerned with immersion in the culture and authentic representation of what the famous anthropologist Malinowski (1922: 25) termed 'the native's point of view ... his vision of his world', still holds sway but has become increasingly controversial. It is clear that observation does not in itself provide the researcher with access to the inner mental states of research subjects, and research which claims to provide a window into the social worlds of staff or patient groups must back this up with supporting evidence that goes beyond inferences about what outward appearances indicate about subjective perceptions. Some naturalistic studies have made a convincing case about the value of examining previously neglected user perspectives, and strongly support this with data (for instance, Daly et al. 1992). However, several influential commentators argue that observational research should be about documenting practices rather than ascribing meanings to participants' action or talk, and advocate a refocusing of analysis to centre on propositions that can be plausibly derived from observational data (see, for instance, Dingwall and Strong 1985; Silverman 1998).

Indeed, for observational researchers with an interest in policy making, organizational processes and practices have been of greater interest than meanings. They have viewed PO as a promising alternative to interviews for seeing inside the 'black box' of health care organizations and understanding service delivery and change. PO can be viewed as a pragmatic way of 'reaching the parts other methods cannot reach' (Pope and Mays 1995). It can reveal routines of which participants are unaware; probe the micro-level behaviours that lie between known differences in outcomes; and shed light on how policies or programmes may be subtly reshaped in the course of implementation. For instance, the following studies in the UK have documented:

- How staff orient to Patient's Charter targets (Sbaih 2002).
- Barriers to medical incident reporting (Waring 2005).
- The implementation of the new GP contract (McDonald et al. 2009).
- The impact of the Quality and Outcomes Framework in general practice (Checkland and Harrison 2010).
- Hard decisions made by individual patient commissioning panels (Hughes and Doheny 2011).

These studies have shown a gap between official policy and actual practices that is highly relevant to the organizational evaluation of health services.

The Challenges of Participant Observation

In the fieldwork phase

Some major disadvantages of PO, particularly in a contemporary British context preoccupied with research outputs and the Research Excellence Framework as an institutional indicator of the quality of research, are the time-consuming nature of fieldwork and the strain of sustained contact with subjects. While some accounts of the research experience may have overdramatized the emotional trauma of fieldwork (see Punch 1986), researchers undoubtedly face taxing challenges in terms of managing their identity in the research setting; mediating between different actors and interest groups; presenting the research in different situations; deciding just how much participation is appropriate; and determining when, and how, to put information into the public domain. There are also well-documented ethical dilemmas concerning trust and disclosure which arise when researchers build up social relationships for research purposes.

Furthermore, given that research funding bodies are often seeking a review of a whole service or population, there is often a temptation to tack a limited observational component on to an interview study covering multiple settings, and to come away with very limited data that are hard to contextualize. Malinowski (1922: 7) emphasized the importance of 'close contact', and cautioned that: 'There is all the difference between a sporadic plunging into the company of natives, and being really in contact with them.' One of the risks associated with contemporary mixed-method studies is that the PO element is so episodic and dispersed across settings that it cannot examine the process aspects of social organization that the method has traditionally coped with so well. This same trend has also affected case studies which in recent times are often of limited scale and of an episodic and truncated nature (Marinetto 2011).

Methodological problems and solutions

The fact that some studies trade wider coverage against some loss of depth often reflects a quest for increased representativeness and generalizability. PO has traditionally been seen to be weak in these areas, but this is a topic about which more than a few misconceptions exist. There are undoubtedly situations where PO studies can illuminate general social patterns affecting a wide range of settings and where sampling may be appropriate (Bryman 1988). Yet the model of statistical inference from sample to population seems unsustainable in real-world situations where the 'population' of organizations from which a researcher might select the sample is itself small and diverse.

For example, some years ago, I was involved in planning a project which required the research team to select three or four study hospitals from all those in Scotland that accommodated teenagers with learning disabilities. Yet the then ten or so candidate hospitals differed on a range of dimensions: some admitted both children and adults while a few were children's facilities; most were specialist learning disability hospitals while at least one also contained psychiatric wards; some provided special education on site while others used outside schools; and some allowed extensive mixed-sex activities, while others did not. Then, there were issues of urban versus rural locations and significant size differences. It took only a little reflection to conclude that any idea of selecting a case to represent a larger group of similar institutions would be flawed.

As a consequence of problems of this kind, examples of conventional sampling in PO studies are thin on the ground. Instead, some PO researchers have opted for purposive samples, intended to facilitate observations and comparisons that will help to build theory. Case studies may permit theoretical generalization rather than statistical generalization (Mitchell 1983), so the issue is not whether the events observed in the case study site precisely represent events elsewhere, but whether the analysis of social processes produced by the research has more general applicability. For Yin (1984) and other exponents of case analysis, the path towards generalizability is not about filling in the gaps by progressively achieving more complete population coverage, but about replication studies which will disconfirm, or leave in place, the theoretical propositions generated by earlier case studies.

The problem of researcher influence

A problem that features prominently in many textbook accounts of PO is 'reactivity' – the possibility that the researcher's presence influences the behaviour observed. This phenomenon, also known as the 'Hawthorne effect', featured centrally in the classic study by Roethlisberger and Dickson (1939) of human relations in the Hawthorne plant of the Western Electric Company in Chicago. Here, a series of 'experiments' carried out by production engineers on a small group of telephone relay assembly workers appeared to show that almost any change in the factory environment led to improved productivity, including both increasing and reducing the lighting (although the data have subsequently been questioned). Clearly, research subjects may very well modify aspects of their behaviour under observation, but arguably this is usually more of a problem in the early stages of a research project than when field relations are well established. Certainly, it is not unknown for a study to be prematurely terminated because of non-cooperation or resistance from subjects (for example, Clarke 1996).

However, even where attempts are made to conceal things from the researcher, many features of social organization are difficult to change without disrupting the work of the setting. In my own experience, the kinds of data that subjects do not want recorded are more likely to involve individual mistakes or indiscretions, such as negative comments about colleagues, than routine work practices. Once the researcher has become familiar to them, subjects may be surprisingly open in discussing sensitive and potentially problematic issues.

Data Coding, Analysis and Interpretation in Participant Observation

Most PO studies rely on some form of thematic content analysis. In line with PO's neo-Chicagoan influences, many observational researchers base their approach to analysis on analytic induction (Becker 1958) or grounded theory (Glaser and Strauss 1967). Both approaches typically start with a general orientation to an issue rather than definitive hypotheses for testing, and move through a process where problems and concepts relevant to an organization are identified, and theoretical propositions for further investigation formulated. Analysis goes on as data are collected and further data collection takes its direction from the provisional analysis. At this stage, the analysis must necessarily remain provisional because of the exigencies of fieldwork, and the final comprehensive analysis will only take place when the fieldwork is completed.

Analytic induction and grounded theory

Analytical induction, as originally conceived by early Chicago researchers, was an approach concerned with the systematic search for falsifying evidence and the progressive refinement of theory until no disconfirming evidence could be found. In the work by Lindesmith (1947), this involved the progressive modification of a hypothesis, set out as a formal proposition at the start of the study. For Znaniecki (1952), analytical induction offered the prospect of producing universal propositions which could then be used to predict future patterns of behaviour. Later writers built on the core notions of inductive inference of theory from data and deviant case analysis, but abandoned the quest for empirical prediction and often avoided any initial hypothesis.

The approach by Glaser and Strauss (1967) to grounded theory emerged out of this period of reappraisal, and represented an extension and elaboration of analytic induction. Grounded theory studies start with a general area of concern rather than a hypothesis, and move to identify the concepts and theoretical connections emerging from the data. Where some contemporaneous qualitative studies (as well as almost all quantitative studies) were concerned mainly with verifying theories, Glaser and Strauss placed primary emphasis on generating theory by discovering relevant concepts and hypotheses through fieldwork. The core ideas of the constant comparative method and theoretical sampling have over time been supplemented by guidelines for a complex system of coding (Strauss and Corbin 1990).

However, the increasing formalization of grounded theory has led to considerable controversy among its exponents (Melia 1996) and may have made the approach less attractive to pragmatically inclined health service researchers. Many contemporary health researchers utilize modified versions of analytic induction or grounded theory. These make use of techniques like thematic coding, constant comparison and deviant case analysis, but do not adhere strictly to the original models (Murphy et al. 1998).

The growth of interest in the use of language has led to the emergence of more sophisticated approaches to the analysis of spoken interaction, such as the ethnography of communication, conversation analysis and discourse analysis. This has led many PO researchers to question whether their field notes adequately represent the interactions they have observed. *The Social Organization of Juvenile Justice* by Cicourel (1968) marked an important step because it encouraged researchers to pay greater attention to language and to produce field notes that were as near verbatim as possible. The emergence of linguistically sensitive forms of PO has changed the way many PO researchers present data (Dingwall and Strong 1985). It has led some to supplement observations recorded in field notes with audio recordings of key events or meetings, and to combine thematic content analysis with sequential analysis of transcribed talk based on conversation analysis or discourse analysis techniques.

Data selection

The process by which a researcher observes and records events, and then analyses them to build descriptions and theories in published form, has led to a good deal of soul searching for several generations of participant observers. There are difficult issues concerning the selection and representation of observations that are not easy to resolve, even when data are presented in considerable detail. There are questions of trust and also about just how ethnographic accounts might be said to represent reality. This quickly leads into the deep waters of epistemology and ontology which are beyond the scope of this chapter.

Many pragmatically inclined researchers have opted for a position of 'subtle realism' (Murphy et al. 1998; Mays and Pope 2000), which accepts that research reports can never encapsulate a single 'truth' but rejects the relativism of postmodern ethnography. They argue that a researcher's aim is to produce a credible account of social processes, which are acknowledged to be representations rather than reproductions of social reality. This may be used to build theories that can be developed in the light of findings from later studies.

Writing Up and Presenting Findings

Different PO studies address different aspects of social organization and rest on different theoretical foundations, and this is reflected in striking differences in how findings are written up and presented. A classic interactionist ethnography like *Boys in White* (Becker et al. 1961) takes a very different form from an anthropology-influenced study like *The Cloak of Competence* by Edgerton (1967), just as the linguistically sensitive study *Medical Talk and Medical Work* by Atkinson (1995) is presented in a different style from the policy ethnography of Flynn and associates (1996). In recent years, styles of writing have come under increasing scrutiny (Hammersley 1993). For example, there is extensive debate about issues such as the viability of realist ethnography (including representational devices such as the invisibility of the author), and the use of alternative forms of textual organization such as chronology, narrative and analytic themes. From a practical perspective, researchers are often required to produce output for multiple readerships, which need to meet the stylistic requirements of different journals. In my own work, straddling sociology, socio-legal studies and health policy, it has been necessary to vary the mode of presentation to suit the particular audience targeted, as highlighted in the case study below.

CASE STUDY

Case study: Participant observation and contracting in the NHS internal market

My research on the NHS internal market with Lesley Griffiths illustrates some of the dilemmas and trade-offs discussed above (see, for instance, Griffiths and Hughes 2000; Hughes and Griffiths 2003). The main component of the research was an observational case study of contracting between a health authority and its main providers, but this was supplemented by an interview study of all Welsh health authorities and NHS Trusts, which provided a context for the case study. We were also aware that the observational data could be utilized to examine both general socio-legal and economic aspects of contracting behaviour, and micro-level issues concerning language and social interaction in contracting meetings. We concluded that we would need to produce different kinds of output to cover our full range of interests.

The study was conceived as a 'policy ethnography' (Strong and Robinson 1990) and took a broadly naturalistic stance to data collection, influenced by interpretive sociology, while also seeking to influence policy. Compared with earlier work, we incorporated a larger observational component and paid more attention to the specifics of discourse by making extensive use of verbatim transcriptions of meetings. Over 80 contracting meetings were observed over two annual cycles, and supplemented with in-depth interviews with key participants. Most meetings and interviews were tape-recorded and transcribed, resulting in a corpus of data amounting to about 2,800 sheets of typescript. Analysis took a broadly inductive form. We sought to identify themes emerging from the transcripts, which were then used to code and index relevant textual segments.

The qualitative data package NUDIST allowed us to automate this process to some extent. However, chronology was an important consideration, and was less amenable to analysis via this 'chunking and coding' approach. It was necessary to read transcripts in context and track issues through a series of meetings.

As fieldwork began, two researchers shared the task of observing weekly meetings of the health authority's core contracting team, and also its negotiation and monitoring meetings with providers. Later, we were also able to negotiate access to the corresponding weekly contracting team meetings in a local trust. This regular round of observations was supplemented by attendance at public health authority meetings, a small number of one-off events and visits to carry out informal interviews with key staff and review documents. Although a policy ethnography of this type centres mainly on a series of timetabled events and appointments, and thus falls short of the full 'immersion' in the field described in classic observational studies, we visited research sites three or four times in an average week.

In retrospect, the key finding emerging from the observational data was the discrepancy that existed between official policy and the actual implementation of the internal market. In several areas, informal social organization was crucial to the operation of the reforms, something that was missed in most interview studies. Although health authorities complied with some high-profile government directives, such as the instruction for purchasers to use contracts to require trusts to reduce surgical waiting times, other 'rules' of the internal market were not enforced to the same extent (Hughes et al. 1997). For example, the Department of Health's 'pricing rules' required that NHS Trusts should calculate the price of treatments on a full-cost basis, with no cross-subsidization of services, and publish standard prices (tariffs) which all purchasers would pay. But our observations revealed that prices were usually not specified in advance, and were often derived during contract negotiations by mechanically dividing the sum available by the agreed number of treatments. Tariffs might be the starting point for negotiations, but were frequently not published at all. This meant that different health authorities frequently ended up paying different prices for the same treatments, depending on historic funding levels and the available monies.

Attempts by health authorities to get trusts to reduce surgical waiting times usually took the form of penalty clauses in contracts, which would lead to a loss of income for the hospital if waiting time targets were not achieved. The official policy in most health authorities was that monetary penalties would be imposed when trusts missed their targets, and that the sanction would apply equally to all providers. However, the informal reality was that penalty clauses were often not invoked when problems arose (Hughes and Griffiths 1999a). Some trusts had confidential 'side letters' containing a promise from the health authority not to impose the penalty specified in the contract. In a few other cases, trusts were able to get the penalty level reduced so that the figures specified in their contract were lower than those in the standard contract.

This led some health authorities and trusts to bend another official rule – the one that said that NHS contracts were public documents, available on request once signed. Health authorities had an incentive to keep secret the concessions forced by individual trusts. Trusts had an incentive not to reveal price differentials and unequal loading of costs between purchasers. In practice, it could be very difficult to obtain complete contracts at the beginning of the financial year. It was common for signing to be delayed for many months, or for certain schedules or price information not to be supplied with the main contractual document (Hughes and Griffiths 1999b; Hughes et al. 2000).

One of the most revealing indications of the nature of a market comes when disputes between buyers and sellers occur. Official policy required that NHS

(Continued)

(Continued)

contract disputes should be settled through special conciliation arrangements, or if these failed, by arbitration by the Secretary of State (a government minister) or an appointee. At that time, this involved 'pendulum arbitration', which meant that a decision would favour one side or the other, rather than proposing a compromise. Actually, the official system was rarely used, largely because purchasers and providers were unwilling to take the risk of losing everything under a pendulum judgement (Hughes et al. 1997). In practice, senior NHS officials devised a variety of informal 'arbitration' arrangements which allowed compromises, and also made frequent use of direct management intervention. One high-profile contract dispute in Wales led to the sacking of the chief executives of the health authority and trust involved, and the preparation of a 'recovery plan' devised by senior NHS managers seconded from other areas to solve the problem.

Our work influenced the then Department of Health and Welsh Office to rewrite their guidance on the resolution of NHS contract disputes. However, the major impact came from a raft of contemporaneous studies that delivered similar messages. Programmes of research with observational components, such as work at Warwick University funded by the Department of Health and the *Contracts and Competition Programme* of the Economic and Social Research Council (ESRC), provided ammunition for policy makers critical of the internal market reforms. Policy on the internal market had been heavily influenced by the discipline of economics, and particularly by principal/agent theory and transactions cost theory.

Observational studies showed that many of the predictions about the likely impact of contracting in the NHS had not taken sufficient account of real-world constraints. The findings highlighted some of the negative features of adversarial contracting and the limited development of health care markets in the NHS. They showed that the early emphasis on complete and binding contracts, close monitoring, and clear incentives and sanctions had not delivered the expected benefits. These findings influenced the decision of the New Labour government after 1997 to discourage annual contracts and move towards longer-term agreements. A number of research teams which had been involved in the ESRC *Contracts and Competition Programme*, including our own, were approached for advice by Department of Health officials tasked with developing guidelines on the new contracting framework.

Reading Health Research Based on Participant Observation

Not all PO studies are created equal. To assess the quality of a particular study, the reader should ask the following pertinent questions:

- Does the author provide sufficient information on fieldwork and data analysis for the reader to be able to construct the main steps in the research process?
- Is the description of the setting presented detailed, plausible and internally consistent?
- Are the data presented sufficiently rich to give a sense of life in the setting and do they support the wider analysis put forward?

- Are the conclusions of the study supported by sufficient corroborating evidence, preferably from more than one data source?
- Are the chosen approaches to data collection and analysis appropriate to the research question?
- Are there indications that disconfirming evidence has been given as much attention as evidence that supports the conclusions presented, perhaps through deviant case analysis?
- Do the theoretical conclusions of the study emerge from the data, or is there a suspicion that the findings have been presented selectively so as to support the theory?

For further discussion of how to assess quality in PO specifically, and in qualitative research more generally, see Mays and Pope (2000) and Seale (1999).

Conclusion

The argument put forward in this chapter is that PO has a number of strengths in addressing particular kinds of research question. In health research, PO can help researchers penetrate social processes and, handled with care, the perspectives of social actors, in particular settings. Most recently, it has been used to penetrate the 'black box' of health care organizations, and probe gaps between public accounts and informal behaviour. Moreover, most PO studies incorporate flexible research designs, which are not derailed by rapid and unpredictable organizational change.

The underlying argument in the chapter has supported the case for a pragmatic selection of methods according to the research question. This runs somewhat counter to recent enthusiasm in health service research circles for enumerating the 'hierarchy of evidence' (see Chapter 3) that favours experiments, particularly randomized controlled trials (RCTs), and the other quantitative methods discussed in the next part of the book. These are the preferred methods of many British funding bodies and tend to marginalize qualitative studies, and to expand the application of experimental methods in programme and policy evaluation (Russell 1996). However, experimental methods do not work well when organizational structures and boundaries are subject to constant rejigging. Indeed, there are no published large-scale studies of this type dealing with the recent health service reforms. This is a less persuasive vision than the one set out some years ago by Illsley (1980) when he called for a multifaceted research programme that includes both RCTs and observational studies. Illsley (1980: 135) notes that there are many real-world situations where:

> The data are not cut and dried in the tradition of the natural sciences, instead they trace and reflect what is and what must be a fragmented, complex process. The data have to be put together and the process reconstructed with various forms of logical analysis but also with judgements about the relative weight and influence of actors and items.

This is what Illsley termed 'illuminative evaluation'. The case study presented above shows that observational research can influence policy, albeit in rather unpredictable ways, and as part of a larger body of research findings. To shed further light on PO as a health research method, a practical exercise based on the use of the method in a health contracting meeting is included below.

Exercise: Participant observation and a health contracting meeting

The following exchange occurred in a health authority contracting team meeting. The first speaker, the finance director (FD), is the team leader. The other speaker, the contracts manager (CM), is the team member with hands-on responsibility for managing provider contracts. Caerbrook is a regional specialist hospital providing children's cancer services – indeed the only hospital offering some treatments in this geographical area. Metro is a regional hospital providing a wider range of tertiary services. The tape recording was made openly with the team's permission. No special assurances were requested after this meeting. Like many Welsh NHS purchasers, this health authority sought to impose a cash penalty on hospitals which 'breached' the guarantees offered by the Patient's Charter – a high-profile government initiative offering a commitment about the maximum surgical waiting times for different categories of patients – and to insert a clause to this effect in service contracts with providers.

> FD: You'll have to be careful how you minute this. What we've agreed with Caerbrook ... is that the penalties for Patient's Charter will only be a thousand pounds this year, not five thousand or ten thousand. The reason for that is that they weren't prepared to sign a contract if we insisted on the other penalties. Their contract is a quarter of a million and they have never incurred a penalty with us.

> CM: We need to be careful George.

> FD: I got a personal assurance from their chief executive, Neil Hayward, that the deal is strictly confidential and not to be leaked to any other East county provider, and that they will not incur any penalties. If they do, we will review. But given that they were only a quarter of a million; given that, well, my figures say, and certainly his were, that they haven't incurred any penalties – that seemed to be confirmed by the budget reports – that we wouldn't ... it's not in our interest not to sign a contract. But we wouldn't want the same to apply to Metro, because Metro is a completely different provider. They have incurred fifty penalties in the last year, and ...

> CM: It's vital that information doesn't get out. Once that gets out we haven't got much of a contract there.

> FD: We've got to hold the line here. Nobody has heard that.

We were already aware from other observed meetings that three local providers had been arguing hard against the inclusion of penalty clauses but had been told that they would be applied in all contracts, and that another regional specialist hospital was also said to be unhappy with penalties.

Answer the following questions:

1 What does this extract show about the use of penalty clauses in the NHS quasi-market?

2 What, if anything, does the extract show about the problem of 'reactivity'?

3 What weight can be attached to a single observation, without corroborating information? How could such corroboration be obtained?

4 What questions does this data extract suggest should be explored in later interviews?

5 What practical problems does knowledge of this arrangement pose, if any, for the research team in managing field relations?

The researchers decided to use this extract, but not until after this health authority was reorganized and the people concerned had moved to new jobs. What ethical problems does this raise, if any?

Recommended Further Reading

Griffiths, L. and Hughes, D. (2000) 'Talking contracts and taking care: managers and professionals in the NHS internal market', *Social Science and Medicine*, 51: 209–22.
This is an article from the case study discussed in this chapter, which illustrates the use of PO and its application to the topical issue of management/professional relations.

Hughes, D., Petsoulas, C., Allen, P., Doheny, S. and Vincent-Jones, P. (2011) 'Contracting in the English NHS: markets and social embeddedness', *Health Sociology Review*, 20(3): 321–37.
This article brings readers up to date by describing the latest episode of NHS contracting research.

Mesman, J. (2008) *Uncertainty in Medical Innovation: Experienced Pioneers in Neonatal Care.* Basingstoke: Palgrave MacMillan.
This is a Dutch PO study carried out in the neo-natal intensive care unit.

Timmermans, S. (2006) *Postmortem: How Medical Examiners Explain Suspicious Deaths.* Chicago, IL: University of Chicago Press.
This is a modern PO study carried out in the Medical Examiners' Offices that uses the classic approach.

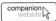 ## Online Readings

Lewis, S., Russell, A. (2011) 'Being embedded: A way forward for ethnographic research', *Ethnography*, 12: 398–416.
What is embedded practice in this context? How does it draw on the principles of PO? What are the challenges of PO as defined by the author?

Carnevale, F., Macdonald, M., Bluebond-Langner, M. and McKeever, P. (2008) 'Using participant observation in paediatric health care settings: Ethical challenges and solutions', *Journal of Child Health Care*, 12: 18–32.
How is PO undertaken in this context? What benefits did this approach bring? Critically evaluate the paper using the checklist provided in PPS 6.5/6.6.

References

Allen, D. (2001) *The Changing Shape of Nursing Practice*. London: Routledge.

Allen, D. (2010) 'Care pathways: an ethnographic description of the field', *International Journal of Care Pathways*, 14: 4–9.

Anspach, R. (1993) *Deciding Who Lives: Fateful Choices in the Intensive-Care Nursery*. Berkeley, CA: University of California Press.

Atkinson, P. (1995) *Medical Talk and Medical Work: The Liturgy of the Clinic*. London: Sage.

Banner, D.J. and Albarrran, J.W. (2009) 'Computer-assisted qualitative data analysis software: a review', *Canadian Journal of Cardiovascular Nursing*, 19(3): 24–31.

Becker, H.S. (1958) 'Problems of inference and proof in participant observation', *American Sociological Review*, 28: 652–60.

Becker, H.S. and Geer, B. (1957) 'Participant observation and interviewing: a comparison', *Human Organization*, 16: 28–32.

Becker, H.S., Geer, B., Hughes, E.C. and Strauss, A.L. (1961) *Boys in White: Student Culture in Medical School*. Chicago, IL: University of Chicago Press.

Bennett, C. and Ferlie, E. (1994) *Managing Crisis and Change in Health Care: The Organisational Response to HIV/AIDS*. Buckingham: Open University Press.

Bosk, C.L. (1979) *Forgive and Remember: Managing Medical Failure*. Chicago, IL: University of Chicago Press.

Bryman, A. (1988) *Quantity and Quality in Social Research*. London: Unwin Hyman.

Caudill, W., Redlich, F.C., Gilmore, H.R. and Brody, E.B. (1952) 'Social structure and inter-action processes on a psychiatric ward', *American Journal of Orthopsychiatry*, 22: 314–34.

Checkland, K. and Harrison, S. (2010) 'The impact of the Quality and Outcomes Framework on practice organisation and service delivery: summary of evidence from two qualitative studies', *Quality in Primary Care*, 18: 139–46.

Cicourel, A. (1968) *The Social Organization of Juvenile Justice.* New York: Wiley.

Clarke, L. (1996) 'Participant observation in a secure unit: care, conflict and control', *Nursing Times Research*, 1: 431–40.

Daly, J., McDonald, I. and Willis, E. (1992) *Researching Health Care: Designs, Dilemmas, Disciplines.* London: Routledge.

Davis, F. (1963) *Passage Through Crisis: Polio Victims and their Families.* Indianapolis, IN: Bobbs Merrill.

Dingwall, R. and Strong, P.M. (1985) 'The interactional study of organisations', *Urban Life*, 14: 205–31.

Edgerton, R. (1967) *The Cloak of Competence.* Berkeley, CA: University of California Press.

Edgerton, R.B., Bollinger, M. and Herr, B. (1984) 'The cloak of competence: after two decades', *American Journal of Mental Deficiency*, 88: 345–51.

Emerson, R. (1981) 'Observational fieldwork', *Annual Review of Sociology*, 7: 351–78.

Fine, G.A. (ed.) (1995) *A Second Chicago School? The Development of Postwar American Sociology.* Chicago, IL: University of Chicago Press.

Flynn, R., Williams, G. and Pickard, S. (1996) *Markets and Networks: Contracting in Community Health Services.* Buckingham: Open University Press.

Fox, N. (1992) *The Social Meaning of Surgery.* Buckingham: Open University Press.

Glaser, B.G. and Strauss, A.L. (1965) *Awareness of Dying.* Chicago, IL: Aldine.

Glaser, B.G. and Strauss, A.L. (1967) *The Discovery of Grounded Theory: Strategies for Qualitative Research.* New York: Aldine.

Gold, R.L. (1958) 'Roles in sociological field observations', *Social Forces*, 36: 217–23.

Griffiths, L. and Hughes, D. (2000) 'Talking contracts and taking care: managers and professionals in the NHS internal market', *Social Science and Medicine*, 51: 209–22.

Hammersley, M. (1992) *What's Wrong with Ethnography?* London: Routledge.

Hammersley, M. (1993) 'Ethnographic writing', *Social Research Update* 5.

Hughes, D. and Doheny, S. (2011) 'Deliberating Tarceva: a case study of how British NHS managers decide whether to purchase a high-cost drug in the shadow of NICE guidance', *Social Science and Medicine*, 73(10): 1460–8.

Hughes, D. and Griffiths, L. (1999a) 'On penalties and the Patient's Charter: centralism v decentralised governance in the NHS', *Sociology of Health and Illness*, 21(1): 71–94.

Hughes, D. and Griffiths, L. (1999b) 'Access to public documents in a study of the NHS internal market: openness vs. secrecy in contracting for clinical services', *International Journal of Social Research Methodology: Theory and Practice*, 2(1): 1–16.

Hughes, D. and Griffiths, L. (2003) 'Going public: references to the news media in NHS contract negotiations', *Sociology of Health and Illness*, 25(5): 571–88.

Hughes, D., Griffiths, L. and Lambert, S. (2000) 'Opening Pandora's box? Freedom of information and health services research', *Journal of Health Services Research and Policy*, 5(1): 59–61.

Hughes, D., McHale, J. and Griffiths, L. (1997) 'Settling NHS contract disputes: formal and informal pathways', in R. Flynn and G. Williams (eds), *Contracting for Health: Quasi-Markets in the NHS*. Oxford: Oxford University Press.

Hume, L. and Mulcock, J. (2004) *Anthropologists in the Field: Cases in Participant Observation*. New York: Columbia University Press.

Illsley, R. (1980) *Professional or Public Health? Sociology in Health and Medicine*. London: Nuffield Provincial Hospitals Trust.

Lambert, E.Y., Ashery, R.S. and Needle, R.H. (1995) *Qualitative Methods in Drug Abuse and HIV Research*, NIDA Research Monograph 157. Washington, DC: US Department of Health and Human Services, National Institutes of Health.

Lee, R.M. and Esterhuizen, L. (2000) 'Computer software and qualitative analysis: trends, issues, and responses', *International Journal of Social Research Methodology*, 3: 231–43.

Lindesmith, A. (1947) *Opiate Addiction*. Bloomington, IN: Principia Press.

Malinowski, B. (1922) *Argonauts of the Western Pacific*. London: Routledge and Kegan Paul.

Marinetto, M. (2011) 'Case studies of the health policy process: a methodological introduction', in M. Exworthy, S. Peckham, M. Powell and A. Hann (eds), *Shaping Health Policy: Case Study Methods and Analysis*. Bristol: Policy Press.

Mays, N. and Pope, C. (1996) 'Observational methods in health care settings', in N. Mays and C. Pope (eds), *Qualitative Research in Health Care*. London: BMJ Books.

Mays, N. and Pope, C. (2000) 'Qualitative research in health care: assessing quality in qualitative research', *British Medical Journal*, 320: 50–2.

McCall, G.J. (1984) 'Systematic field observation', *Annual Review of Sociology*, 10: 263–310.

McDonald, R., Harrison, S. and Checkland, K. (2009) 'The new GP contract in English primary health care: an ethnographic study', *International Journal of Public Sector Management*, 22: 21–34.

Melia, K.M. (1982) 'Tell it as it is: qualitative methodology and nursing research – understanding the student nurse's world', *Journal of Advanced Nursing*, 7(4): 327–35.

Melia, K.M. (1996) 'Re-discovering Glaser', *Qualitative Health Research*, 6: 368–78.

Mitchell, J.C. (1983) 'Case and situation analysis', *Sociological Review*, 31: 187–211.

Murphy, E., Dingwall, R., Greatbatch, D., Parker, S. and Watson, P. (1998) 'Qualitative methods in health technology assessment: a review of the literature', *Health Technology Assessment*, 2: 16.

Olesen, V.L. and Whittaker, E.W. (1968) *The Silent Dialogue: A Study in the Social Psychology of Professional Socialization*. San Francisco, CA: Jossey-Bass.

Pope, C. and Mays, N. (1995) 'Qualitative research: reaching the parts other methods cannot reach – an introduction to qualitative methods in health and health services research', *British Medical Journal*, 311: 42–5.

Porter, S. (1995) *Nursing's Relationship with Medicine: A Critical Realist Ethnography*. Aldershot: Avebury.

Punch, M. (1986) *The Politics and Ethics of Fieldwork*. London: Sage.

Roethlisberger, F.J. and Dickson, W.J. (1939) *Management and the Worker: An Account of a Research Program Conducted by the Western Electric Company, Hawthorne Works, Chicago*. Cambridge, MA: Harvard University Press.

Roth, J.A. (1963) *Timetables*. New York: Bobbs Merrill.

Roth, J.A. (1999) 'Hired-hand research', in A. Bryman and R.G. Burgess (eds), *Qualitative Research, Volume One: Fundamental Issues in Qualitative Research*. London: Sage.

Russell, I. (1996) 'Methods of health service evaluation: the gospel of Archie Cochrane after 25 years', *Journal of Health Services Research and Policy*, 1: 114–15.

Sbaih, L.C. (2002) 'Meanings of immediate: the practical use of the Patient's Charter in the accident and emergency department', *Social Science and Medicine*, 54: 1345–55.

Seale, C. (1999) 'Quality in qualitative research', *Qualitative Inquiry*, 5(4): 465–78.

Silverman, D. (1998) 'Qualitative research: meanings or practices?', *Information Systems*, 8: 3–20.

Strauss, A.L. and Corbin, J. (1990) *Basics of Qualitative Research: Grounded Theory Procedures and Techniques*. Newbury Park, CA: Sage.

Strong, P. and Robinson, J. (1990) *The NHS: Under New Management*. Milton Keynes: Open University Press.

Sudnow, D. (1968) *Passing On: The Social Organization of Dying*. New York: Prentice Hall.

Timmermans, S. (1999) *Sudden Death and the Myth of CPR*. Philadelphia, PA: Temple University Press.

Timmermans, S. (2006) *Postmortem: How Medical Examiners Explain Suspicious Deaths*. Chicago, IL: University of Chicago Press.

Waring, J. (2005) 'Beyond blame: cultural barriers to medical incident reporting', *Social Science and Medicine*, 60: 1927–35.

Yin, R. (1984) *Case Study Research: Design and Methods*. Beverly Hills, CA: Sage.

Znaniecki, F. (1952) *Cultural Sciences*. Urbana, IL: University of Illinois Press.

Zussman, R. (1992) *Intensive Care: Medical Ethics and the Medical Profession*. Chicago, IL: University of Chicago Press.

Zussman, R. (1993) 'Life in the hospital – a review', *Milbank Quarterly*, 71(1): 167–85.

7

The Use of Focus Groups in Research into Health

JUDITH GREEN

Introduction

- Focus groups are a widely used qualitative research method in researching health. Some authors use the term 'focus group' specifically to describe one specific research technique, in which a number of strangers are brought together by the researcher to discuss a topic in a 'focused' way. The roots of this kind of focus group lie in market research where the aim is to gather consumers' views of new products and services as an aid to marketing. However, it can be used as another term for a group interview, which has a long history in social research. Since the 1980s, focus groups have become increasingly popular as a data generation technique for a range of purposes, with health researchers being some of the most enthusiastic proponents. Focus groups have been used in projects with aims as broad ranging as needs assessment, users' perceptions of services and sociological studies of the understanding of health by the public.
- This chapter examines the typical structure of a focus group and the kinds of questions that can be explored in a focus group setting. It then examines the different types of resource required for running a focus group and the strengths and weaknesses of the method covering methodological and ethical considerations. Questions of data management, analysis and presentation are a particularly challenging issue when using the focus group method and the chapter argues that the researcher must keep in mind that it is the group, rather than individuals within it, that is the focus of the analysis. A case study example demonstrates the various stages of a project using a focus group method in practice.

Focus Group Size and Structure

Although there are many variations, a focus group typically consists of between six and ten people brought together to discuss a topic, with one or more facilitators (sometimes called 'moderators') who introduce and guide the discussion and record it in some way. Sometimes the group is also asked to carry out exercises together, such as sorting a set of cards with statements on them, or ranking a list of priorities. A typical focus group might include the following stages, as set out in Box 7.1.

Box 7.1   The stages of a focus group

- *Welcome:* the facilitator(s) welcome the participants, ask for consent forms to be completed, and perhaps provide refreshments
- *Icebreaking exercise:* once the group is together and seated, and the aims of the group outlined, an introductory exercise is used to introduce the participants to each other and establish a relaxed, informal atmosphere. This might be an invitation for each participant to say their name and one thing about themselves (such as their favourite food, or something related to the topic in question)
- *Introductory exercise:* this is designed to introduce the topic, and get participants discussing it. Examples would be inviting participants to sort or rank pictures or phrases
- *Group discussion:* a series of questions (the topic guide) is used to 'focus' the discussion. These usually move from the general to the more specific. For instance, here are some prompts from a study to explore women's views of taking folic acid supplements before and during pregnancy, from a study by Rose Barbour and colleagues (2011):

  - Can I start by asking you what your thoughts are about taking supplements during pregnancy?
  - What other changes did you make either in the run-up to or during your pregnancy?
  - What about folic acid specifically?
  - Why do you think women might decide not to take folic acid supplements or to stop taking them?
  - Can you please have a look at this leaflet [from the Health Education Board for Scotland]. Do you remember seeing this – or something similar before you got pregnant/in early pregnancy/during pregnancy?

- *Summing up:* the facilitator summarizes the key issues raised, and asks for any additional comments.

Source: Barbour et al. (2011)

Why Focus Groups for Health Research?

Focus groups provide an opportunity to research not only people's experiences and attitudes, but how these are communicated in a relatively 'naturalistic' setting (see, for instance,

Barbour 2007). As health topics are often readily discussed in everyday contexts such as workplaces and social environments, a group setting often works well for generating talk about health and health services. One rationale for using focus groups follows the market research tradition, in which focus groups are used to ask users about their views of health services. Where there are policies to develop health services that are more user-centred, focus groups are a useful tool for proactively seeking the views of users and potential users. Unlike user surveys, focus group discussions allow participants to frame their concerns in their own terms rather than that of the researcher, and to bring issues to the agenda that researchers might not otherwise have considered. Analysing discussion, rather than single opinions, allows the complexity of views to be studied. Bringing together people with something in common, such as using the same hospital services or having similar health problems, can be a direct way for service providers and commissioners to find out how satisfied users are with services.

The potential for discussion also means that focus groups have advantages for studies of broader views about health and illness, such as investigating what people know, how they know it, and how this knowledge is communicated in social interaction (on the role of interaction, see Morgan 2010). Health researchers have therefore made extensive use of focus groups either on their own, or in combination with individual interviews or other methods, to explore the public understanding of health and how accounts of health and illness are used in everyday talk. One example is from Evans et al. (2001), who explored parents' decisions about accepting the combined measles, mumps and rubella (MMR) immunization for their children. In the wake of considerable media coverage of controversy about the safety of the MMR vaccine in the UK, there was concern that rates of immunization were falling to dangerously low levels.

The study is an example of the role of focus groups in exploring beliefs about these kinds of controversial issues. The researchers used group interviews to explore in detail how parents made decisions, and asked about the sources of knowledge they drew on. They found that most parents considered the decision of whether to immunize their children or not very stressful, and that they were dissatisfied with the information available. Parents wanted more open and informed discussion with health professionals about the risks and benefits. By bringing together groups that included only parents who had immunized or only those who had not, Evans and her colleagues provided a safe environment in which parents could discuss their views.

One advantage of focus group methods cited by some researchers is their potential for redressing some of the traditional power imbalances between researchers and research participants. A group may be able to exert more control over the research agenda than a single interviewee and, if focus groups are used as part of a participatory approach, being a focus group participant may encourage individuals to become involved in the research. At the end of a project, focus groups can be a very useful way of getting feedback from participants on draft reports. However, focus groups in themselves are not inevitably more, or less, likely to lead to participation. Critical factors are:

- How far participants are involved in the early stages of setting the research agenda.
- How committed the research commissioners are to implementing recommendations.

If commissioners are committed to a participatory approach, deliberative methods such as citizens' juries may be more appropriate than one-off focus groups. These involve a greater time commitment from participants, who have the task of developing a consensus view in the light of expert witness presentations and structured discussions.

Finally, focus group discussions are widely used in preparatory work within larger health research projects, when they may be used to generate data to help in survey design or in the development of patient-reported outcome measures. Thomas et al. (1995) used focus groups, as well as individual interviews, in this way as part of their development work on the measure of patient satisfaction with nursing care. Focus groups were held with groups of patients in medical and surgical wards and with one group of post-discharge patients in a family doctor's surgery. The aim was to use the data from these groups and interviews to develop a multidimensional concept of satisfaction with nursing care, which could then be used on a scale of satisfaction that was patient based. The researchers identified key elements of satisfaction from these focus groups and interviews, such as availability, attentiveness and information.

Resources Required for Focus Groups in Practice

Focus groups are often selected in health research because they appear to be a relatively cost-effective data generation method, compared with alternatives such as individual interviews or ethnography. A small number of groups can certainly generate a large data set, without the labour-intensive commitment of long-term ethnographic fieldwork. However, it is perhaps a mistake to assume that focus groups are necessarily a cheap option. Identifying participants and organizing the groups is resource-intensive, and there are a number of hidden costs. Some of the key issues to consider when thinking about resources are:

- How participants will be recruited.
- Identifying a suitable location.
- Whether professional facilitators will be needed.
- Making payments to participants.
- The cost of data preparation.

Recruitment

Depending on the aims of the study, participants can be recruited through advertising for volunteers; working with personal contacts or established gatekeepers for particular groups, such as community leaders, school heads or trade unions; or by paying for professional recruitment, for instance, through a market research company. The advantages and disadvantages of these recruitment methods depend on the aim of the study, but all incur some costs. Advertising is relatively cheap, but rarely effective; few people respond to calls for volunteers unless there are financial or other incentives. Moreover, developing relationships with gatekeepers in the community takes up considerable researcher time. Professional recruitment agencies are often very effective, especially if the participants come from very specific sub-populations, with expensive additional direct payments.

Location

The location for a focus group needs careful consideration. A relatively neutral location with good facilities for refreshments, seating and transport access is necessary to maximize attendance and goodwill – see also Chapter 17 for a discussion of recruiting ethnic minority groups. In practical terms, choosing a convenient location is crucial: Barbour and colleagues (2011) report poor attendance from those invited to attend a focus group at a hospital, but better from those invited to pre-existing mother and toddler groups. The specific location also shapes the kind of data collected (Green and Hart 1999), and a range of locations may be required. People's accounts are context-dependent and if you talk to them in the workplace, for example, they are more likely to be in work roles and their accounts will reflect this. In their study of children's views of risk around accidental injury, Green and Hart (1999) found children gave very different accounts depending on whether the group was held in school premises or in youth club premises. Those in the school-based groups were more likely to stress 'sensible' views, and in the youth club groups more likely to tell stories in which they had taken risks.

Facilitators

Facilitating a focus group discussion is a skill, and not one all researchers have developed, so a professional facilitator may be needed. For most groups, two people will be needed to run the discussion. One leads the discussion, making sure the topic guide is covered. The other has responsibility for practical issues such as meeting and greeting participants, organizing refreshments, checking that tape recorders are working and perhaps taking notes or summarizing at key points. In addition, professional help may be needed for translation, childcare or other special needs.

Payments to participants

Participants recruited by a market research company will usually expect payment for their time, in addition to travel expenses. Professionals will often expect payment to cover locum costs. This can be expensive if a study has to include large numbers of health care workers. There is some debate about both the ethical and methodological implications of paying participants. Offering an incentive may make it difficult for low-income people to decline, and paying people may make them more likely to say what they think the researcher wants to hear. It is difficult to judge these concerns empirically, but there is some justification for paying focus group participants, who will usually turn up at a time and place of the researcher's choosing, devoting several hours to a study. There are ways of minimizing any potential impact of payment on the quality of data by not advertising the payment, but offering store vouchers at the end of the group as a 'thank you'.

Costs of data preparation

Most social research in health adopting this research method uses transcripts of focus group discussions as the basis for the analysis. The costs of producing transcripts vary considerably, but a skilled audio-typist can take four to six hours to transcribe each hour of focus group discussion. If a more detailed transcript is required or the discussion is difficult to hear, this obviously takes longer.

Other resources

Other costs incurred will include refreshments; travel for participants; audio-recording equipment; and pens, paper and flip charts for exercises and summing up. Some groups will have special needs that have to be considered, such as crèche facilities or interpreters. If the topic is a sensitive one, it may be appropriate to provide facilities for debriefing.

Focus group research is, then, rarely a cheap option, but it is cost-effective if the data generated address the research question. Costing obviously also depends on how many groups are to be included. There may be a trade-off between a perfect research design, such as a method that continues sampling groups until theoretical saturation has been reached, and a design that is acceptable within the resources available.

Focus Groups in Health Research: Methodology

The first issue to be considered here is the strengths and weaknesses of focus groups as a method in health research. The decision to use focus groups should be based primarily on methodological considerations. Are the data that a focus group generates likely to address the research question posed? Like other qualitative data generation techniques, focus groups are appropriate when there is a need to identify participants' perspectives, and to understand their frames of meaning. The key methodological advantage of using group rather than individual interviews is that they provide access to interaction between participants. Analysing this interaction allows the researcher to explore the underlying assumptions, norms and cultural beliefs of the participants. Bloor et al. (2001: 90) suggest that focus groups are the method of choice when

> researching topics relating to group norms, the group meanings that underpin those norms and the group processes whereby those meanings are constructed ... Focus groups are a particularly advantageous method where these group norms, meanings and processes are hidden or counter-cultural.

Other issues will also influence the decision to use focus groups, including the resources available and the topic – is it one, for example, which is easier for participants to talk about in a group setting? Like all methods, the strengths and weaknesses of focus groups relate to the specific research question, topic and setting: what is a strength for one study may be a weakness for another. Three particular issues illustrate how strengths and weaknesses need to be considered in the light of a specific research project. These are access to interaction, naturalism and talking about sensitive issues.

Access to interaction

The main methodological advantage of using group interviews compared with individual interviews is that the researcher has access to interaction between participants, rather than just to talk between the researcher and one participant. This potentially allows access to rather more 'naturalistic' talk about the topic of interest, which (it is assumed) might reflect the ways in which people discuss issues in everyday life. This advantage is maximized when the focus group consists of people who might ordinarily interact in work, domestic or other settings. Khan and Manderson (1992: 60) note how useful it is to tap into social networks such as kin groups or neighbours when doing research on health:

> Such natural clusterings of people represent, in a loose fashion, the resources upon which any member of the group might draw, both in material terms and with respect to information and advice ... It is precisely this natural social network which provides the scripting for the management of an illness event – what to do with a child with bloody diarrhoea, for example, or how to nurse a high fever, or who to call in the case of a threatened miscarriage. As a result, discussions with such groups provide fairly accurate data regarding the diagnosis and treatment of illness, choices of health services and so on.

Although Khan and Manderson are discussing informal interviews in rural settings, this captures neatly the advantage of utilizing 'natural' groups in more formal focus group research. To some extent, the researcher has access to the kinds of discussions that might happen in non-research settings about treatment decisions, or health services, rather than the supposedly more artificial 'opinions' that are more readily offered in one-to-one interviews. Kitzinger (1994: 105) used natural groups in a study of how media messages about HIV/AIDS were understood by various audiences in a UK context, noting:

> We chose to work with pre-existing groups – clusters of people who already knew each other through living, working or socialising together. We did this in order to explore how people might talk about AIDS within the various and overlapping groupings within which they actually operate. Flatmates, colleagues and friends – these are precisely the people with whom one might 'naturally' discuss such topics. The fact that research participants already knew each other had the additional advantage that [they] could relate each other's comments to actual incidents in their daily shared lives. They often challenged each other on contradictions between what they were professing to believe and how they actually behaved.

Focus groups allow exploration of interaction and this has great advantages for many of the kinds of questions health researchers wish to address. We are often interested not just in the content of knowledge, but in how decisions come to be made, or how information about health is transferred between people within social networks. Individual interviews are often criticized for providing information on what people say, but not on what people do. As Kitzinger (1994) suggests in the quote above, in focus group discussions between people who know each other, stories about how people say they behave are challenged, corroborated or undercut, giving some information on the relationship between behaviour and how people talk about it.

A good example of how focus groups can generate data on the gaps between professed beliefs and behaviour comes from a European study on attitudes to food risk, discussed further later in the chapter (Green et al. 2003). In the focus groups held with adolescents, some of the young people in both the UK and Italy talked during the discussions about how they avoided 'fast food' as 'unsafe'. However, as the group discussion progressed, friends challenged each other, with reminders of how they had eaten burgers from street stalls, especially when they were returning late from clubs or concerts. In analysing focus group data, the researcher can contrast what might be called a 'public' account, such as 'we don't eat fast food', with stories drawn from everyday experience. This can provide data on normative ideas about health: that is what people think they should do, as well as accounts of situations in which these normative ideas do not, in practice, shape behaviour.

Naturalism

However, the 'naturalism' that generates such useful interaction for analysis also presents both practical and methodological problems. There is a trade-off between facilitating the kind of natural discussions that happen in everyday life, with people interrupting and talking over each other, and generating a discussion in which people's talk can be heard, transcribed and analysed. The researcher has to make a decision about the main aim of the study: is it to reproduce 'natural' talk, in order to analyse how ideas are transmitted and knowledge about health is discussed? If so, the facilitator will allow discussion to continue in a more natural way. If the main aim is to access a range of views, and ensure that the group's views on every topic are heard, then the discussion may have to be more tightly controlled.

A more methodological limitation is the seductiveness of a natural focus group discussion; it appears like 'everyday talk' and it is tempting to treat it as such. Nonetheless, even if relatively informal, a specially constituted focus group is still an artificial setting. People's talk is contextual. It is shaped by, and for, specific contexts and we cannot assume that what is said in a research setting reflects what might be said in the home, the workplace or other environment. The stories recounted in focus groups may be different from those recounted in one-to-one interviews, but they are not necessarily more valid as representations of 'what really happened'. It cannot be assumed that accounts provided in a focus group setting reflect in any simplistic way 'real life'. For this reason, focus groups are not a substitute for detailed ethnography. If the aim of the study is to research social practice in context, a design that uses long-term observational methods would be a more appropriate choice.

Talking about sensitive issues

A practical strength of a group setting is that it can offer a more supportive environment for participants to discuss sensitive issues. One example is dissatisfaction with health services. In a one-to-one interview, it may be difficult to express dissatisfaction, especially if the interviewer is known to be a health professional, or associated with the provider service. In a group, other participants can legitimate negative views, and one participant's story about their experiences can trigger other participants' recollections.

However, this has the potential disadvantage of over-emphasizing negative experiences. There are also some topics for which a focus group might not be an appropriate setting, unless the participants all share a particular experience. Using focus groups to explore deviant behaviour, or socially stigmatizing experiences, may be inappropriate if some participants are likely to feel uncomfortable. If an understanding of the views of those marginalized in particular settings is needed, individual interviews may be a more appropriate method.

Sampling Groups and Participants

When sampling, both the selection of groups and the selection of individual participants have to be considered. As in most qualitative research, the sampling strategy is usually purposeful. It does not aim to be statistically representative of a larger population, but is dictated by identifying what Patton (1990) describes as 'information-rich' cases. These are the groups that are most likely to furnish the data needed to address the research question. However, more pragmatic concerns are also likely to influence both the sample size and who is included. Often, focus group research is done with an aim of influencing policy, whether at the immediate local level (such as improving service provision) or at a more national level. To provide convincing data for policy makers, the sample also has to be credible. It should include representatives of all the constituencies in which policy makers are likely to be interested.

The number of groups needed depends largely on how many constituencies there are within the population of interest. In a local study of health care users, it may be enough to convene two groups of patients, perhaps segregated by gender as men and women tend to talk very differently in mixed as opposed to single-gender groups. In a study with a broad research question, such as the case study reported at the end of this chapter on how consumers in four European countries choose safe food, there might be a large number of population segments in terms of characteristics such as gender and age. This is especially the case if the researcher also wants to include both homogeneous and more heterogeneous groups. Rather than including groups that reflect every possible combination of factors, it is worth designing a sampling grid and selecting groups across the grid. The sampling grid for the study of European consumers is shown in Table 7.1 later in this chapter.

Within each group, a key decision is whether to sample participants for homogeneity, where some characteristics are shared, or heterogeneity. Traditionally, market researchers sample for heterogeneity, in order to generate a range of views within each group. The advantage of homogeneity is that shared experiences can provide a more supportive environment for discussing a difficult or sensitive issue. However, including a range of participants can also be a useful way to trigger participants' accounts of issues that they may consider too 'common sense' to mention unless prompted by someone who does not share their perspective. In practice, of course, researchers may have little control over the individuals who participate, especially if recruitment is undertaken by inviting volunteers or through gatekeepers.

Ethical Considerations

In a focus group, participants outnumber researchers and this can be an important element in shifting the balance of power towards participants. In projects that aim to listen to communities, or to access the voice of groups that are traditionally marginalized in the public arena, this can be an important ethical advantage. In work with young people, for instance, using group, as opposed to individual, interviews can be a very useful way of redressing the power imbalance between interviewer and interviewee (Green and Hart 1999). However, Michell (1999) found, in the context of her study of young people's peer groups, that the hierarchical relations of the friendship group were reproduced in the focus group and the voices of those low down in the pecking order were not heard. Experiences of bullying and victimization were only accessible through individual interviews. So the group setting may facilitate access to marginalized communities, but at the same time it may reproduce local hierarchies and limit access to marginalized individuals within those communities (see also Chapter 17).

Focus groups differ from interviews in that the researcher cannot guarantee the confidentiality of what is said. Participants are reliant on other members to treat them with respect and keep their contributions confidential. The facilitator should consider setting ground rules at the beginning of the discussion, but also be aware that the supportive environment of a group can lead people to 'over-disclose' and perhaps talk about issues in a way that they regret later. This is a particular risk if the group is a natural group that exists outside the research setting. Vissandjee et al. (2002), in their report of how they used focus groups in a study of women's health behaviour in rural Gujarat in India, discuss this as a particular problem in doing research in small communities. People have to interact with each other long after the research team has gone home. There is an ethical obligation therefore to make sure that participants do not reveal information they had not intended to. This might make them vulnerable in their everyday lives so facilitators need to discuss how to deflect over-disclosure within natural groups.

Discussions of ethics tend to focus on informed consent, and ensuring that participants have not been cajoled or bullied into taking part. This is of course crucial, particularly if working with gatekeepers who may have pressurized people to take part. However, there are also ethical concerns about those who do not get the opportunity to take part. For young people, the need to secure parents' consent may mean that some children are disenfranchised (Green and Hart 1999). Similarly, if using community leaders to aid recruitment, it is worth considering who is not being asked to participate, as well as ensuring that those who do have provided their genuine consent.

Finally, researchers have an ethical duty to consider what happens to the data from focus groups. Those invited to a group to discuss an issue may have more investment in the research than those who fill in a survey, or take part in a brief interview. Where possible, it is good practice to feed back summaries of the findings to those who took part. Indeed, focus groups can be a useful forum for disseminating findings as well as for generating data. Researchers can use the comments of participants to check on their findings and their interpretation of the data.

The Management, Analysis and Presentation of Focus Group Data

Managing focus group data can be challenging. In particular, 'naturalistic' data can be difficult to transcribe and to understand. A key decision is whether to work with full transcripts. In social research, it is usual to transcribe fully all group discussions and use these as a basis for analysis. However, in many projects it may be enough to use notes of the discussion, transcribing only those sections of the tape that are most relevant. This is justifiable if only a summary of key concerns is needed or if the aim is to access a group's consensus view on a particular topic, rather than to identify how they came to that decision. If it is not possible to tape and transcribe the discussion – and this may be impossible for practical or political reasons – facilitators should ensure that detailed notes are taken and that the group's opinions are summarized at key points during the process.

If there are complete transcripts of all, or most, of the groups, there are a number of strategies for analysis. Essentially, these are no different from techniques for analysing any other qualitative data set and there are various textbooks that provide advice (see Miles and Huberman 1994; Strauss and Corbin 1998; and Silverman 2011 who offer different approaches). As in any other type of study, choosing a strategy for analysis depends on the aim of the study in terms of the research question, the requirements of the funding body and the methodological orientation of the researcher. If the focus groups were convened to provide a broad-brush overview of community views or to identify some common issues to feed into later studies, then a fairly simple content analysis of transcripts of the discussion or notes taken will suffice.

Thematic content analysis

A thematic analysis involves identifying recurring themes within the data; exploring typologies of these themes; and looking at variations relationships between, and within, themes. Analysis is an iterative process that begins with the first data collected, and continues into the writing up of the project. It involves moving between the data and the empirical and theoretical literature in a way that helps to make sense of the data and aids discussion within the research team about 'what is going on here'. This is not just a technical exercise in coding extracts of talk, but one that involves some analytical imagination. However, there are some steps that can help with a simple thematic analysis, which are set out in Box 7.2 below.

Box 7.2   Steps for thematic analysis

- *Familiarization with the transcripts:* reading and rereading the transcripts and listening to the tapes to get an overall sense of key issues for participants. For example, what made participants angry, enthusiastic or nervous? A summary can be written of each group discussion.
- *Developing a coding frame:* it is worth doing this in a group, with either a team of researchers or colleagues. Read early transcripts in detail, identifying in each segment the key concept: what the participant is 'talking about'. Try to label these concepts in as abstract a way as possible. Rather than merely summarizing the content, think about what the extracts are an example of and then build these into a coding frame. A coding frame is essentially a list of concepts and their labels (the 'codes').
- *Coding:* when you have a coding framework, the entire set of transcripts can be 'coded' by identifying each segment as an instance of a code. This will be modified as more data are analysed.
- *'Cut and paste':* all the instances of the same code can now be gathered together, either manually by literally cutting up the transcripts or using a word processor or specialized software. Now look at the list of extracts under each code to identify the range of talk about each topic.

This kind of thematic content analysis is suitable for mapping out the range and strength of views and comparing the kinds of issues that arise across the group. To exploit the strengths of focus group data and maximize the chance of producing useful policy-relevant findings, a more detailed and sociologically informed analysis will probably be needed, which takes interaction into account.

Social interaction: analysis and presentation

A common criticism of much focus group research is that researchers often stress the advantage of interaction, but rarely show in published papers how this has been used in the analysis. One exception is Wilkinson and Kitzinger (2000) who, in their study of women's talk about 'thinking positive' in the context of cancer, provide a good illustration of how analysing interaction in focus groups can generate a much more sophisticated understanding of health knowledge than merely identifying some common themes. They note that their data on women's talk could have furnished a number of quotes such as 'You just have to think positive'. In a superficial content analysis, these could be identified as 'evidence' of the importance of 'thinking positive' in cancer patients' lives.

However, a more subtle analysis of this talk as discourse enabled Wilkinson and Kitzinger (2000) to reflect on how and why such comments are used in talk. First, they argue that such comments as 'thinking positive' are a common idiom in English: a taken-for-granted summary of common-sense knowledge that is used as a general purpose statement within everyday talk to move the conversation along and to take it from a personal to a general frame. Participants invoke such idioms when they want to cite a shared norm, something with which the audience can agree, and turn a conversation from a potentially difficult one about personal difference into an inclusive one about affiliation. Thus, through paying attention in the analysis to the content of what is said (through stripping out phrases or paragraphs without any sense of context) and to how interaction works discursively, Wilkinson and Kitzinger are able to specify much more precisely what participants are doing when they invoke such phrases as 'thinking positive'. By so doing, they uncovered the social context in which such statements might be made. In this case, a broad cultural norm was expressed in a setting where 'thinking positive' was the expected and morally required response.

The group as the unit of analysis

Given that focus group studies often include a large number of individual participants, it can be tempting to treat any data as derived from individuals quantitatively. This is a mistake: individuals are not selected as representatives of a broader population, but as a group, and the group should properly be the unit of analysis. When writing up, it is inappropriate to report on the characteristics or beliefs of individuals as if they were a population sample. The focus should be on the group, with sufficient context given about their composition to enable the reader to judge how the data were generated. This might include details of how the groups were recruited; what social characteristics they shared and what they were asked to discuss. A description of the discursive context should also be provided, to indicate how particular utterances were used within the discussion, rather than merely using individuals' statements as indicators of their beliefs. This might include details of the issues over which participants agreed or disagreed; which topics were difficult to discuss; and how persuasive particular kinds of accounts were in interaction.

Case study: Exploring accounts of food risk using focus groups

As part of a large European study of the public perception of risk associated with bovine spongiform encephalopathy (BSE), we wanted to explore public concerns about food risk in general, and to identify what kinds of information on food safety were trusted (Green et al. 2003, 2005). The aim was to include people from four European countries, which had been chosen to represent a range of 'food cultures' (Germany, Italy, the UK and Finland), and to include people from different stages in the life cycle theoretically associated with different approaches to food choice – adolescents, young single people, those responsible for shopping for young children and older citizens.

In addition to providing detailed data on how these population groups talked about their food choices, we also aimed to compare findings across the four countries and the four life cycle stage groups. An international study presents particular challenges (see Chapter 21 of this book), but many are typical of the kinds of issues with which researchers in any focus group study have to deal.

The first was selecting an appropriate sample of groups. For comparative purposes, we wanted a similar range of groups in each of the four countries. However, within each country, the meaning of the life cycle groups and other population groups differed. As an example, young single men in Italy had rather less experience of choosing their own food than those of similar age in other countries. In some countries, moreover, regional or rural/urban differences were more pronounced than in others.

The second issue was that focus group methodologies have to resonate with local cultural norms about interaction. In some countries, it became clear that it would not be productive to run single-gender groups, as there are few situations in which men would interact normally in this way. The focus group setting simply would not reproduce 'natural' talk in the way that it might for other groups. We therefore created a sampling grid, which aimed to select a range of life cycle groups in each country and a range representing other factors theoretically linked to food cultures,

(Continued)

CASE STUDY

(Continued)

such as geographical location or social class. A total of 36 groups were sampled to generate a data set that would enable us to compare countries and life cycle groups, and within each country to take account of differences in location or social class, as illustrated in Table 7.1.

TABLE 7.1   Sampling grid for the food risks study focus groups

Country and location	Adolescents	20-25s	Family food purchasers	55+
Finland:				
Kuopio	X	XX	XX	XX
Germany:				
Kiel	X	X	XX	X
Eckernförde	X	X	X	X
Italy:				
Bologna	X	X		X
Naples		X	X	
Trento	XX		X	X
UK:				
London and environs	X	X	XX	X
Midlands	XXX	X	X	X

Note: X = one focus group
Source: Green et al. (2005)

The aim was to recruit natural groups wherever possible, to maximize the methodological advantages discussed above. The research teams used a mixture of methods to do this, including contacting community groups such as church-based or local associations and working with schools to recruit friendship groups of adolescents. However, for the 'young single' groups, which may consist of relatively mobile individuals with few obvious community allegiances, we relied on market research companies to recruit these.

The protocols for running the groups also had to balance comparability with flexibility. We used icebreaking exercises, asking participants to rank pictures of foodstuffs in terms of their 'riskiness' to generate discussion in all groups, with the pictures reflecting the kinds of food eaten locally. The list of topics to cover in each group was the same, but facilitators worded prompts appropriately for local participants.

Typically, health research is done by teams of people rather than individual researchers. In this project, we had research teams in each of the four countries and had to coordinate the analysis of data collected in four languages. First, pilot data from each country were transcribed and translated into English so all the project teams could carry out an initial thematic analysis. At a project meeting, these transcripts and the initial thematic analyses were discussed and we then generated a combined coding scheme to aid a comparative analysis across all countries. This was used within each country to generate a country report and provide a more detailed analysis. These reports were then subject to a 'meta-analysis' to produce integrated results across the study.

Access to interaction in the groups provided useful accounts of choosing safe food and how food was used in everyday life. In the transcripts, we could see to which sources of knowledge people referred and also how effective these sources were in persuading others. In interaction, personal anecdotes about food risk were much more effective for convincing others. Analysing interaction, rather than just individual accounts, also enabled us to look at the social consequences of talk about risk. We were interested in how 'risk' has become a relatively neutral discourse for discussing social difference. We looked at how talk about 'differences', such as ethnicity and religion, was reframed in many group discussions into talk about how aspects of risk illustrated some of the social uses of the rhetoric of risk in a multicultural society. This example is from a group of women in the UK, who quickly reframed one participant's religious rationale for avoiding pork into a frame of 'hygiene':

A: *We don't eat pork in any case ... for religious reasons.*

B: *A lot of the religious things to do with meat come from the hygiene aspect anyway, like Jewish people, they won't store meat in the same fridge as dairy produce – a lot of that is down to hygiene.*

C: *They are dirty, pigs.*

D: *Absolutely, it has been proved apparently, many years ago.*

B: *So it all comes down to hygiene.*

Source: Green et al. (2003: 42)

However, as suggested above, we cannot assume that the interaction we record is in any unproblematic way 'natural'. First, recruiting people within particular life cycle segments raises some methodological problems. In a group consisting only of those responsible for household shopping, for instance, participants arrive already attuned to one particular social role, usually that of 'mother', and we are to some extent generating the kinds of discourse we analyse as an artefact of our sampling strategy. The same individuals, if recruited as part of a group with some other characteristic in common such as profession, or political affiliation, may focus on different aspects of food choice and risk. Second, the process of taking part in a focus group on 'food risk' is in itself one way in which participants learn about the topic. Indeed, many of the participants in the groups said they had enjoyed themselves because they had learnt a lot, or commented that the discussion itself had changed their opinions. While this is very useful data, in that we can explore what kinds of talk are likely to lead to people saying they will change their behaviour, it does suggest that the setting (an hour and a half devoted to one topic) is not one that really reflects the kinds of everyday talk people are likely to have.

Reading Health Research Based on Focus Groups

When reading reports of focus group studies, the criteria used to assess usefulness or quality will depend on the reader's needs. For instance, readers may want an insight into the views of a population or to understand in greater depth the barriers to service uptake. Journal editors, particularly for biomedical journals, now require authors of qualitative studies to conform to guidelines for reporting on focus group and other qualitative methods (see Tong et al. 2007). Although there is debate about the appropriateness of such criteria, they suggest some questions to ask when assessing the quality of focus group studies. These questions include:

- Is the rationale for the use of focus group (rather than, say, individual interview) data clear?
- Have the authors been clear about their strategy for sampling groups and their rationale, such as the selection of natural groups and deciding on homogeneity or heterogeneity?
- Have the author(s) said how participants were recruited? Is there some evidence of reflexivity about the role of the research team and the choice of setting?
- Is there enough evidence for the reader to judge how context may have shaped the data generated?
- Are interactive data extracts reported, rather than just utterances from single participants?
- Does the analysis take interaction into account?

Conclusion

It has been argued that the focus group method has a number of advantages in gaining access to the way in which people discuss issues and deal with problems related to health in everyday life. Particularly if people in a focus group already share a common background and know each other, this can enable the researcher to understand frameworks of meaning, what resources people use and how they draw on social networks to deal with matters that arise on a day-to-day basis. Focus groups based on population samples that deliberately seek to bring together a group of people from different backgrounds to discuss a particular topic can also serve to demonstrate the range of views about a specific issue. However, using the focus group method can be challenging in terms of management, resources, process, data recording and analysis, particularly for the lone researcher. It is also important for researchers using the method and analysing the data to concentrate their attention on aspects of social interaction within the group in terms of understandings, views and attitudes and lines of agreement and divergence.

The case study demonstrates how focus groups can be used in relation to exploring people's understanding of food risk. The exercise below provides the opportunity for readers to consider employing the method in finding out about people's experience of maternity services and their priorities in any reorganization. There is also discussion of focus group research in Chapter 17 where the method has been used in a range of studies on service development for ethnic minority communities and in Chapter 20 where focus groups were used as one method in a study of user involvement in cancer services.

Exercise: Planning a focus group study of maternity services

There are plans to reorganize local maternity services, and a research programme has been commissioned to find out the views of staff and users on what could be improved in the new system. You have been asked to carry out some focus groups, with professionals and users, to explore their views of current service provision and their priorities for change. Write a brief (500 word) proposal for a focus group study. This should cover the following issues:

1 Sampling:

- Which groups of users and professionals should be included?
- How many will be needed to cover the main constituencies of interest?
- Are there particular sub-groups of the population that should be included?
- Will the groups be homogeneous or heterogeneous, and what is the rationale for your decision?

2 A protocol for running the groups:

- Think of an introductory exercise that would be appropriate for the groups of professionals and users.
- List 5–6 prompts for a topic guide.

3 Resources:

- What resources are needed to conduct your study?

4 Ethical issues:

- What particular ethical issues are raised by your proposed study?
- How will these ethical issues be addressed?
- Consider ethical issues in conducting the study and disseminating the findings.

5 Assessment:

- What are the main advantages and disadvantages of using focus groups for this study?

Recommended Further Reading

Barbour, R. and Kitzinger, J. (eds) (1999) *Developing Focus Group Research: Politics, Theory and Practice*. London: Sage.

This collection of papers stimulates more thoughtful use of focus groups by addressing methodological and practical issues, including researching sensitive topics, ethical considerations and different styles of analysis.

Bloor, M., Frankland, J., Thomas, M. and Robson, K. (2001) *Focus Groups in Social Research*. London: Sage.

This book usefully discusses the more methodological issues raised by employing focus groups in social research in health and is particularly strong on issues of analysis and interpretation.

Kreuger, R. and Casey, M.A. (2009) *Focus Groups: A Practical Guide for Applied Research*, 4th edition. London: Sage.

The authors of this text use their experience of a range of studies/participants to provide excellent practical advice on all stages of an applied focus group study – planning and recruiting, moderating, coping with problems and managing and reporting data.

 ## Online Readings

Janke, M., Jones, J., Payne, L. and Son, J. (2012) 'Living with arthritis: Using self-management of valued activities to promote health', *Qualitative Health Research*, 22: 360–72.

How is the focus group adopted in this context? What benefits did this approach bring? Critically evaluate the paper using the checklist provided in PPS7.7.

Clavering, E. and McLaughlin, J. (2007) Crossing multidisciplinary divides: Exploring professional hierarchies and boundaries in focus groups, *Qualitative Health Research*, 17: 400–410.

How is the focus group adopted in this context? What benefits did this approach bring? Critically evaluate the paper using the checklist provided in PPS7.7.

References

Barbour, R.S. (2007) *Doing Focus Groups*. London: Sage.

Barbour, R.S., Macleod, M., Mires, G. and Anderson, A.S. (2011) 'Uptake of folic acid supplements before and during pregnancy: focus group analysis of women's views and experiences', *Journal of Human Nutrition and Dietetics*, 25: 140–7.

Bloor, M., Frankland, J., Thomas, M. and Robson, K. (2001) *Focus Groups in Social Research*. London: Sage.

Evans, M., Stoddart, H., Condon, L., Freeman, E., Grizzell, M. and Mullen, R. (2001) 'Parents' perspectives on the MMR immunisation: a focus group study', *British Journal of General Practice*, 51: 904–10.

Green, J. and Hart, L. (1999) 'The impact of context on data', in R. Barbour and J. Kitzinger (eds), *Developing Focus Group Research*. London: Sage.

Green, J., Draper, A. and Dowler, E. (2003) 'Short cuts to safety: risk and "rules of thumb" in accounts of food choice', *Health, Risk and Society*, 5: 33–52.

Green, J., Draper, A., Dowler, E., Fele, G., Hagenhoff, V., Rusanen, M. and Rusanen, T. (2005) 'Public understanding of food risks in four European countries: a qualitative study', *European Journal of Public Health*, 15: 523–7.

Khan, M.E. and Manderson, L. (1992) 'Focus groups in tropical diseases research', *Health Policy and Planning*, 7: 56–66.

Kitzinger, J. (1994) 'The methodology of focus groups: the importance of interaction between research participants', *Sociology of Health and Illness*, 16: 103–21.

Michell, L. (1999) 'Combining focus groups and interviews: telling how it is; telling how it feels', in R. Barbour and J. Kitzinger (eds), *Developing Focus Group Research*. London: Sage.

Miles, M. and Huberman, A.M. (1994) *Qualitative Data Analysis: An Expanded Sourcebook*, 2nd edition. Thousand Oaks, CA: Sage.

Morgan, D.L. (2010) 'Reconsidering the role of interaction in analysing and reporting focus groups', *Qualitative Health Research*, 20: 718–22.

Patton, M.Q. (1990) *Qualitative Evaluation and Research Methods*, 2nd edition. Newbury Park, CA: Sage.

Silverman, D. (2011) *Interpreting Qualitative Data*, 4th edition. London: Sage.

Strauss, A. and Corbin, J. (1998) *Basics of Qualitative Research*, 2nd edition. London: Sage.

Thomas, L., MacMillan, J., McColl, E., Hale, C. and Bond, S. (1995) 'Comparison of focus group and individual interview methodology in examining patient satisfaction with nursing care', *Social Sciences in Health*, 1: 206–20.

Tong, A., Sainsbury, P. and Craig, J. (2007) 'Consolidated criteria for reporting qualitative research (COREQ): a 32-item checklist for interviews and focus groups', *International Journal for Quality in Health Care*, 19: 349–57.

Vissandjee, B., Abdool, S. and Dupere, S. (2002) 'Focus groups in rural Gujarat, India: A modified approach', *Qualitative Health Research*, 12: 826–43.

Wilkinson, S. and Kitzinger, C. (2000) 'Thinking differently about thinking positive', *Social Science and Medicine*, 50: 797–811.

8

Action Research and Health

HEATHER WATERMAN

Introduction

- Action research is a participative method of research that seeks to gain more knowledge and to change people's circumstances for the better by engaging them in the research process. The process of action research is therefore complex and requires participants to develop skills in research, practice, education and change management. This chapter outlines some of the challenges of action research and how difficulties can be overcome. Despite the pitfalls, the literature on action research shows that this approach can have a positive impact on people's health and health services.

- From a personal perspective as an action researcher, I have shifted from a position of viewing action research as a technical approach to solving problems in health care, to seeing the method as one that aspires towards empowerment and democracy. In this case, empowerment refers to enabling research participants to take action, often in difficult situations, and democracy, to encouraging people from diverse backgrounds to debate freely and work towards improving their circumstances through research. As a practitioner, a ward manager, I was enthusiastic about the immediacy of action research and challenged by the idea of studying a situation and changing practice at the same time. Later, after participating in several action research projects, I came to appreciate the significance of critical reflection within groups and joint decisions on action, thus empowering participants, both practitioners and patients, in health care settings. The increased knowledge and confidence that occurs enables changes to be made by those who are experiencing a problem, whether they are patients or staff, in areas related to direct patient care, management, administration or education. Action research by its nature is an exercise of democracy as it encourages a group of people who normally may not be heard or enabled, to change their lives, to work together actively and take responsibility for changing their situation. However, over time, I have become more realistic and critical of the method. In this chapter, I will expand on these issues by:

o Examining the main characteristics and rationale for action research in health care settings and the resources required to apply it in practice

o Considering the strengths and weaknesses of action research and the challenges of data analysis and report writing

o Providing an example of action research still in progress and an exercise to help the reader understand the interrelationships between theory, method and data.

Action Research: Rationale, Principles and Resources

Definition and methods

Action research is defined by Kemmis and McTaggart (1988: 5) as

> ... simply a form of collective self-reflective enquiry undertaken by participants in social situations in order to improve the rationality and justice of their own situations, their understandings of these practices and the situations in which these practices are carried out.

This definition captures the essence of action research in highlighting its participatory and action-oriented goals. It also underlines that learning is an important part of the process. In practice, action research has been variously interpreted and applied depending on the research paradigm and discipline base of the action researcher (Kemmis and McTaggart 2005). For example, action research in a health education setting will tend to play out differently to that found in commercial organizations (Hart and Bond 1995). The former is likely to focus on a single teacher who has chosen to improve the quality of their teaching, and the latter will tend to concentrate on institution-wide problems as identified by senior managers.

Research may be undertaken using a range of methods: surveys, interviews with patients and practitioners, focus group interviews, observation of practice and the secondary analysis of previous research. Qualitative and quantitative research methods are employed depending on the nature of the problem and the scope of the project. The research should aim to provide insight into different perspectives on a problem and may be undertaken throughout the process of action research in order to help assess what needs to be done and to monitor and evaluate any changes introduced. In the study to be discussed, patients' perspectives were sought through letters and focus group interviews; staff views were gathered via interviews;

clinical nursing care was observed; and the effect of different posturing regimes was measured (Waterman et al. 2005a, 2005b).

The principles of action research: improving practice, critical reflection, participation and implementation

In discussing the principles of action research, and its strengths and weaknesses, illustrative examples will be drawn mainly from this one study, referred to throughout the chapter as the Posturing Study (for full details, see Waterman et al. 2005a, 2005b). This action research study was undertaken at a regional eye hospital in the UK. The study aimed to encourage patients to maintain a regime of 'face-down posturing' following retinal surgery. This had been recommended as a regime to maintain healing, but there was uncertainty about how best to support patients in following the regime at home. The first phase of the action research project consisted of interviews with nurses and doctors from both inpatient and outpatient settings to learn about current practice and how this could be improved. This led to consensus among staff that the best way forward was to make 'take-home' specialist equipment available for patients to help them to 'posture' for longer and, in consequence, achieve more cost-effective treatment.

Improving practice

The study illustrates the first principle of action research in health care: the overriding purpose is to improve practice and the experience and outcome of patient care (Koch et al. 2002). Action research aims to assist both practitioners and patients to understand their problems better and to enlighten and inform them so that they can decide on action. The research moves beyond describing the 'status quo' as in traditional research to speculating on what 'might or ought to be', introducing changes and assessing the results. Thus, the research is about producing knowledge for action (Winter and Munn-Giddings 2001).

Critical reflection

A second important ingredient in action research is critical reflection. Critical reflection, while presented for the purposes of explanation as separate from research method, has an interdependent relationship with it. It binds together all activities associated with the research process and leads to empowerment and action. In practice, critical reflection in a group setting refers to the process of identifying and examining assumptions that underpin daily activity and asking whether the ideologies and attitudes that influence practice are those that best serve the interests of patients and staff. It means examining critically professional values and assumptions and assessing whether these are carried into practice (Koshy et al. 2011).

Professionals will have their own views of what actually happens in practice and a further test is to investigate the views of patients. Critical reflection aims to examine the (power) relationships between practitioners and patients and between, and within, professional groups. Different perspectives on a problem are deliberately sought to help illuminate an issue and to prevent one viewpoint from taking precedence. Some techniques are to enable patients and practitioners to discuss issues together and for professionals from different disciplines to share their experiences with one another. An example of this process is described by Waterman et al. (2005a, 2005b) in the Posturing Study. Here, the key stakeholders in the project on post-retinal surgery – namely, nurses, a specialist registrar and managers – watched a number of videos of patient focus group interviews. These showed that patients were critical of the lack of warning about, and information on, posturing. This provoked discussions critical of the ethos, practicalities and effects of existing forms of nursing and medical care.

A synthesis of different perspectives occurs over time, both in the group and individually. By drawing on experiences and integrating these with other types of evidence, conclusions can be drawn about how, and why, practice could be changed. The main result of the critical reflection in this study led to the setting up of nurse-led, pre-operative clinics so that patients could be provided with detailed information about 'posturing' two weeks in advance of their surgery. The process of critical reflection is challenging. It takes time and, as indicated later, may not always be successful.

Participation

A third important principle in action research is participation. This is linked to ideas of democracy and the belief that people should be able to inform the health care service and participate in or be consulted about health care decisions defined in the broadest sense. Compared with traditional approaches to research where research participants may play a passive role, in that they do not tend to determine the research questions or affect practice, participants in action research are active (McNiff and Whitehead 2011). Cornwall and Jewkes (1995) argue that action research was born out of methodological critiques of conventional research that ignored issues of power in the research process, especially with regard to the subjugated position of the research subject. A partnership between researchers and participants is seen as equitable and liberating in action research (Stringer and Genat 2004). Action research can therefore address the contemporary NHS agenda for patient and public involvement in research (National Institute for Health Research 2011). However, resources are required to achieve participant participation, as discussed later.

The level of participation may vary within a project, and between projects. Cornwall (1996) identifies six types of participation ranging from co-option and token representation with no real input, to collective action where local people set, and carry out, the research agenda without assistance from professional researchers. In many action research projects in health, participants have been practitioners – that is, mainly nurses and doctors (Waterman et al. 2001). This has parallels in educational action research and the teacher-as-researcher movement (Elliott 1991). In health and social care, clients and carers are consulted and may cooperate with a project but they tend not to be placed in an equal position with health care practitioners in making decisions about the research. As Cornwall and Jewkes (1995) describe, they are 'participants in a process' over which they have no real control.

Research by Bradburn and Mackie (2001) is an exception. In their project, clients with cancer jointly led an action research project where the aim was to raise awareness of the needs of cancer service users in cancer service planning meetings of the local health authority. The clients were directly involved in determining the course of the project – further examples are given in this volume in Chapters 17 and 20. One hazard of research with patients who have a particular illness is that some patients may be, or become, too ill to participate actively. Researchers in these circumstances must take care to respect the wishes of participants.

Implementation

A fourth fundamental aspect of action research is the inclusion of a change intervention. The process is often described as a 'spiral' (Kemmis and McTaggart 1988) or 'cycle' (Lewin 1947) of different phases that incorporate fact finding (also known as reflection or reconnaissance), planning, action and evaluation, reflection, planning, action, and so on. Each phase is the foundation for the next. Readers from a nursing or quality assurance background will find the outline of this process similar to the nursing process and the audit cycle respectively. However, it is fundamentally different to both as there is iteration between reflection, action and research, and an ethos of empowerment and democracy that is fundamental to action research. Action may come in several forms, as set out in Box 8.1 below.

Box 8.1   Forms of action

There may be:

- *Technical advancement:* this was the case referred to above where new equipment was purchased to encourage patients to maintain 'face-down postures' following retinal surgery (Waterman et al. 2005a, 2005b).
- *The development of educational programmes for staff:* an example is the project to develop a multisensory environment for patients with dementia (Hope and Waterman 2004).
- *Developments in professional roles:* for example, nursing roles were developed to improve the social rehabilitation of patients with neurological disorders (Portillo et al. 2009).
- *Service reorganization:* for example, participatory action research was employed to develop recommendations to improve the evacuation of individuals during major disasters (Gershon et al. 2008).

Box 8.1, however, does not take into account the more subtle changes in thinking and behaviour that will occur through participating in research and critical reflection.

When to Choose Action Research

Action research may be an appropriate choice of research methodology when the problem being addressed is complex, poorly understood, culturally bound, causes conflict, gives rise to ethical issues, or when resolution is required. Complexity typically refers to the different factors which may influence a problem. For example, poor pain management on a ward may be a result of poor assessment, lack of staff knowledge on analgesia, lack of empathy, poor leadership or poor communication. To improve pain management, a holistic strategy including action research may be needed. Action research may also be suitable in situations where there is conflict between groups or one occupational group dominates another. Meetings and forums for critical reflection can allow for the discussion of ethical and cultural issues and help to empower all participants (Koshy et al. 2011). Again, to draw on the Posturing Study referred to above, the iterative action research process demonstrated differences in perception between staff. Nurses felt they were doing their best to encourage patients to posture. Patients, however, found it difficult to carry out the instructions given by doctors, while doctors themselves thought that their post-operative instructions were being ignored. Through meetings and research, the nurses and doctors realized that their discussions with patients on posturing in the outpatients' clinic had been too superficial to convey to patients the importance of following a face-down posturing regime. Furthermore, the lack of information given to patients on their responsibilities on discharge prevented them from preparing themselves properly for post-operative face-down posturing at home.

Resources: human, technical and support staff

Action research is resource-intensive. For instance, the action research project described above involved eight members of staff in the core action research team, as well as costs for the author as research director. Costs were also incurred in the development and implementation of changes in practice, although these costs were later absorbed by the hospital. A systematic review on action research projects suggests that the majority do not secure external funding (Waterman et al. 2001). Funding is essential as participants must be released from their day-to-day activities to attend meetings and undertake research, and resources are required to implement changes (Stringer and Genat 2004). Action researchers often have to seek resources as part of their task, and some examples of strategy follow.

Webb et al. (1990) were invited to carry out an action research project by nurses on a ward caring for elderly people. Their aim was to move from a drug-round administration of medicines to a system where patients were permitted to take medicines without supervision. They managed to secure funding to replace staff who were then able to attend meetings to develop a strategy. In contrast, in the project on posturing following retinal surgery, we had to meet on a side ward so that the nurses were accessible in an emergency. Although there was strong internal support for the project, no external funding was secured. This meant that meetings occurred less frequently and, when they did take place, they were sometimes hurried or interrupted. Generally, funding should be gained prior to the commencement of a project so that planning and implementation can take place within a budget (Koshy et al. 2011).

External funding may be gained from health authorities, charities and research funding agencies, or government agencies. However, action researchers face certain barriers. Proposals for action research may not fit the conventional research template. Ways of overcoming such problems are to ensure that there is a match between what action researchers want to do and the objectives of the organization from which they hope to obtain funding, and to work closely with others experienced in developing research applications for a particular funding body.

Table 8.1 outlines the main resources needed to carry out an action research project and for what they are likely to be needed. The budget should be worked out between participants so that all their costs are accounted for. Sometimes full economic costing is required, including overheads and costs of supervision. Action researchers should seek advice on what they need to cost from research accountants, business managers and experienced action researchers.

TABLE 8.1   Resources typically required for an action research project

Item	Purpose
Research assistant	To facilitate the research and the process of critical reflection. To work closely with the clinical team
Time for all stakeholders	To pay for staff replacements
Travel expenses including accommodation	To pay for travel costs incurred – for example, by clients to attend meetings and to pay for a hotel
Tape recorder and transcribing machines	To record meetings/interviews and to speed up the process of transcribing
Transcribing costs	To pay for a typist for checking by participants
Costs for educational qualification	To pay for MSc, MPhil or PhD fees
Miscellaneous costs	To pay for unforeseen costs that may occur in action research including implementation costs

The Strengths of Action Research

The main characteristics and rationale for action research indicate three main strengths. First, it can lead to contextually relevant changes or innovations in practice, education or management that will have a positive effect on clients' experiences and the outcome of health care interventions. Second, the knowledge and theory gained are directly relevant for action. Third, participants are helped to take responsibility for their own circumstances. Each of these strengths will now be explored in turn.

Action research: change and innovation

The rhetoric of action research focuses on how it can improve people's situations. There are many examples of action research where this ultimate goal has been achieved. These include the reorganization of inpatient and outpatient services; the identification and development of new professional roles for nurses and allied health professionals; new care planning documentation; better assessment and management of patients; and the development of educational packages for students and educational videos for patients. However, not all projects bring about successful changes, as defined by researchers and participants (for positive and negative examples, see Waterman et al. 2001). There is no single cause for a lack of success, which is likely to be a combination of the following factors: over-ambition; the imposition of researchers' goals upon participants; a high staff turnover so that group cohesion is lost; power relations where one professional group dominates another; poor or no external supervision; a lack of research skills; poor interpersonal skills on the part of the researcher; a lack of, or withdrawal of, organizational support; and, lastly, deliberate sabotage. Action research is more likely to succeed when realistic expectations are set; where there are good collaborative relationships; when there is supervision of the researcher; when the researcher has been educated in action research and has good people management skills; and where the organization is supportive of the project.

It has been argued that action research can also promote professional development (Koch et al. 2002), as staff can reflect critically on their situation and participate in various activities. This is thought to lead to:

- Greater self-confidence as the process is self-validating.
- Enhanced competence as it is a learning exercise.
- Reassessment and consolidation of professional values as these are dissected and reconstructed.

However, it is not easy to demonstrate whether and how these changes in practice have taken place, let alone attribute them to action research. A self-reflective diary and interviews may record personal views of changes in understanding, or observations of nursing care in practice may demonstrate that changes have taken place.

Action research, knowledge and theory development

Another of the main advantages of action research is that it produces knowledge and theory that are relevant to a particular context (Coghlan and Casey 2001). Typically, knowledge and theoretical ideas are identified in the first phase of a project and then tried out and evaluated.

Findings are reflected upon and action plans amended. In other words, practice is studied in order to change it and then to change it again in the light of this assessment (Winter and Munn-Giddings 2001). The interaction between reflection, research and action broadens the developing theory and makes it more applicable to the particular research setting. As Hope and Waterman (2003) argue, the dialectical process of action research prevents premature closure and provides opportunities for further study to enhance the depth and breadth of analysis. Again, the Posturing Study may be used to illustrate this process of change and reassessment. While initially research participants thought that the purchase and use of specialist equipment would facilitate adherence to post-operative posturing instructions, as the equipment was utilized it became apparent that there were other issues. An analysis suggested that both better communication with patients and further education were also necessary.

The theory that is generated through action research may be informal or formal. Informal theory development takes place within individuals as they expand their understanding and experience of the issue under study. The 'theory' is locally bound, unwritten, practical and experiential, and could be described as helping to develop personal explanatory frameworks for action. For example, in the Posturing Study, discussions among nurses of how they could help patients' posture showed they felt competent in what they were doing to help patients and the reasons that underlay their practice. This was tantamount to an informal explanatory theory (Waterman et al. 2005a, 2005b).

Theory may also be formal, communicable and generalizable beyond the specific setting. An example may be taken from a study of HIV/AIDS home-based care coordinators in an action research project in Kenya (Waterman et al. 2007) that is described more fully below. The care coordinators applied sociological theories on how to reduce stigma in the analysis of qualitative interview data collected as part of the project. As this analysis was presented in a theoretical framework, it could be transferred to assist HIV/AIDS work in other settings in Africa.

Findings from quantitative data may also be generalizable beyond a specific action research setting. For example, Waterman (2002) undertook a pilot randomized controlled trial (RCT) as part of the Posturing Study described above. The hypothesis stated that a group of patients who held a face-down posture for 45 minutes with a 15-minute break would comply with instructions to a greater extent and feel less depressed, than a group who postured for 55 minutes and had a 5-minute break. The aim of this research was to generate information on the sample which would be useful in the development of a full RCT that could test the hypothesis.

In action research, most theory development is of the informal variety. It is practical and based on experience. This could be perceived as a missed opportunity to make the findings more widely accessible. However, formal theory development requires good supervision as well as education and training in research methods.

Within action research, there is undoubtedly a tension between undertaking rigorous research to develop theory that is generalizable and the pragmatic concerns of the staff group or institution to improve practice. In the Posturing Study, for example, managers wanted changes to practice to be made before we had completed the research into patient experiences of face-down posturing. We carried on with the research knowing that some changes were taking place, so we documented these parallel changes and noted their effect. This meant that the research was used as a basis for change and as a tool for monitoring the changes. However, there was some loss of rigour and this reduced the possibilities for generalizability to other settings as discussed further below. Both Coghlan and Casey (2001) and Williamson and Prosser (2002) underline the importance of understanding the institutional context in action research to identify potential hazards early on in a project.

Action research and empowering participants

A common justification for action research is the empowerment of those who are oppressed or marginalized in society. As practitioners, Koch et al. (2002) argue that this is a key advantage of the approach. Empowerment is a subtle process that occurs as participants gain in confidence, knowledge and understanding of their situation. However, it takes time to gain sufficient insight to decide on the best action to take in ways that are likely to be sustainable. Again, an example can be drawn from the Posturing Study. It took a number of phases in the project and a variety of practical difficulties had to be overcome before finally introducing nurse-led instruction in outpatient pre-operative clinics.

Limitations and Dilemmas in Action Research

As well as strengths, there are a number of limitations and dilemmas in action research, which include empowerment and management issues; the challenge of data collection and analysis; ethical issues; and writing up and presenting findings. These will now be considered in turn.

Empowerment and management issues

Empowerment is not always achieved in action research (Kemmis and McTaggart 2005). For example, Sturt (1997) attempted to carry out action research in a primary health care trust in a study to improve health promotion practices for smoking cessation. She reports that the practice nurses were effectively disempowered by the doctors who took a decision to halt the project without negotiation. This led to frustration and dissatisfaction for all concerned. Ironically, although empowerment is thought to be useful in conflict resolution, when power relations hitherto hidden are revealed, this may lead to surprise, shock or even explicit conflict. Cornwall and Jewkes (1995) suggest that while action researchers may be enthusiastic about empowerment, participants may prefer the status quo of hierarchical relationships. Inevitably, empowerment means going outside one's 'comfort zone', provoking anxiety and uncertainty. It is important also for the researcher not to raise expectations at the beginning of the study by discussing possibilities of empowerment. The starting point of any project is a careful analysis of the original problem and an assessment of how the project fits into the wider organization (Coghlan and Casey 2001).

Closely connected to the issue of empowerment is the question of whether a project should be managed by an insider or outsider. Action researchers may be insiders holding a formal position of employment in the research institution, or they may be outsiders who are facilitating a project in an organization where they have no formal position. In practice, the two positions are often blurred. For example, a researcher may be an employee – that is, an insider – but an outsider to the group taking part in the research. Both situations have advantages and disadvantages in terms of empowerment. An insider will have knowledge of the organizational structure and this is useful in getting support and approval for the project. On the other hand, they may be constrained by unwritten organizational rules and may have to live with the consequences of the action research process (Coghlan and Casey 2001). In contrast, an outsider will have to spend time getting to know formal organizational structures and informal social relationships. However, they may be in a better position to see the opportunities for change.

Titchin and Binnie (1993) suggest ways in which the advantages of the insider and outsider roles are combined in a 'double act'. They argue for shared responsibility between an insider and outsider, with the former responsible for the clinical component of the action research and the latter facilitating and leading the research and critical reflection. This was a model adopted in the Posturing Study already described. Initially, I led the research and the changes in clinical practice, but subsequently the roles were split.

The challenge of data collection and analysis

A further challenge in action research is how to collect and analyse data. Winter and Munn-Giddings (2001) identify three reasons for undertaking data analysis in action research:

- Data may be analysed to provide insights into what changes can be made in the future.
- Data interpretation helps to make findings generalizable.
- Data can be used to provide a baseline to explore what learning has taken place.

If participants discuss and plan their approach to data analysis in advance, then any tension between these objectives will be reduced.

In a conventional research project, the researcher is 'detached' from the research setting and has sole responsibility for data collection and analysis. In action research, not only are there difficult and possibly conflicting purposes for data collection, but priorities may shift over time. Moreover, there may be various sources of data that will be available at different points in the life of a project. How data are to be analysed, by whom and for what purpose, will require active management in a participative manner (Christensen and Atweh 1998; Winter and Munn-Giddings 2001). In the Posturing Study, for example, a staff nurse and I undertook most of the detailed analysis of patient focus group interviews. Then, the team as a whole participated in reflective discussions based on the results. In the subsequent RCT, a research student undertook all the statistical analysis so that the results could be presented for discussion.

As indicated, action researchers may collect both qualitative and quantitative data over the course of an action research project. Using a mixed-methods approach is advantageous as it provides multiple perspectives of the issue under consideration but, on the other hand, it can be challenging. Westhues et al. (2008) aimed to improve practice in a community mental health organization. They carried out an extensive literature review, set up focus group interviews (a qualitative method) and undertook an online survey (a quantitative method). The research took place in two geographic locations, had four sub-projects and a multidisciplinary team, and provided multiple perspectives. The data collection in the different arms of the study was conducted in parallel, which was useful in terms of a timely triangulation of data. However, had the researchers carried out a sequential form of data collection, they would have had the opportunity to explore unexpected issues that emerged more thoroughly. They report that the process of reaching a shared understanding within the team of the findings from the different data sets was time-consuming and intellectually challenging. Moreover, engagement with practitioners and patients in the study was not constant, so their interest waned, particularly when the researchers were undertaking the analysis and synthesis of data. In summary, participants including researchers also found it difficult to fully grasp all the research findings. The challenge of using a mix of methods is discussed further in Chapters 2, 22 and 23.

Ethical issues

Ethical issues arise in the course of action research – and while some can be predicted in advance, others arise during the process. In either case, these matters require discussion and negotiation. When conducting action research, it cannot be assumed that patients, carers and practitioners can participate to the same degree as action researchers. Participating in action research may lead to additional burdens for participants who may be ill, or who face difficulties in their daily lives (Salmon et al. 2010). It should be recognized that participation in the action research will need to take into account other life issues of the people concerned and, as a consequence, it will fluctuate during the course of the project (Salmon et al. 2010).

For example, a number of difficulties arose during the course of the Posturing Study. There were eight core patient members of the action research group, but because of commitments to family and/or work only 4–6 were present at meetings. The numbers reduced during the course of the project. Additional support costs were needed to provide material and psychosocial support to help participants take part (Salmon et al. 2010). However, there is a fine line between fair recompense and coercion to participate. Confidentiality was an issue. It could not simply be assumed that the patient participants would want the contents of their interviews and observations to be shared by other participants, whether colleagues or clients. The matter required discussion in advance. Maintaining the anonymity of participants is also an issue. It should not be assumed that identities are hidden by using anonymous quotes (Williamson and Prosser 2002). Acknowledgements and contact details can give away information that can lead to the identification of participants. On the other hand, it has been my experience of the Kenyan action research study (Waterman et al. 2007) that participants want to be identified in any report, as participation in a research project that is acknowledged may give recognition and status, but they do not want to be individually cited in quotations.

The websites for INVOLVE, which is part of the NIHR and is a national advisory group that supports greater public involvement in the NHS, public health and social care research (INVOLVE 2011), and the National Research Ethics Service (2011) provide guidance on what is reasonable to provide in terms of financial and other types of support when involving participants in research – see also Chapters 15 and 20 for further discussion.

Writing up and presenting findings

Christensen and Atweh (1998) rightly suggest that writing a report is an essential stage in action research. This represents the final and formal end of reflective activities in which all strands of the study should be pulled together. The submission of a report to a funding agency is a significant act of closure. The public distribution of a report and papers is also important in the external validation of the work and usually involves external peer review (McNiff et al. 1996). Yet, there may be different interests in what kind of report should be written and for what audience.

In preparing to write the report, McNiff et al. (1996: 134) identified four different audiences for a research project: 'your boss, your colleagues, your tutor, and your academic peers'. These may require different kinds of report. Managers will want a report that emphasizes organizational and change issues; colleagues will be interested in practical issues and health care outcomes; participants studying for a higher degree and their tutors will want a focus on the value of the research for learning; while academic peers will be interested in how the research has contributed to knowledge. Most reports are presented chronologically to tell a 'story' of the different cycles of the project (Henderson 1997). Academic papers may report on the whole project or focus on one part of it (Harker et al. 2002), or discuss methodological issues (Meyer 1993).

In keeping with the rest of the process of action research, writing up should be participative. However, as Christensen and Atweh (1998) identify, this is not always straightforward. If a number of researchers undertake different parts of the research, deadlines will have to be coordinated. Some participants may not have the experience or confidence to write, but nevertheless may feel excluded if they are not included in some way. To maintain the integrity of the project and to prevent conflict, writing up and authorship should be discussed openly in the early stages of the project and revisited often. Christensen and Atweh (1998) present three strategies for participative writing:

- One person takes responsibility to write the full first draft, which is then passed around other participants for comment. This is progressive writing.
- Accounts may be written by different groups and placed together in a final report.
- A small group of people plan and write together. This is 'shared writing'.

In all of these situations, agreement must be reached on whose 'voice' is given priority. This is tied into issues of power and the importance of retaining a sense of shared ownership. Such matters are linked to empowerment. Sharing and learning skills requires time and patience, but can be rewarding (McLauchlan et al. 2002). These matters are discussed in more detail in Chapter 23, which explores writing up research and getting published. This brings us to the presentation of a practical case study in action research in countries with limited resources.

Case study: Action research and HIV/AIDS in resource-limited countries

The following provides an example from the author of how action research can be applied in resource-limited countries. Sub-Saharan Africa has been affected by the AIDS epidemic disproportionately, when compared with Western and Central Europe. There have been 2.4 million deaths from AIDS in Sub-Saharan Africa, and only 12,000 in Western and Central Europe (UNAIDS 2005). In Nyanza Province, Kenya, the prevalence rate of HIV/AIDS is 20.2 per cent (Nyanza Provincial Medical Office 2005).

A key strategy to deal with HIV/AIDS in Sub-Saharan countries is home-based care. Home-based care is a form of comprehensive community-based care that includes social, economic and health services. In practice, it encompasses hands-on nursing care in people's homes, which helps to reduce stigma; setting up and sustaining health care clinics; finding refuge and adoptive parents for orphans; facilitating income-generating activities for widows and people living with HIV/AIDS; establishing referral mechanisms for clients needing counselling and testing for HIV/AIDS; and treating clients with anti-retroviral therapy.

(Continued)

CASE STUDY

(Continued)

Little information is available to practitioners and policy makers on how to implement these forms of care. The objectives of our research, therefore, were to clarify the concept of home-based care; to articulate its key constituents; to identify a framework for the introduction of home-based care; and to examine contextual factors that facilitate or hinder its development.

Action research was selected as the preferred method by the lead HIV/AIDS health care personnel of a non-governmental organization, Mildmay International, based in Kisumu, Nyanza. This was because it fulfilled the need to document, reflect and research on practice while at the same time endeavouring to deliver the best possible home-based care. The research team consisted of three researchers from the University of Manchester, who worked closely with personnel from Mildmay and the HIV/AIDS home-based care coordinators in Nyanza. The relationship had parallels with the 'double act' as described earlier. The study took place across the 12 districts of Nyanza Province and the main participants were the coordinators and members of the District Health Management Team who became known as co-researchers.

Data were collected from 27 focus group interviews and notes were made on 16 field visits to the community. The topics of focus group interviews varied over the course of the project but included discussions on the significance of stigma, poverty, nutrition and gender for people with HIV/AIDS, and the importance of volunteers and the linkages between organizations in delivering care. The action research consisted of two interrelated cycles: the implementation of a plan to integrate HIV/AIDS home-based care into the existing health system based on a prior needs assessment and the embedding of policies to provide home-based care.

The focus group interviews encouraged critical reflection and empowerment among the co-researchers, as they provided the opportunity for the exchange of information between participants and the identification of different perspectives. Among other issues, the reasons why some implementation strategies worked and others did not were explored. The co-researchers reported that discussions helped to provide some answers to their difficulties so that they could agree on ways forward for their work.

The findings suggest that there is a process through which home-based care may be implemented through preparation, needs assessment, establishing services, mobilizing the community, and embedding and sustaining. There are several barriers to implementation, including poverty, stigma, a lack of food, gender issues and a lack of resources. Nevertheless, the action-based approach enabled a critical approach to the introduction of home-based care in Nyanza and led to findings that will be of interest and use to settings beyond this particular context.

Reading Health Research Based on an Action Approach

There are general aspects to appraisal that can be applied to any method including action research – for example, is an adequate justification provided for the design, sample, data collection methods and analysis? Waterman et al. (2001) argue that the following questions will assist researchers in discriminating between action research and other approaches to research and help them to assess the quality of the action research:

- Were the phases of action research clearly outlined? This question helps reviewers to assess whether the process of action research was apparent, including fact-finding, planning, action, evaluation and re-assessment.
- Were participants and stakeholders clearly described and justified? The selection process of those participants closely involved in the action research project needs to be articulated and justified.
- What considerations were given to the local context while implementing change? With this question, reviewers are examining whether the researchers have explored the impact of local context on the research, such as the effect of the local culture on introducing change.
- Was the relationship between the researchers and participants adequately considered? Here, reviewers are appraising whether the level and extent of participation was appropriate, how relationships evolved over the course of the action research and how they reflected critically on their perspectives and roles.

Conclusion

The argument underlying this chapter is that the action research method is an appropriate tool where the aim is to change practice or behaviour. A key aspect of achieving this change is to include the range of professionals who provide a service; those who are the clients or patients using a service; people in groups or communities who stand to benefit from improved practice; and researchers with relevant skills. Depending on the nature of the project, all members of such groups or their representatives should be included. The role of the lead researcher in an action research project is a challenging one; not only are research skills required, but also the ability to play a number of roles as an educator, facilitator and mediator. Furthermore, unlike other forms of research where the researcher tends to act as a detached observer, in action research they should be committed to achieving the outcomes of the research while not allowing this commitment to cloud their judgement in evaluating data and findings.

The case study on action research and HIV/AIDS in resource-limited countries shows that action research is a flexible method that may be used in a variety of settings. It is followed by a brief practical exercise, focusing on applying action research to a health-related work setting with which you are familiar.

Exercise: The use of action research in a health-related work setting

This exercise is intended to help readers critically explore the issues raised in this chapter, and particularly to explore the interrelationship between theory, method and data in action research. On the basis of the practical advice provided in this chapter, draw up a proposal for an action research project based on your own experience in a work setting in which you either operate, or of which you have some knowledge. First, identify an area of practice that you think causes problems. This may, for example, give rise to conflict among professional groups or relate to an aspect of practice that is not up to standard. You should then answer the following questions:

1 Where would you obtain funding to carry out the project?
2 What methods could be used to understand the problem better?
3 Who will be the key participants in the action research team and what is the rationale for inclusion?
4 How will you promote and maintain participation in the project?
5 How will you apply the action research process to your issue and context?
6 What process of critical reflection might be implemented and what part will it play in moving the research project forward?
7 Will you be an insider or outsider to the research setting and what effect will your position have on the project?
8 What ethical issues will be encountered in the course of the project and how will they be addressed?
9 What knowledge and theory will be generated for participants and service users planning to improve the care of patients in your area of interest?
10 What will be the limitations of your project?

Recommended Further Reading

Hart, E. and Bond, M. (1995) *Action Research for Health and Social Care: A Guide for Practice.* Milton Keynes: Open University Press.
This book offers a good introduction to action research, containing a useful typology and history of the methodology involved.

Kemmis, S. and McTaggart, R. (1988) *The Action Research Planner*, 3rd edition. Geelong, Victoria: Deakin University.
This classic book provides a detailed framework for the first phase of action research, providing much helpful advice.

Koshy, E., Koshy, V. and Waterman, H. (2011) *Action Research for Healthcare: A Practical Guide.* London: Sage.
This recent publication contains useful guidance for novice action researchers on all aspects of action research.

Winter, R. and Munn-Giddings, C. (2001) *A Handbook for Action Research in Health and Social Care.* London: Routledge.
This text is a handbook for action researchers, describing and exploring the theoretical issues underpinning action research.

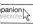 ## Online Readings

Crow, J., Smith, L. and Keenan, I. (2010) 'Sustainability in an action research project: 5 years of a Dignity and Respect action group in a hospital setting', *Journal of Research in Nursing*, 15: 55–68.
How is action research defined in this context? How sustainable has this project been? What benefits has the project bought? Critically evaluate the paper using the checklist provided in PPS8.8.

Davies, J., Lester, C., O'Neill, M. and Williams, G. (2008) 'Sustainable participation in regular exercise amongst older people: Developing an action research approach', *Health Education Journal*, 67: 45–55.
How is action research defined in this context? How sustainable has this project been? What benefits has the project bought? Critically evaluate the paper using the checklist provided in PPS8.8.

References

Bradburn, J. and Mackie, C. (2001) 'A foot in the door: a collaborative action research project with cancer service users', in R. Winter and C. Munn-Giddings (eds), *A Handbook for Action Research in Health and Social Care*. London: Routledge.

Christensen, C. and Atweh, B. (1998) 'Collaborative writing in participatory action research', in B. Atweh, S. Kemmis and P. Weeks (eds), *Action Research in Practice: Partnerships for Social Justice in Education*. London: Routledge.

Coghlan, D. and Casey, M. (2001) 'Action research from the inside: issues and challenges in doing action research in your own organization', *Journal of Advanced Nursing*, 35(5): 674–82.

Cornwall, A. (1996) 'Towards participatory practice: participatory rural appraisal and the participatory process', in K. De Koning and M. Martin (eds), *Participatory Research in Health: Issues and Experiences*. London: Zed Books.

Cornwall, A. and Jewkes, R. (1995) 'What is participatory action research?', *Social Science and Medicine*, 41: 1667–76.

Elliott, J. (1991) *Action Research for Educational Change*. Milton Keynes: Open University Press.

Gershon, R.R., Rubin, M.S., Qureshi, K.A., Canton, A.N. and Matzner, F.J. (2008) 'Participatory action research methodology in disaster research: results from the World Trade Center evacuation study', *Medicine and Public Health Preparedness*, 2(3): 142–9.

Harker, R., McLauchlan, R., MacDonald, H., Waterman, C. and Waterman, H. (2002) 'Endless nights: patients' experiences of posturing face down following vitreo-retinal surgery', *Journal of Ophthalmic Nursing*, 6(2): 11–15.

Hart, E. and Bond, M. (1995) *Action Research for Health and Social Care: A Guide for Practice.* Milton Keynes: Open University Press.

Henderson, C. (1997) *Changing 'Childbirth' and the West Midlands Region 1995–1996.* London: Royal College of Midwives.

Hope, K.W. and Waterman, H. (2003) 'Praiseworthy pragmatism? Validity and action research: methodological issues in nursing research', *Journal of Advanced Nursing*, 44(2): 120–7.

Hope, K.W. and Waterman, H. (2004) 'Multi-sensory environments (MSEs) in clinical practice – factors impeding their use as perceived by clinical staff', *International Journal of Social Care and Practice*, 3(1): 45–68.

INVOLVE (2011) www.invo.org.uk/

Kemmis, S. and McTaggart, R. (1988) *The Action Research Planner*, 3rd edition. Geelong, Victoria: Deakin University.

Kemmis, S. and McTaggart, R. (2005) 'Participatory action research: communicative action and the public sphere', in N.K. Denzin and Y. Lincoln (eds), *The SAGE Handbook of Qualitative Research*, 3rd edition. London: Sage.

Koch, T., Selim, P. and Kralik, D. (2002) 'Enhancing lives through the development of a community-based participatory action research programme', *Journal of Clinical Nursing*, 11: 109–17.

Koshy, E., Koshy, V. and Waterman, H. (2011) *Action Research for Healthcare: A Practical Guide.* London: Sage.

Lewin, K. (1947) 'Frontiers in group dynamics: social planning and action research', *Human Relations*, 1: 143–53.

McLauchlan, R., Harker, R., MacDonald, H., Waterman, C. and Waterman, H. (2002) 'Using research to improve ophthalmic nursing care', *Nursing Times*, 98(27): 39–40.

McNiff, J., Lomax, P. and Whitehead, J. (1996) *You and Your Action Research Practice.* London: Routledge.

McNiff, J. and Whitehead, J. (2011) *All You Need to Know about Action Research*, 2nd edition. London: Sage.

Meyer, J. (1993) 'New paradigm research in practice: trials and tribulations of action research', *Journal of Advanced Nursing*, 18: 1066–72.

National Research Ethics Service (2011) www.nres.nhs.uk/

National Institute for Health Research (2011) www.nihr.ac.uk/awareness/Pages/default.aspx

Nyanza Provincial Medical Office (2005) Unpublished report. Nyanza Provincial Medical Office, Kisumu.

Portillo, M.C., Corchon, S., Lopez-Dicastillo, O. and Cowley, S. (2009) 'Evaluation of a nurse-led social rehabilitation programme for neurological patients and carers: an action research study', *International Journal of Nursing Studies*, 46(2): 204–19.

Salmon, A., Browne, A.J. and Pederson A. (2010) '"Now we call it research": participatory health research involving marginalized women who use drugs', *Nursing Inquiry*, 17(4): 336–45.

Stringer, E. and Genat, W.J. (2004) *Action Research in Health*. Upper Saddle River, NJ: Merrill Prentice Hall.

Sturt, J. (1997) 'Placing empowerment research within an action research typology', *Journal of Advanced Nursing*, 30(5): 1057–63.

Titchin, A. and Binnie, A. (1993) 'Research partnerships: collaborative action research in nursing', *Journal of Advanced Nursing*, 18: 858–65.

UNAIDS (2005) 'HIV/AIDS statistics and features in 2003 and 2005', *UNAIDS Epidemic Update: Sub-Saharan Africa*, UNAIDS/WHO AIDS, December.

Waterman, C. (2002) 'A randomised controlled trial to evaluate the effects of two facedown posturing regimes following vitreo-retinal surgery with internal gas tamponade', MSc dissertation, University of Manchester.

Waterman, H., Tillen, D., Dickson, R. and De Koning, K. (2001) 'Action research: a systematic review and assessment for guidance', *Health Technology Assessment*, 5(23): iii–157.

Waterman, H., Harker, R., MacDonald, H., McLaughlan, R. and Waterman, C. (2005a) 'Advancing ophthalmic nursing practice through action research', *Journal of Advanced Nursing*, 52(3): 281–90.

Waterman, H., Harker, R., MacDonald, H., McLaughlan, R. and Waterman, C. (2005b) 'Evaluation of an action research project in ophthalmic nursing practice', *Journal of Advanced Nursing*, 52 (4): 389–98.

Waterman, H., Griffiths, J., Gellard, L., O'Keefe, C., Olang, G., Obwanda, E., Ayuyo, J., Ogwethe, V. and Ondiege, J. (2007) 'Power brokering, empowering, and educating: the role of home-based care professionals in the reduction of HIV-related stigma in Kenya', *Qualitative Health Research*, 17(8): 1028–39.

Webb, C., Addison, C., Holman, H., Saklaki, B. and Wager, A. (1990) 'Self-medication for elderly patients', *Nursing Times*, 86: 46–9.

Westhues, A., Ochocka, J., Jacobson, N., Simich, L., Maiter, S., Janzen, R. and Fleras, A. (2008) 'Developing theory from complexity: reflections on a collaborative mixed method participatory action research study', *Qualitative Health Research*, 18(5): 701–17.

Williamson, G.R. and Prosser, S. (2002) 'Action research: politics, ethics and participation', *Journal of Advanced Nursing*, 40(5): 587–93.

Winter, R. and Munn-Giddings, C. (2001) *A Handbook for Action Research in Health and Social Care*. London: Routledge.

PART III
Quantitative Methods and Health

9

Health Research Sampling Methods[1]

PETER DAVIS, ALASTAIR SCOTT AND
MARTIN VON RANDOW

Introduction

Sampling a smaller number of respondents so that generalizations can be made about a larger population is an important tool to master for the researcher carrying out a quantitative investigation. In a properly constructed sample, the costs of the research in time and money are kept to a minimum without loss of generalizability. This chapter outlines the basic features of sampling in health research. The emphasis is on probability sampling, both because this is the most widely used approach and because there is a well-established body of theory and practice on sample design and inference. In the chapter, we discuss the rationale of sampling and introduce key terms. Different forms of non-probability sampling and the techniques employed in probability sampling are discussed together with issues that arise in sampling and ways of reducing error. The chapter draws examples from four studies undertaken in New Zealand by the authors and others, and there is a case study that illustrates the use of sampling in practice.

(Continued)

(Continued)

The studies shown in Table 9.1 are all based on national sample surveys under-taken in New Zealand: a socio-dental survey based on an area sample; an investigation of partner relationships, using telephone interviewing; a patient safety study drawing on a sample of medical records held by public hospitals; and a survey of patients attending general practitioners (GPs), which required us first to select a sample of medical practitioners. Throughout the chapter, we will draw on these studies selectively for illustration. The details of the studies are found in Table 9.1, including reference to measurement issues. A user-friendly website teaching resource is cited. The terminology and concepts used are standard in the literature and are drawn mainly from Aday and Cornelius (2006) and Groves et al. (2009).

Sampling and Its Rationale

Why sample?

The topic of 'sampling' goes to the methodological heart of drawing inferences about human populations. In the cases outlined in Table 9.1, the populations were national in scope and the topics diverse. Typically investigators, whether they are health practitioners, social scientists, managers, clinicians or interested citizens, want to gain information about the features of a particular population group. Yet information gathering has to be selective, and the process of selection raises issues about the representativeness and accuracy of the knowledge and insights gained from the sample. Thus, sampling is the science and practice of selecting information from populations in a manner that allows defensible inferences to be drawn from those data.

The focus of this chapter is on sampling that takes place in a well-defined setting where the probabilities of selection can be attributed to elements in the population. However, it is worth noting that systematic empirical work of any kind requires the analysis of samples of information drawn from a larger universe or population. In the case of qualitative research, the selection of information is based on informed human judgement rather than under-taken through a technical procedure, and one of the judgement criteria may well be based on a claim to representativeness or typicality (Murphy and Dingwall 2003). In principle, it should be equally possible for qualitative investigators to justify inferences based on samples selected on judgement criteria as for quantitative researchers who draw on probability sample designs.

Basic terminology

The starting point for a sampling scheme is the definition of a 'target population'; this is the population 'of interest' to the proposed investigation. In the case of the four studies outlined in Table 9.1, in the first two the target populations were all adult New Zealanders with an age restriction for the partner relations survey. In the third and fourth, the focus was on hospital patients and GP patients respectively. In identifying these four populations 'of interest', the aim was to ensure that the results of our sample selection and the subsequent analyses of the data were reflective of, and could be applied to, the four defined sets of adult and patient populations.[2]

TABLE 9.1   Examples of surveys to illustrate sampling techniques

Survey topic	Dental health	Partner relations	Hospital safety	Primary care
Target population	Adult population,1975	18–54-year age group, 1991	Hospital inpatients, 1998	All GP patients, 2001–02
Sampling frame	Household enumeration of areas	Random digit dialling	Central admissions register	Telephone page listing of GPs
Sample stages	68 Primary Sampling Units (PSU),136 Secondary Sampling Units (SSUs), 28 adults	1,750 clusters of 3,1 eligible each	13 hospitals,575 patient admissions	350 GPs, 1 in 4 patients
Size and response rate	3,231 (84%)	2,361 (63%)	6,731 (91.5%)	8,258 (68.5%)
Number of strata	Two (rural and urban)	14 dialling zones	Three (hospital size)	Seven (type of practice, practitioner)
Weighting criteria	Self-weighting	Number of eligibles per household	By hospital size	By practice type
Measurement issues	Interviewer variation http://tinyurl.com/saoh-intvar	Item sensitivity http://tinyurl.com/prs-method	Reviewer variation http://tinyurl.com/nzqhs-var	Electronic collection http://tinyurl.com/natmedca-e
Website sources	http://tinyurl.com/nzssds-saoh	http://tinyurl.com/nzssds-prs	http://tinyurl.com/nzssds-nzqhs	http://tinyurl.com/nzssds-natmedca

A member of the target population is known as a sampling unit or element. In probability sampling, each one of these units or elements has a specifiable chance of being selected. It is on account of this characteristic that we are able to apply statistical techniques of estimation and inference to the data collected. In many research designs, this chance of selection is equal across all units, or self-weighting. However, in others it is not. In the dental health study, for example, larger territorial local authorities had a higher chance of being selected because, at the first stage, these units were selected with probability proportional to size, as were two second-stage units in each selected territorial local authority. The overall respondent likelihood of selection then equalled out because of the constant sample size at the third stage (28 respondents in each of the two units in each selected territorial local authority).

Conversely, in the case of the primary care study, GPs had different chances of selection depending on what kind of practice they were in, but the final number of patients chosen, one in four in each case, was not uniform but proportionate to workload. This meant that the data had to be reweighted in the analysis. This process is illustrated in an example given later in the chapter.

Sample Selection Using Non-probability Designs

Quota sampling is a non-probability technique commonly used in market research. It involves selecting sample elements according to a predetermined distribution across certain defined categories. For example, respondents may be recruited in such a way as to ensure that there is a roughly equal distribution between males and females, or to cover certain age bands or socio-economic positions, or to obtain an area spread such as rural and urban. This is a form of stratified sampling as the predetermined categories are the strata that ensure a predicted sample distribution. However, it is not possible to estimate the probability of selection within those strata because the actual selection process is not a random one. It can involve working in selected streets or suburbs and trying to accost cooperative respondents (Yoon and Kim 2011), but is more typically by phone contact.

The distinctive characteristic of non-probability sampling is its non-random basis for selecting sample elements using judgement criteria. This is also a distinctive feature of sampling in qualitative research. The main types are set out in Box 9.1 below.

Box 9.1   The main types of non-probability sampling

- *Convenience sampling*: this is the most rudimentary selection technique. Selection may be based on the ease of recruitment, for example those attending an outpatient clinic or decision makers who can be easily accessed (Hedt and Pagano 2011).

- *Calling for volunteers:* this is a version of the convenience method and is widely used in experimental research (Yusoff et al. 2011).
- *Snowball sampling:* this is a further refinement of the convenience method that requires explicit judgements. With this technique, the investigator starts with an initial group, such as those known to have a particular health condition, and then increases the size of this initial sample by referrals from this group (Adamson et al. 2012).
- *Purposive sampling:* this increases the deliberative or judgemental element by selecting all sample elements according to certain criteria. For example, extreme or unusual cases may be selected to pre-test a questionnaire. In certain study designs, explicit inclusion criteria may be used (Kirton et al. 2012).
- *Quota sampling:* uses judgement criteria in a more systematic way, by selecting sample elements according to a pre-determined distribution across defined categories (typically gender and age).
- *Theoretical sampling:* this is a method of selection that is informed by a particular philosophy of qualitative research involving the generating and testing of empirical hypotheses (Ryan et al. 2011).

Probability Sample Designs

There is a wide range of probability sample designs that vary along two dimensions – the number of sampling stages and the extent of departure from a simple random selection strategy. The most rudimentary design combines these two features: a single sampling stage with a simple selection strategy (Fealy et al. 2011). The simplest random sample can be picking names out of a hat, or using a table of random numbers. Where the elements are not returned to the pool after selection, this is called sampling without replacement. According to a strict interpretation of sample theory, this requires a correction factor in estimating standard errors. The impact of this factor reduces as the proportion of the population sampled decreases.

Two departures from the simple random strategy are systematic, or list, sampling and stratification. In the case of the former, a sample is drawn from an existing list that has a degree of organization or ordering of the target population (Bellón et al. 2010). Approached in the right way, this can be a helpful feature since it ensures a better spread of the sample across implicit strata within the population. For example, an alphabetical ordering by names can ensure a good spread across ethnic groups. We used this method to identify patients by date of admission in the hospital safety study. The New Zealand Health Information Service was able to order patients by date of admission throughout the year for each selected hospital and then set an interval that would generate the required 575 cases with a random start point, working from January to December. In this way, we ensured a spread of cases that was representative of the mix and volume of workload through the year.

Stratification is a more explicit method for ensuring a desired distribution of a sample across important groups in the population (Muñoz et al. 2011). It requires a certain amount of prior knowledge of the population since subsections of the sample will be allocated to predefined strata, usually on a proportionate, that is a representative, basis. There are, however, cases where disproportionate sampling might be used, such as to ensure larger numbers in the sample for a particular ethnic minority group or for more variable strata. In the partner relations survey, we knew from census information how many people in our target age groups there were in the different dialling zones and we allocated our sample to reflect that distribution. In the case of the primary care study, however, we wanted to ensure a minimum number of practitioners and their patients within different practice types. We therefore under-sampled doctors in heavily populated strata, such as private GPs, and over-sampled in sparsely populated strata, such as GPs in community-governed practices.

Stages in sample design

In terms of design, cost and logistics dictate whether there should be more than one stage of sampling, which is needed for any but the most concentrated and easily accessible population (Botman et al. 2000). This helps to localize the requirements of data collection into what are called clusters that are usually geographically defined. Another advantage of this approach is that the frame, or list, of individual population units is required only for the selected clusters, which may be a consideration where there is no simple master frame for the entire population. Both of these considerations were important in the dental health study. First, we wished to interview 3,000 adult New Zealanders throughout the country. For reasons of both cost and logistics, therefore, it was essential to concentrate our interviewing efforts. Second, there was no master list of the adult population. We needed to compile such a list, which we did door to door, but only for the 136 geographical areas selected at the second stage.

The trick with constructing an efficient multi-stage sample design is to strike the right balance between the number and size of clusters (De Hoop et al. 2012). The larger and fewer the clusters, the easier the logistics and the lower the costs tend to be. There is also a slightly greater chance that such clusters will be internally more heterogeneous. Although smaller clusters will be internally more homogeneous, there will be more of them. This should assist representativeness, but the management task and costs will increase with the degree of dispersal.

Frame and coverage

The sampling frame is the list of units or elements that are assumed to define best the target population, or survey population, if there is a discrepancy or incompleteness in this list. It is from this list that the sample is drawn. A good frame is one that is up to date and includes all units in a way that ensures they are distinguishable from one another and are only counted once. Physical lists are commonly used, like the electoral roll or telephone book. Area frames, the enumeration of an area to compile a list, may also be used, as, for example, a conceptual list of people booking an airline ticket. In the primary care survey, there was no complete list of GPs, so we used the electronic White Pages to compile a list, on the assumption that every practice would have to be listed for business purposes. In the dental health survey, we listed household members in the selected areas by going door to door and used an agreed selection procedure for those adults identified.

More complex lists can be constructed by dual or multiple frames and screening surveys (Guterbock et al. 2011). A dual or multiple frame is one in which more than one list is used in order to achieve adequate coverage of the target population by incorporating a frame that includes a higher concentration of a hard-to-reach group. For example, in order, say, to over-sample some identifiable group, a combination of the electoral roll and an area sample in which the particular group lives may be used. Another approach for identifying a hard-to-reach population is to use, either by design or opportunistically, an initial survey to screen a larger population. For example, a survey of people with disabilities could be mounted on a much larger survey of the population, as long as the relevant screening questions for disability were embedded in the first study. New Zealand's official statistical agency conducted two such special post-census surveys following the 2001 Census, to identify two hard-to-reach populations: Māori and disabled people (Statistics New Zealand 2006).

Under-coverage

A complete list is one in which every individual in the target population appears and can be assigned a calculable non-zero probability of selection. This is rarely achieved because usually there are at least some members of the population not entered on the list. This is often due to some systematic bias in the list rather than random error. Such a shortcoming in a list is called incomplete coverage or under-coverage.

Non-response, the failure to collect data on sampled units, is another source of incomplete coverage. Although this occurs at a later stage of the survey process and requires a quite different response, such as through improving contact rates, technically this is a coverage issue. For instance, in our partner relations survey those members of the population without phones could not be contacted using our methodology, which was telephone interviewing. This was an example of incomplete coverage in the list, and nothing could be done about it. At the same time, there were a good number of phone numbers for which there was no reply or a refusal. This contributed to our non-response rate. Here, modifications to the approach might have reduced under-coverage.

The impact of under-coverage depends on the proportion of the population that is missing due, for example, either to failures of the list or to non-response, and on the difference in the values of key study variables for these missing units, compared with those that are adequately covered. This is the degree of systematic bias (Kypri et al. 2011). There are a number of methods for trying to correct for the impact of under-coverage. These include weighting, post-stratification, ratio estimation and imputation (He and Zaslavsky 2012). However, none of these methods are as effective as getting the right sample in the first place, and therefore strenuous efforts need to be made to ensure both a complete frame and low non-response rate, concentrating particularly on eliminating bias. Indeed, it may be worth settling for a lower initial sample size if this achieves cost savings that can then be allocated to gaining a higher response rate.

Sample Size and Distribution

Sample size is a central consideration when it comes to minimizing the error of sample estimates and maximizing study value for a given cost. There are two components to the error term associated with a sample-based estimate of a population parameter: accuracy (how close is it to the 'true' value?) and precision (how tightly bunched are the estimates?). Sample size affects precision, but not accuracy. Generally speaking, the larger the size of the sample, the more precise the estimates derived from that sample are likely to be. Indeed, it is possible to work out the size of sample required to achieve a given level of precision (Biau et al. 2008). For example, in the dental health survey we were able to estimate from other studies the size of sample we needed to get reasonably precise estimates of what we considered a key parameter, namely the average number of teeth that were affected by dental disease and are decayed, missing or filled.

However, achieving a high level of precision is unlikely to be the only consideration, because the larger the sample, the higher the cost of the study. Usually, an investigator is faced with a relatively fixed envelope of field costs, and therefore the objective is to try and maximize sample size to a point where precision is good, while at the same time minimizing costs through sample design. This can be done by clustering and choosing a low-cost method of data collection such as telephone contact as opposed to face-to-face interviews. Again, in the dental health study, precision could be attained by a certain sample size, but that in turn had to be distributed nationally in such a way as to meet a budget. This allowed for three teams working across a prescribed number of geographical clusters in three broad regions: the South Island, the lower and central North Island, and Auckland and the north. For the partner relations survey, a similar sample size calculation around a target measure of precision was made to include the proportion of units with multiple partners in the last year. In this case, moving from face-to-face to telephone interviews halved the cost of data collection and allowed a doubling of the sample size.[3]

For more complex sample surveys, an important consideration is the design decisions that need to be made about the way in which the sample is distributed. Again it is important to balance the minimization of error and the maximization of study value for a given cost. At this point, the issue is not so much the sample size as the sample distribution across, say, clusters or strata.

In the case of strata, from the point of view of precision there should be a disproportionate allocation of sample numbers to strata containing units with high diversity or variability (Cardozo et al. 2004). For example, in both the dental health survey and the hospital safety study, sample numbers were allocated proportionately to the size of these units. The reasoning was that large territorial local authorities, such as cities and their associated hospitals, were likely to be the most diverse. On the other hand, there may be other considerations that dictate a strategy that points away from size. Thus, a stratum that is cheap to sample may, other things being equal, justify a higher sampling fraction. There may also be analytical considerations. A stratum of particular interest may justify greater attention. In the primary care survey, we had a higher sampling fraction in the stratum of practices that were community governed.

For sample allocation across clusters, in order to optimize error reduction and cost control, the key questions are the number of clusters and the number of units in each cluster. The optimal cluster sample size increases both with 'within-cluster' heterogeneity or variability and with the cost of adding an extra cluster relative to the cost of obtaining an extra element within a cluster. For a fixed cluster sample size, the ideal is to maximize the number of clusters for a given fieldwork budget (Agarwal et al. 2005).

Sampling and Non-Sampling Error

The central concern of theory and practice in sampling is reducing overall survey error as far as possible. There are two types of error, random and systematic, and two sources of error, sampling and non-sampling. Usually, effort is focused on sampling error, particularly the random element. This is easy to estimate and to control for. Systematic error, or bias, is harder to identify. The theory and practice for non-sampling error are also much less developed than in the case of sampling.

The primary criteria to be assessed in probability sample designs are set out in Box 9.2.

Box 9.2 Primary criteria of assessment in probability sample designs

- *Precision:* the minimal random or variable sampling error.
- *Accuracy:* the lack of bias in estimates.
- *Complexity:* the amount of advance information required and the number of stages.
- *Efficiency:* the minimization of cost for given precision and accuracy.

Generally speaking, stratified designs increase precision and clustering erodes it, but also reduces cost. List sampling should have higher precision, although this could be severely eroded if there is a periodic or recurrent pattern in the ordering of the units. Simple random sampling is less complex, but may have lower precision and efficiency.

The main components of non-sampling error are coverage, the frame and non-response rate, and measurement error. Coverage error or bias is hard to estimate and control. In the case of measurement error, there are well-established models for assessing the properties of scales and similar instruments (Diehr et al. 2005), but theory and practice have been less fully developed for questionnaire, respondent and interviewer sources. For each of our studies, we have identified measurement issues in Table 9.1.

Controlling for non-sampling error

Some techniques for controlling for non-sampling error, such as the pilot-test questionnaires, concern approaching respondents in a uniform way with realistic expectations on information recall, and it is better to have more interviewers with smaller workloads than the reverse. Interviewers are able to attend better to a smaller load and any bias affects fewer respondents. For example, in the dental survey all these points were illustrated (Davis and Scott 1996). First, one item in particular elicited a very large variation in response across interviewers. This was mainly because it asked about an unusual activity, the use of disclosing solution, and interviewers had not been provided with a standardized coding response to reflect the lack of knowledge of interviewees. Second, the component of interviewer error was higher for items that aimed to elicit attitudes and they required a recall. Third, although the errors of interviewers were small, as reflected in the small intra-cluster correlation of their respondents, their workload was high and this small interviewer-specific error therefore translated into quite a major impact across the entire sample.

Stratification and weighting

As already discussed, stratification is a technique whereby information about the structure of the population of interest is used in advance in the design of the sample. Stratification can also be used after the event – that is, after sample selection. This is called post-stratification, and is applied in association with the weighting of sample outcomes. In a typical case, key sample outcomes are compared with known population distributions and weights are then applied to sample units in order to achieve a closer correspondence between the sample and the population.[4] This approach was used in the partner relations survey to correct for the fact that women were heavily over-represented in the sample.

Although such discrepancies between sample and population could be due to the normal workings of random or variable error, it is far more likely that they are due to bias or systematic error in coverage (such as frame and non-response), and therefore such a practice can be controversial. While weighting in this case may be controversial, its use to correct for features of sample design is completely acceptable; indeed it is desirable. For instance, in the primary care study the sampling fraction, that is the proportion of GPs sampled, varied between different practice types and this had to be accounted for in any analysis that pooled data across these strata in order to ensure that practices were given the same weight that they had nationally.

In summary, it is possible to see sample weights, as applied after selection, as consisting of three elements:

- The base weight, which accounts for different probabilities of selection.
- The non-response adjustment, correcting for differences in collecting information on individuals in the population.
- The post-stratification, correcting for bias in the population representativeness of the frame or list.[5]

Drawing inferences

The central strength of probability sampling is the much greater confidence we have in drawing inferences about the population to which we wish these results to apply. Ideally, we should be in a position to draw conclusions that are both precise (there should be a narrow band around our estimates) and accurate (they should be close to the true value of the parameters in the population). The base case is one in which a simple random sample has been drawn with replacement and a single parameter, like a proportion or a mean, estimated. These are the conditions for the typical 'test of significance' using standard packages.

Once the sample design becomes more complex, and particularly if any weighting is required, a more elaborate approach is needed. In the case of sample designs that are more elaborate than the simple random sample, the 'design effect' captures the impact of this design complexity (Agarwal et al. 2005).

For instance, a design effect of four means that the standard error is twice that for a similarly sized simple random sample of the same population and that the sample size needs to be four times that of a simple random sample in order to achieve the same accuracy (overcoming the extra burden of sampling error introduced by the more complex sample design). The consequence is that, in technical terms, the standard error needs to be twice that for a similarly sized simple random sample of the same population. Rather than increasing the sample size four-fold – which would generally not be practical – the confidence interval would have to be doubled and the value of a statistical test would need to be increased before reaching significance.[6] In the dental health survey, we estimated the impact of a multistage sample with clustering. We went further and determined how this design effect might vary according to the kind of item. Thus, very little adjustment was required in the case of gender, because of the uniform distribution of men and women across clusters, but the design effect was quite marked in the case of ethnicity as there was extensive clustering on this variable (Davis and Scott 1996).

CASE STUDY

Sampling in practice in primary health care

The National Primary Medical Care Survey (NatMedCa) was undertaken to describe primary health care in New Zealand, including the characteristics of providers and their practices, the patients they see, the problems presented and the treatment management proposed. Although the study covered community-governed organizations, Accident and Medical (A&M) Clinics and Emergency Departments, as well as private general practices with 'family doctors', this case study will concentrate on this last group.

A nationally representative, multistage sample of private GPs, stratified by place and practice type, was drawn. Each GP was asked to provide data on themselves and on their practice, and to report on a 25 per cent sample of patients in each of two week-long periods. A pad of forms, structured to select each fourth patient, was provided. On the first page, the visits of four patients could be logged; on the second, a detailed record of the visit of the fourth patient was to be entered. The process was repeated on each subsequent pair of pages.

A sampling frame of all active GPs was generated from telephone White Pages listings. Other sources included the Medical Council Register and laboratory client lists. A comparison of the Medical Register with the White Pages listings showed a poor match. In particular, many individuals entered on the Medical Register did not appear to be in active practice in New Zealand. Conversely, some practitioners listed in the telephone book did not appear on the Medical Register. Another data source, the laboratory client list, was not freely available and only included practitioners receiving results electronically.

Seven strata were used in the sample selection of GPs for the National Medical Care Survey. While the first stratum covered those GPs working in community-governed practices, GPs in private practice were sampled through the strata 2–7 shown below. The strata for sample selection were defined as follows:

1   A single stratum of GPs working in community-governed non-profit organizations, who were sampled with certainty wherever they were located
2   GPs who had participated in the earlier Waikato Medical Care (WaiMedCa) Survey study
3   Independent GPs in metropolitan and city areas
4   Independent Practitioner Association (IPA) GPs in metropolitan and city areas
5   GPs paid on a per capita basis in metropolitan and city areas
6   GPs in areas surrounding the big cities
7   GPs in towns and rural areas.

(Continued)

(Continued)

In order to generate adequate, and approximately equal, numbers of GPs in strata 2–7, different sampling fractions were chosen. In the analysis presented below, the results are weighted to compensate for the different likelihood of being sampled. It should be noted that the GPs in stratum 7, towns and rural areas, were sampled in two stages: (a) a representative 4 out of 11 areas were first selected on judgement criteria; (b) a sample of 59 GPs was selected randomly from these four areas. Account was taken of the two-stage sampling process in stratum 7 in the calculation of standard errors in all subsequent analyses.

In Table 9.2, the sampling probabilities used in weighting the results for all strata are shown: the weighting factor is the inverse of the sampling probability. It should be noted that for Auckland and the cities, the sampling probability differed by practice type, while for the towns and rural areas a single sampling probability was applied across types. The number sampled was calculated to allow for a 30 per cent refusal/ineligible rate.

TABLE 9.2   Sample size and sampling percentage, all strata

Stratum	Description	Population of GPs	Sample drawn	GP weights	GPs in sample
1	Community governed	66	63	1.00*	63
2	WaiMedCa	118	58	2.03	38
3	City independent	444	50	8.88	23
4	City IPA	886	72	12.31	51
5	City capitated	71	40	1.78	21
6	Areas around the big cities	367	55	6.67	33
7	Remaining towns and rural areas	831	59	14.08	33
Total		2,783	397		262

* Sampled with certainty.

Table 9.2 shows the GP weights associated with each stratum calculated as the inverse of the sampling probability. Visit weights were calculated as GP weight × 4 (where 4 is the inverse of the sampling probability of each patient visit). The weight for each practice was calculated approximately by multiplying the GP weight by the inverse of the number of GPs in the practice, to compensate for the increased likelihood of sampling large practices.

When attempts were made to contact a GP, it was sometimes found that they were on sabbatical, had moved or had retired. In such cases, if a new practitioner had been appointed specifically to take on the departed person's workload, the new practitioner was asked to participate. Where there was no direct replacement, the sampled GP was marked ineligible. The other cause of ineligibility was the discovery that the individual was in speciality practice.

(Continued)

(Continued)

It was anticipated that additional practitioners who had not appeared on the sampling frame might be discovered when the practice of a sampled practitioner was approached. This might be because the practitioner had newly arrived or was an assistant, trainee or locum. When such people were identified, they were added to the overall sample and 13 per cent, matching the average sampling ratio, were asked to join the study.

Recruitment of selected practitioners included the following steps:

- A letter was sent from the project team requesting participation, accompanied by a letter of support from the local Professor of General Practice.
- A telephone call was made by the Clinical Director or the Project Manager requesting an interview.
- A practice visit was made, at which an information booklet was presented and, with agreement, a time for data collection was set; an estimate of weekly patient numbers was obtained and practitioners signed a consent form.
- The visit record pad and other questionnaires were delivered by courier.
- A telephone call was made to the practice early in the week of data collection as a reminder.
- Follow-up telephone call(s) were made if the data pack was not returned.
- A telephone call was made prior to the second week of data collection.
- The second visit record pad was delivered by courier.
- Follow-up telephone call(s) were made if the second data pack was not returned.
- A short questionnaire was sent to GPs who felt unable to contribute to the research.

A small payment was made to practitioners based on the number of completed visit forms. This was seen as recognition of the opportunity cost of contributing to the research, and was based on an hourly rate similar to the after-cost earnings of GPs. The Royal New Zealand College of General Practitioners agreed to recognize participation as a practice review activity able to be submitted for postgraduate education credit (MOPS). All these features of the recruitment process probably contributed to the achievement of a relatively high response rate for surveys of this kind.

Reading Health Research Based on Sampling Methods

The key questions to ask in reading and appraising health research in relation to sampling methods include:

- Is the sampling frame reported and open to scrutiny?
- Are intra-class correlations and design effects provided?
- Is the sample design structured so as to ensure coverage of sub-populations?
- Is the sample size large enough to permit precise estimates of key parameters?

- Is the response rate high enough to have confidence about sample representativeness?
- Is there information about non-responders? Are they systematically different?
- Is there information about how the investigators have tackled non-sampling error?
- Is there information on measurement error and its estimation and control?

Conclusion

This chapter has outlined the basic principles of probability and non-probability sampling. Although probability sampling is the more reliable method in statistical terms as it is based on the theory of random numbers, the decision about how to sample will depend on a number of factors such as cost, convenience and whether a reliable sampling frame exists from which the researcher can draw a sample. Researchers who are developing their probability sampling skills should seek advice from a statistician if they are uncertain about how many subjects to sample. This will make sure that their results are generalizable. Researchers should also be mindful of ethical issues, including consent – see Chapter 11 in Groves et al. 2009 and Chapter 15 in this volume.

Whatever the choice of method, when writing up results the researcher should explain clearly in the text or a methodological appendix why they have chosen a particular approach; how the sample has been drawn; and the limitations of the inferences that can be made from the findings. Further discussion on writing up research results is given in Chapter 23, while the next chapter deals with other aspects of survey research. An exercise for the reader follows on developing effective sampling strategies.

Exercise: Planning for health with a sampling strategy

Below are outlined three plausible scenarios of research settings in which a social scientist might be involved in helping to formulate a plan, an essential part of which would be the development of an effective sampling strategy. These scenarios, developed for teaching by Andrew Sporle, have been selected because they require engagement with communities and target populations that might be seen as outside the standard range for orthodox sampling theory and practice. Therefore, aside from the more conventional considerations of sample design, frame and coverage, sample size and distribution, and sampling and non-sampling error, you will also need to think about how to engage with key stakeholders and keep them supportive of your research goals.

Scenario A: An industrial area has recently had a spate of cancers among residents in a nearby neighbourhood. Most of those affected had worked at a timber treatment plant, recently closed. Those living in the community are concerned

(Continued)

(Continued)

that the cancers may be the result of chemical poisoning from the timber plant. They have approached you as a social researcher for help in investigating a possible association between the chemicals and the recently diagnosed cancers.

Scenario B: Your market research firm has been approached to undertake a study for a large telecommunications company. This company is interested in exploring the potential for the expansion of the 'pink dollar' (gay and lesbian) sector of their market, due to its perceived high disposable income and lifestyle expenditure. A survey is proposed to assess how telecommunications are used by gay and lesbian people in order to target this market.

Scenario C: You are a member of a research team that has developed a new type of follow-up and self-management plan for managing diabetes symptoms among those diagnosed as having chronic diabetes. This system has proved effective in the UK, but you are interested in implementing it in predominantly Māori, rural communities where diabetes is rife (or in the UK context in an area with a predominantly South Asian population). Your research team are interested in improving the management of diabetes in this group.

In each of these scenarios, develop a written plan, outlining the proposed sampling strategy.

Notes

1 The four illustrative examples used in this chapter were funded either by the Health Research Council of New Zealand or by its predecessor, the Medical Research Council.

2 A term that is also used to identify the same concept is 'study universe'. Population and universe are used interchangeably, and refer to the pool of elements from which a sample is drawn. A related, but distinct, term is that of 'survey population'. This is not universally applied in the literature, but can be a useful distinction. The survey population refers to that subset of the target population that has a chance of being selected for the sample. For very good practical reasons, it may be that not all units in the target population can be accessed. For example, if the survey involves telephone interviewing, then people in the target population who do not have a telephone will have no chance of selection.

3 In both the dental health and partner-relation surveys, the sample size and precision calculations were made around a single parameter (mean and proportion respectively). It should be noted that for complex sample designs, the standard formula for the simple case will underestimate the required sample size. The most straightforward way to correct this is to calculate the so-called design effect and multiply the estimate for the simple case by this value.

4 This technique is used widely in the commercial world to correct for sampling shortcomings (for instance, quota selection and non-probability designs).

5 It should be noted that, although weighting may assist in correcting an overall potential bias, it is also inefficient because it wastes information on those units that are weighted downwards.

6 A further refinement occurs in the case of 'complex statistics'. These are parameters that are much less straightforward than a mean or proportion – for example, a regression coefficient or a difference between two means (or proportions). Again, the sample size will usually need to be greater to achieve the same level of precision as that attained for a simple parameter. This means that confidence intervals and levels of significance have to be adjusted accordingly.

Recommended Further Reading

Aday, L.A. and Cornelius, L.J. (2006) *Designing and Conducting Health Surveys: A Comprehensive Guide*, 3rd edition. New York: Jossey-Bass.
This is a standard reference written with the non-technical user in mind, drawing substantially on recent methodological research on survey design and cognitive research on question and questionnaire design and presenting a total survey error framework.

Groves, R.M., Fowler, F.J., Couper, M.P., Lepkowski, J.M., Singer, E. and Tourangeau, R. (2009) *Survey Methodology*, 2nd edition. Hoboken, NJ: Wiley.
This book provides a concise overview of the entire survey research process, using clear and easy-to-understand language.

Korn, E.L. and Graubard, B.I. (1999) *Analysis of Health Surveys*. New York: Wiley.
This is a more advanced book dealing with the technical aspects of the analysis of data from complex surveys, illustrated with many examples from real health surveys.

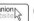 ## Online Readings

Emery, S., Lee, J., Curry, S., Johnson, T., Sporer, A., Mermelstein, R., Flay, B. and Warnecke, R (2010) 'Finding needles in a haystack: A methodology for identifying and sampling community-based youth smoking cessation programs', *Evaluation Review*, 34: 35–51.
How is sampling defined in this context? Critically evaluate the paper using the checklist provided in PPS9.6.

Lindström, M. (2011) 'Social capital, political trust, and health locus of control: A population-based study', S*candinavian Journal of Public Health*, 39: 3–9.

How is sampling defined in this context? Critically evaluate the paper using the checklist provided in PPS9.6.

References

Adamson, S.J., Deering, D.E.A., Sellman, J.D., Sheridan, J., Henderson, C., Robertson, R., Pooley, S., Campbell, S.D. and Frampton, C.M.A. (2012) 'An estimation of the prevalence of opioid dependence in New Zealand', *International Journal of Drug Policy*, 23(1): 87–9.

Aday, L.A. and Cornelius, L.J. (2006) *Designing and Conducting Health Surveys: A Comprehensive Guide*, 3rd edition. New York: Jossey-Bass.

Agarwal, R., Girdhar, G., Awasthi, S. and Walter, S.D. (2005) 'Intra-class correlation estimates for assessment of Vitamin A intake in children', *Journal of Health and Population Nutrition*, 23(1): 66–73.

Bellón, J.A., De Dios Luna, J., Moreno, B., Montón-Franco, C., GildeGómez-Barragán, M.J., Sánchez-Celaya, M., Díaz-Barreiros, M.A., Vicens, C., et al. (2010) 'Psychosocial and socio-demographic predictors of attrition in a longitudinal study of major depression in primary care: the predictD-Spain study', *Journal of Epidemiology and Community Health*, 64(10): 874–84.

Biau, D.J., Kernéis, S. and Porcher, R. (2008) 'Statistics in brief: the importance of sample size in the planning and interpretation of medical research', *Clinical Orthopaedics and Related Research*, 466(9): 2282–8.

Botman, S.L, Moore, T.F., Moriarity, C.L. and Parsons, V.L. (2000) *Design and Estimation for the National Health Interview Survey, 1995–2004*. Vital and Health Statistics, Series 2, No. 130. Hyattsville, MD: National Center for Health Statistics.

Cardozo, B.L., Bilukha, O.O., Crawford, C.A., Shaikh, I., Wolfe, M.I., Gerber, M.L. and Anderson, M. (2004) 'Mental health, social functioning, and disability in postwar Afghanistan', *Journal of the American Medical Association*, 292(5): 575–84.

Davis, P. and Scott, A. (1996) 'The effect of interviewer variance on domain comparisons', *Survey Methodology*, 21: 99–106.

De Hoop, E., Teerenstra, S., Van Gaal, B.G.I., Moerbeek, M. and Borm, G.F. (2012) 'The "best balance" allocation led to optimal balance in cluster-controlled trials', *Journal of Clinical Epidemiology*, 65(2): 132–7.

Diehr, P., Chen, L., Patrick, D., Feng, Z. and Yasui, Y. (2005) 'Reliability, effect size, and responsiveness of health status measures in the design of randomized and cluster-randomized trials', *Contemporary Clinical Trials*, 26: 45–58.

Fealy, G.M., McNamara, M.S., Casey, M., Geraghty, R., Butler, M., Halligan, P., Treacy, M. and Johnson, M. (2011) 'Barriers to clinical leadership development: findings from a national survey', *Journal of Clinical Nursing*, 20(13–14): 2023–32.

Groves, R.M., Fowler, F.J., Couper, M.P., Lepkowski, J.M., Singer, E. and Tourangeau, R. (2009) *Survey Methodology*, 2nd edition. Hoboken, NJ: Wiley.

Guterbock, T.M., Diop, A., Ellis, J.M., Holmes, J.L. and Le, K.T. (2011) 'Who needs RDD? Combining directory listings with cellphone exchanges for an alternative telephone sampling frame', *Social Science Research*, 40(3): 860–72.

He, Y. and Zaslavsky, A.M. (2012) 'Diagnosing imputation models by applying target analyses to posterior replicates of completed data', *Statistics in Medicine*, 31(1): 1–18.

Hedt, B.L. and Pagano, M. (2011) 'Health indicators: eliminating bias from convenience sampling estimators', *Statistics in Medicine*, 30(5): 560–8.

Kirton, J. A., Jack, B. A., O'Brien, M.R. and Roe, B. (2012) 'Care of patients with neurological conditions: the impact of a Generic Neurology Nursing Service development on patients and their carers', *Journal of Clinical Nursing*, 21: 207–15.

Kypri, K., Samaranayaka, A., Connor, J., Langley, J.D. and Maclennan, B. (2011) 'Non-response bias in a web-based health behaviour survey of New Zealand tertiary students', *Preventive Medicine*, 53(4–5): 274–7.

Muñoz, R.A., Pisani, M.J. and Fullerton, T.M. (2011) 'Exchange rate premia and discounts for retail purchases using Mexican pesos in El Paso, Texas', *Social Science Journal*, 48(4): 612–20.

Murphy, E. and Dingwall, R. (2003) *Qualitative Methods and Health Policy Research.* New York: Aldine de Gruyter.

Ryan, A., McKenna, H. and Slevin, O. (2011) 'Family care-giving and decisions about entry to care: a rural perspective', *Ageing and Society*, 32: 1–18.

Statistics New Zealand (2006) *Introduction to the Census.* Wellington: Statistics New Zealand.

Yoon, C., Ju, Y.S. and Kim, C.Y. (2011) 'Disparities in health care utilization among urban homeless in South Korea: a cross-sectional study', *Journal of Preventive Medicine and Public Health*, 44(6): 267–74.

Yusoff, N., Taib, N.A.M. and Ahmad, A. (2011) 'The health seeking trajectories of Malaysian women and their husbands in delay cases of breast cancer: a qualitative study', *Asian Pacific Journal of Cancer Prevention*, 12: 2563–70.

10

Quantitative Survey Methods in Health Research

MICHAEL CALNAN

Introduction

- This chapter explores the use of survey methods in research into health and health care which are widely used in this and other fields of research (see, for example, Fowler 2001; Bryman 2012). It begins by defining and explaining what quantitative survey methodology is; describing the techniques and resources required for carrying out a survey; and discussing the role of theory. It then outlines the process of translating concepts into indicators and assesses the strengths and weaknesses of different survey techniques for collecting data. It identifies the major issues in managing a survey, and in analysing and presenting data. The chapter concludes with a description of how different survey methods are put into practice, illustrated through examples drawn from my own research.

- Survey methods can be defined in a number of different ways but the most cogent is provided by De Vaus (2002), who argues that the two defining characteristics of a survey are: how data are collected and the method of analysis used. In a survey, data should be collected on the basis of the same characteristics – such as social position, beliefs, attitudes and behaviours – from a number of cases or units of analysis to provide a structured data set. Analysis in survey methods involves a comparison of cases. This can be descriptive, for example by trying to identify among a group of people the level of satisfaction with health care, or it can be taken further analytically to locate cause. For instance, the level of public satisfaction with health has been systematically associated with age: older people have higher levels of satisfaction than younger people. Causal inferences may then be drawn by a careful comparison of the characteristics of cases to try to explain why age may affect public assessments of satisfaction. However, it is important to avoid the mistake of attributing a causal link to age and satisfaction. Showing that two variables are associated does not, in itself, provide sufficient evidence to prove a causal link.

Types of Survey

Surveys can be of different types (Czaja and Blair 2005). An ad hoc survey is carried out for a one-off purpose, such as a local survey of health care users to find out the level of satisfaction with a particular organization or service. Cross-sectional surveys are regular surveys that monitor trends over time, such as the British Social Attitudes Survey (Park et al. 2003). This national survey is carried out annually and consists of a set of core questions with new questions added that relate to a current problem area. These regular surveys are useful for monitoring general trends such as public satisfaction with the NHS and the various services it provides in the UK. A longitudinal study, that is a survey repeated on the same cohort or population at different points of time, would show the proportion of those over time who took out a new subscription to private health insurance; the proportion who maintained their subscription to private health insurance; and the proportion that let their subscription lapse.

It should be stressed, though, that national surveys may not be able to identify certain aspects of change. For example, the British Social Attitudes Survey can show people's attitudes to private health care, the level of coverage and the level of subscriptions to private health insurance, and how these change over time. Thus, during the 1980s, this survey showed a gradual increase in the proportion of the population covered by private insurance. However, as the overall figure did not identify the proportion of lapsed subscribers, which in the case of private health insurance was high, the data could not show whether the increase reflected a large or small increase in new subscriptions (Calnan et al. 1993). So surveys carried out on a regular basis can be useful for measuring gross change but longitudinal designs, using cohort or panel studies, are more appropriate for understanding individual and within-group net change.

Survey methods are often associated with the use of a questionnaire where data are collected through interview, face to face, by telephone, or are self-completed through postal or other means. However, surveys can draw on a wide range of techniques. They may, for instance, have a qualitative element when the interview schedule includes both open-ended and semi-structured questions, and some surveys include structured observation where specific activities are recorded. For example, if the aim is to explore practitioner–patient encounters, activities may be recorded in a hospital ward or general practice. Another technique for data collection is the structured record review where the researcher uses a specially created form to elicit information, for example from patients' medical records. Qualitative data in a survey may be organized and analysed quantitatively, using a content analysis method (Fink 2003). This might involve counting the frequency that topics occur in respondents' narratives, as discussed in Chapter 4. Thus, a survey is not synonymous with using a questionnaire, as various methods can be used to collect and analyse data as in other case study and experimental designs.

The Rationale for Employing Survey Methods

The previous discussion has hinted at the type of research question where it may be appropriate to employ quantitative survey methods. The sample survey using different data collection techniques can be used to address descriptive questions, such as what, who, when and how questions. It can also look at variations in the characteristics of different groups, as discussed above. Furthermore, surveys may be used for explanatory research to explore 'why?' questions where the aim is to try to impute cause or consequence. In cross-sectional surveys, information is collected at one point in time to take a 'snapshot' to explore such questions. However, this approach lacks a time dimension that can hinder the exploration of causal influences. Surveys that are repeated or that are repeated at intervals can better explore changes in relationships and the strength of interrelationships between variables. They will also identify naturally occurring variation, although it is generally difficult to pinpoint a specific cause of such variation and impossible to eliminate a range of confounding or contaminating factors. In these circumstances, an experimental or quasi-experimental design could attempt to control, or allow for, a range of possible confounding influences.

In summary, survey methods are distinguishable from other research methods, in terms of the form of data collection and methods of analysis adopted. However, surveys are not necessarily distinguished by the techniques of data collection that may also be used in other methods. Survey methods tend to address questions that are both descriptive and analytical, although they have limitations in relation to exploring specific causal influences.

The Techniques and Resources Required for the Survey Method in Practice

What resources are required in terms of time and money to carry out the survey method? Fink (2003) suggests that to estimate the resources necessary, the following questions should be addressed: What are the major tasks of the survey? What skills are needed to complete each task? How much time does each task take? How much time is available to complete the survey? Who can be recruited to perform each task? What are the costs of each task? What additional resources are needed? These questions may be addressed by quantifying and listing basic information on the direct and indirect costs and expenses incurred by the survey:

- Decide on the number of days (or hours) that constitute a working year.
- Formulate survey tasks or activities in terms of the number of months it will take to complete each task.
- Estimate how long, in a number of days (or hours), you will need for each person to complete their assigned task.
- Decide on the daily (hourly) rate for each person that will need to be paid.
- Decide on the cost of benefits (such as superannuation).
- Decide on other expenses that will be specifically incurred in the study, such as questionnaire piloting or focus groups.
- Decide on the indirect costs that will be incurred to keep the survey team going, such as overheads and accommodation.

Translating Concepts into Indicators

Operationalizing concepts

Survey research should be informed by theory, and the impact of theory, as with most other research methods, helps to focus questions and enhance the value of findings. Once a theoretical framework is constructed, an important issue is deciding how concepts should be translated into questions or indicators – in other words, how theory can be operationalized in the survey. This, according to De Vaus (2002), involves three essential steps that are: clarifying concepts, developing indicators and evaluating indicators. Concepts have been seen by De Vaus as abstract summaries of sets of behaviours, attitudes and characteristics that share something in common.

Three steps assist in the process of conceptual clarification. These are set out in Figure 10.1 which uses 'deprivation' to illustrate the different elements involved in operationalizing a concept. First, obtain a range of definitions. In the case of deprivation, five different definitions are identified: physical, economic, social, political and psychic. Second, decide upon a particular definition, which in the case of deprivation might be the 'social' aspect. Third, the dimensions of the concept must be delineated.

For deprivation, three have been identified: social isolation, the absence of socially valued roles and a lack of social skills. The process of moving from abstract concepts to the point where they can be operationalized via a specific questionnaire item is called 'descending the ladder of abstraction'. Clarifying concepts involves descending this ladder.

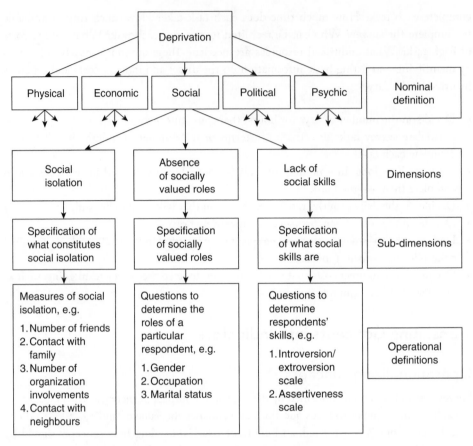

FIGURE 10.1   Clarifying concepts: descending the ladder of abstraction
Source: De Vaus (2002)

How many indicators should be used?

There is no definite or clear-cut answer to the question of how many indicators should be used, but the following points provide a guideline for indicator development:

- Where there is no agreed way of measuring the concept, it is helpful to develop indicators for a range of definitions in order to see the effect on the results.
- If the concept is multidimensional, it is necessary to decide if there is interest in all, some or any one of these dimensions.
- The researcher must be able to develop measures of key concepts.
- Complex concepts are best measured via a number of questions so as to capture the scope of the concept.

- Piloting indicators is an essential way of eliminating unnecessary questions.
- The number of items will be affected by pragmatic considerations (for example, the length of the questionnaire and the method of administration).

How should indicators be developed?

For certain concepts, it is simple to identify indicators as they are well established, as is the case with age or marital status. However, other more abstract concepts are more difficult, although there are a number of different ways of approaching the problem. First, a well-established measure from previous research may be used. This makes it possible for a direct comparison to be made between the results of the research and previous research findings. However, the danger of using an 'off-the-shelf' instrument is that it may not be tailored to measure the specific concept that one wishes to explore. A second approach, which is less convenient and more time consuming, is to use a qualitative method such as informal face-to-face interviews or focus groups initially to develop relevant questions. A third approach is to interview key informants or interest groups to provide clues or pointers to what the most appropriate questions might be.

Figure 10.1 shows how the three dimensions of social deprivation might be operational-ized. To assist further, see De Vaus (2002: 49) for a discussion of how the concept of social capital could be operationalized. Chapter 17 in this volume also describes an approach to conceptualizing ethnicity.

Evaluating indicators: reliability and validity

How should indicators be evaluated to ensure that they are reliable and valid before the survey is conducted? Reliability is where a similar result is obtained in response to a particular question or indicator on repeated occasions. Sources of unreliability stem from a range of factors, such as poorly worded or ambiguous questions and the effect of different interviewer characteristics or styles on responses. Reliability can be tested for single items by the method of test–retest and by item-to-item correlation for multiple-item scales, which involves examining the strength of the statistical relationship between items. Using multi-item indicators and removing the unreliable item after testing should increase reliability. Other ways of improving reliability are through using well-tested questions, training interviewers prior to embarking on the research and reading, and re-reading questions, preferably with colleagues to find unambiguous wording for questions.

The question of validity is more complex and involves the extent to which the operation-alized indicator is really measuring the concept it is intended to measure, and whether it is a valid empirical indicator of the theoretical concept. There are various methods of judging validity but the four outlined in Box 10.1 are the most common (see, for instance, Litwin 1995; Fink 2003).

Box 10.1   Methods of judging validity

- *Content validity:* this refers to the extent to which a measure thoroughly and appropriately assesses the characteristics or skills it is intended to measure. A concept should be derived from a conceptual framework or set of theoretical ideas and the indicator should closely match the concept.
- *Face validity:* this refers to how a measure appears on the surface and whether all the required questions are framed in the appropriate language. In this case, it may not necessarily have been informed, at least explicitly, by theory.
- *Criterion validity:* this refers to the degree of convergence or divergence with a tried and tested indicator of the concept. Criterion validity may be concurrent or predictive. Concurrent refers to the validity of a measure, for example for current health status, while predictive validity is the extent to which a measure forecasts future health status: for example, a general health examination, or a particular indicator, may predict health status over the coming years.
- *Construct validity:* this refers to examining whether or not a proposition that is assumed to exist is actually confirmed when the new indicator is tested. For example, there is strong evidence of a positive relationship between health status and affluence/deprivation. Thus, the development of an indicator of deprivation could have its validity tested by examining its relationship with a robust measure of health status.

Strengths and Weaknesses of the Survey Method

This section of the chapter evaluates the specific techniques used in surveys to elicit information. At a general level, as the earlier discussion suggested, survey methods are valuable in examining comparisons and variations between groups, particularly in large populations. The standardization of the data collected is believed to be another distinctive strength of survey research (Babbie 2008). Surveys can provide a broad overview of a social phenomenon and a general, if sometimes superficial and artificial, picture. What are the weaknesses? One possible weakness is that surveys are incapable of capturing the meanings and perceptions of social actors and the context in which action is taking place. Qualitative methods, such as informal interviews and observation, are more appropriate in addressing this type of research question as they provide greater flexibility. Surveys have also been seen to be tied to a more positivistic school of thought (see Chapter 2), which emphasizes the importance of structural forces or 'causes' and neglects the importance of human action or agency. Certainly, survey methodology is associated with measurement and not all social phenomena are measurable. In general, it is suggested that 'survey research is comparatively weak on validity and strong on reliability' (Babbie 2008: 309).

What then of the strengths and weaknesses of data collection techniques commonly used in surveys? The question will be addressed by first looking in Box 10.2 at the shortfalls of the most common forms of data collection through questionnaires administered by postal, telephone, face-to-face and web-based methods.

Box 10.2   Shortfalls of other methods of data collection

- Postal questionnaires are poor in avoiding response bias, do not tend to use open-ended questions, do not control question sequence, cannot motivate people to answer 'boring' questions and may not produce high-quality entries.
- Telephone interviews are more costly than postal surveys, more difficult to implement and tend not to be useful for exploring sensitive topics.
- Face-to-face questionnaires are difficult to implement in that they are costly, slow and involve recruiting suitable staff. There may also be difficulties with the quality of the answers, particularly the distortion of response due to interviewer characteristics that may subvert the questions, and they may be more likely to be intrusive and make it more difficult to protect anonymity.
- Web-based questionnaires are becoming more common – as indicated by the example in Chapter 2.

On the positive side, all three techniques can achieve good response rates. However, telephone surveys consistently have been found to produce significantly higher response rates than postal surveys, but lower response rates than face-to-face interview surveys (Bourque and Fielder 2003). Web-based surveys are becoming increasingly popular, not least because of perceived ease of access (Couper 2008). However, response rates are rarely above 50 per cent (Wilson et al. 2010) and tend to be lower than in postal surveys and other survey methods of data collection (Lozar et al. 2007; Shih and Fan 2008).

The Management of the Survey and Survey Data

Data collection and fieldwork

The management of the survey and the fieldwork are important for the quality of the data collection and adherence to the proposed design. For example, the tasks involved with a telephone interview survey will include ensuring that all questions are asked; the response rate at each follow-up is recorded; the interviewer stays within the time limit set; the interests of the respondents are respected; and ethical guidelines are agreed prior to interview.

Managing a postal survey places more responsibility on survey coordinators. The coordinators must develop identifiers and package questionnaires to include self-addressed, pre-paid envelopes for respondents to return. They must have a method for identifying and sending out follow-up letters or reminders to those who did not respond by the due date. Non-response to questionnaires can affect the validity of surveys and introduce bias. It is important that survey coordinators record the reasons for non-response so that a distinction can be made between those who refused to take part and those who did not do so because, for instance, they moved away or were too ill. For surveys in general in the UK, it is becoming difficult to gain a high response rate and researchers increasingly use rewards and incentives to try to encourage respondent participation and therefore boost response rates. Survey coordinators may therefore have to manage the distribution of incentives such as prizes or shopping vouchers. A crucial element in organizing an interview survey is ensuring that interviewers are well trained and that training is standardized. This is generally the responsibility of the researcher or project manager.

The offer of financial incentives has been widely used as a method to increase response rates to postal questionnaires. A Cochrane systematic review of 481 randomized controlled trials (RCTs) evaluating different ways of increasing response rates to postal questionnaires in a wide range of populations found that the odds of response can be doubled through the use of monetary incentives (Edwards et al. 2009). Other factors that increase response included a topic of interest, pre-notification, follow-up contact, unconditional incentives, shorter questionnaires, providing a second copy of the questionnaire at follow-up, mentioning an obligation to respond and university sponsorship. However, this evidence base relates to postal questionnaires and, although a number of systematic reviews (Van Geest et al. 2007) have been conducted, available evidence relating to the use of incentives in other methods of data collection, such as electronic questionnaires, is less substantive. The Cochrane review included 32 RCTs evaluating 27 different ways of increasing response rates to electronic questionnaires in a wide range of populations (Edwards et al. 2009). Despite one RCT that evaluated monetary incentives finding no significant effect, a further six RCTs found that use of other financial incentives, such as gift vouchers, doubled the chance of response.

However, the relationship between incentives and participation is not straightforward, as illustrated by evidence from a recent study which used an RCT design to test whether knowledge of a financial incentive would increase the response rate to an online questionnaire (Wilson et al. 2010). The RCT included 485 UK-based principal investigators of publicly funded health services and population health research. Participants were contacted by email and invited to complete an online questionnaire via an embedded URL. Participants were randomly allocated to receive either 'knowledge of' or 'no knowledge of' a financial incentive (a £10 gift voucher) to be provided on completion of the survey. At the end of the study, gift vouchers were given to all participants who completed the questionnaire, regardless of initial randomization status. Reminder emails were sent out to non-respondents at one-, two-, three- and four-week intervals; a fifth postal reminder was also undertaken. The primary outcome measure for the trial was the response rate one week after the second reminder. The response rate was also measured at the end of weeks one, two, three, four and five, and after a postal reminder was sent. A total of 243 questionnaires (50%) were returned (with 232 completed and 11 declining to participate). One week after the second reminder, the response rate in the 'knowledge' group was 27% (n = 66/244) versus 20% (n = 49/241) in the 'no knowledge' group (x^2: $P = .08$). The odds ratio for those responding with knowledge of an incentive was 1.45 (odds ratio [OR]: 95%, CI: 0.95 to 2.21). At the third reminder, the 'no knowledge' group members were informed about the incentive, ending the randomized element of the study. However, all respondents were followed up from reminder three onwards and no significant differences were observed in responses between the two groups. The authors concluded that knowledge of a financial incentive did not significantly increase the response rate to an online questionnaire, suggesting that other factors such as the salience of the topic may be more important. The data is presented graphically in Figure 10.2 below.

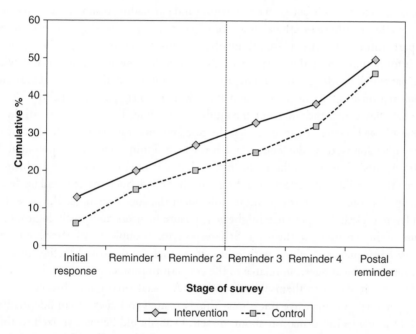

FIGURE 10.2   Does knowledge of a financial incentive increase the response rate to an online questionnaire?
Key: Intervention = knowledge of incentive; Control = no knowledge of incentive; vertical dotted line signifies point at which control group were informed about incentive.
Source: Wilson et al. (2010)

Ethics and survey research

Social inquiry as a whole can result in a range of ethical dilemmas that need to be considered before research is undertaken (Babbie 2008; Bryman 2012). Ethical decisions arise when a decision needs to be made between one course of action and another by reference to standards of what is morally right or wrong. Social surveys are no different and formal ethical approval is required if human subjects are involved, which they will be if a survey is being used as a primary data source. Ethical and governance approval from an NHS Committee will be required if the study is being carried out in the English NHS and involves collecting data from patients and/or staff. Researchers need to note a number of issues, including:

- The right to autonomy and self-determination, which involves the right to agree or not agree to take part in the survey.
- The right to be informed about the study, encompassing the right to informed consent.

A balance has to be made between encouraging and persuading respondents to participate in the study and the less ethical practice of coercing or harassing the respondent to take part. Informed consent usually involves a prospective respondent being supplied with information about the purpose of the research, how it is funded and whether participants will be identified by name. Researchers must also give potential participants an information sheet about the research and ask them to sign a consent form. This must state that they can withdraw from the study at any time. This option of withdrawal is made available because of concerns that the research might cause harm to participants – the key question is, does the 'benefit' from research findings justify the potential 'harm' to participants? Sometimes 'harm' or 'risk of harm' is obvious, for example in medical research the possible side-effects of a drug must be stated. Such matters will be discussed by the ethics committee but it is more difficult in the social sciences. The potential for harm from a research experience might be exposure to stress and psychological damage because of the sensitivity of the topic. Self-respect, for example, may be undermined with negative consequences – along with other issues that are discussed further in Chapter 15. A further ethical question relates to the concern to protect privacy and the right for people to limit access to themselves by others. A social survey may breach privacy by asking personal and intrusive questions. This is related to issues of confidentiality and the right to control information about oneself. Data should be anonymized so they are 'non-attributable' to specific persons and stored carefully to follow the requirements of the Data Protection Act. Each and all of these questions are usually addressed in the decision to grant ethical approval or not.

Coding/analysis of survey data

Data management begins when the first batch of survey questionnaires is returned, and a key task is developing the coding frame. The coding frame contains the definition of all the variables (such as age); the categories for each variable (for example, one way of dividing up an age group would be in 10-year intervals: 10 years or younger, 11–20 years, 21–30 years, and so on); and the location of the variables and their values (often expressed as numbers in columns). The development of the coding frame, as well as its operationalization, is the method whereby the data are translated from the respondent's answer to the survey questions to a database where aggregate data can be analysed. The development of the coding frame is based on the questions asked. The complexity of the coder's task will depend on the extent to which the questions are pre-coded, that is codes have been allocated already in the questionnaire, or are open-ended, with no pre-codes attached.

For some variables, such as marital status, educational qualifications, socio-economic status, sets of codes exist, and, where possible, these may be used as they are well worked out and enable comparison with other studies. However, the open type of question requires the development of specific codes to accommodate the range of answers. This can be done by coding a sample of responses to identify the answer most frequently reported. The provisional coding categories can be refined if new categories emerge as the main body of the questionnaires are coded. Given the possibility of variation in interpretation of response, particularly to open-ended questions, it is important that those coding the questionnaires are well trained, as the codes they enter represent the data. It is also important to double-code the data, or at least a sample of them, to test for reliability and consistency, but also to identify problematic questions and possible variations in interpretation.

One common problem in surveys is that some questions are better answered than others and hence there are sometimes marked variations in the response rate to specific questions. Thus, the overall response rate to a questionnaire will not always reflect usable questions. Data entry is also a major activity in data management. Survey data can be entered into a computer spreadsheet or statistical program. Statistical programs can verify accuracy, although it is important, once again, that those entering data are well trained and directed during the project. Data entry tends to be automatic with computer-assisted, online or scanned surveys that have used pre-coded, closed questions.

There are a number of computer programs available but one of the most popular and widely used is SPSS (originally Statistical Package for the Social Sciences), now in its 20th version (IBM SPSS Statistics, 20.0 -2011). It aids data management, data documentation and statistical analysis. The latter include: descriptive statistics (frequency), bivariate (correlation), linear regression and predictions for identifying groups such as factor analysis (see Bryman 2012 on how to get started with SPSS).

Issues of data analysis and presentation

The approach to data analysis will depend upon the specific research questions or objectives being examined. For example, the five objectives outlined below in Box 10.3 have different implications for data analysis (see Chapter 11 for further background on statistical analysis).

Box 10.3 The objectives of data analysis and their implications

The main objectives considered here are to:

- Describe the background of the respondents who took part in a 'satisfaction with health care' survey: here, a frequency count may be appropriate or percentages calculated of the proportion of respondents who were men or women or who owned or did not own a car. This could be used as a possible indicator of deprivation.
- Describe responses to specific questions: for example, on average how many times did respondents consult their GP in the past year? The average might have been 4 with the range between 0 and 20. Average refers to the measure of central tendency and range to the measure of dispersion.
- Determine the relationship between recent use of the GP and level of satisfaction: this would involve estimating the relationship between the level of use of GPs and the level of satisfaction. One way of estimating the relationship between the two would be through correlation. The expected result would be a positive relationship or correlation, with levels of satisfaction increasing with higher use.
- Examine whether there were any differences between men and women in terms of levels of satisfaction with care received in general practice: this would involve comparing the average satisfaction scores for men and women, and using a test of statistical significance to see if any differences observed are statistically meaningful, rather than simply due to chance. The statistical test used will depend, at least in part, on whether the survey data being analysed are nominal (that is, with no numerical preferential values), ordinal (the rate or order of a list of items) or numerical (numbers, such as age in years or height in metres).
- Find out if gender, age or income predict the level of satisfaction: to answer this question, an appropriate design is needed, but a distinction needs to be made between independent and dependent variables. Independent variables are usually applied to explain or predict a result or outcome – in contrast to the dependent variable. In the case of a patient satisfaction survey, the independent variables are gender, age or income and the dependent variable is level of satisfaction. However, to choose an appropriate statistical method of analysis, it is necessary to specify the purpose of the analysis and identify the number of independent and dependent variables and whether the data being analysed are nominal, ordinal or numerical. Once these questions have been addressed, then a choice of statistical method can be made. The appropriateness of choice depends on the extent to which the assumption about the characteristics and quality of data associated with the method can be met (Fink 2003).

Writing up and presenting survey findings

Survey findings can be written up in reports, articles and scientific/academic papers and in books or monographs. Whatever the medium of dissemination, it is important that the findings are clearly presented. However, if the aim is to publish a scientific or academic paper, a number of points should be addressed. The paper format, at least for quantitative surveys, usually consists of an introduction, methods, results and discussion ending with a concluding paragraph (as discussed in Chapter 23). The methods section should contain a concise rationale for the use of a particular method of data collection and why survey methods were used to address the research objectives. It should also contain details of the response rate and possible biases, particularly estimates of non-response bias and details of the statistical analysis and packages used, on which Chapter 11 further elaborates.

The following chapter on statistical methods also underlines the notion that the presentation of an accurate report of survey results is facilitated by the use of such aids as lists, charts and tables that are more fully described than in this context. Lists are useful for stating survey objectives, methods and findings. Presenting data in graphic form is becoming increasingly popular, perhaps because of the ease with which this can be undertaken electronically through word-processing packages. Pie, bar and line charts provide different kinds of figures:

- Pie charts are useful for describing proportions or slices that make up the whole.
- Bar charts are common because they are relatively easy to read and interpret and useful for purposes of comparison.
- Line charts are helpful when plotting trends and changes over time.

Figure 10.3 below provides an example of data presentation using a bar chart. In order to address the question of whether GPs experience higher levels of job stress than other

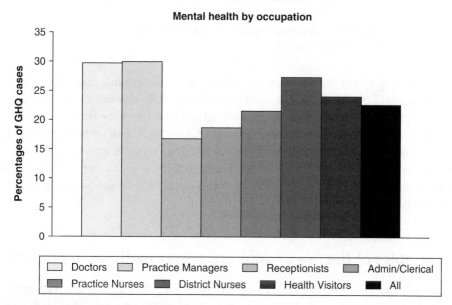

FIGURE 10.3   Stress in the general practice workforce
Source: Calnan and Wainwright (2002)

members of the health workforce, Calnan and Wainwright (2002) examined stress levels among various groups in a primary care setting, such as doctors, nurses, managers, administrators and clerical staff. The bar chart in the Figure presents comparisons and shows that practice managers have the highest levels of stress, followed by GPs.

Figure 10.4 is an example of a line chart used to plot trends over time. It examines changes in levels of public satisfaction and dissatisfaction with the NHS over the last 20 years. It shows that differences have tended to decrease with levels of satisfaction generally falling and dissatisfaction generally increasing.

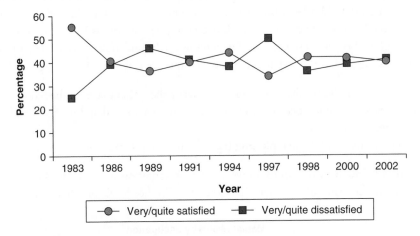

FIGURE 10.4   Changes in levels of public satisfaction with the NHS
Source: Appleby and Rosete (2003)

Tables can complement charts and are particularly useful for providing detailed information and the results of statistical analyses about patterns of findings that other researchers might wish to replicate. The number of tables presented will depend on the length of the article and are more commonly used in research reports. Charts, on the other hand, are useful in oral presentations for maximizing visual impact. Finally, in terms of writing up, it is important for the discussion and conclusion to be based on the results presented. The limitations of the methods and design should be identified and explained, followed by an interpretation of the findings and their significance.

CASE STUDY

Examples of the use of different survey methods in practice

Examples of survey methods in the area of health and health care are numerous. The following examples illustrate different types of survey methods based primarily on the author's own research.

(Continued)

(Continued)

Postal surveys

Calnan and Sanford (2004) aimed to examine how the public assess trust in health care in England and Wales. This formed part of an international study including the Netherlands and Germany, which compared levels of trust in different health care systems (Van der Schee et al. 2007). A postal survey was used because it was the most efficient means of eliciting information from a national sample. It contained a common core of structured questions derived from a survey instrument developed in the Netherlands that could assist international comparison. One of the problems with carrying out national surveys is finding an easily accessible, comprehensive and up-to-date sampling frame. One of the most popular, at least until recently, has been the Electoral Register. The Electoral Register provides an accessible and up-to-date source of information but is biased towards those who are more likely to register and under-represents those who do not register. Registers may also be out of date.

In the study in question, pilot work suggested it would be necessary to allow for at least 10 per cent inaccuracy when estimating sample size. There was also the added problem that no information was available from the Electoral Register about non-respondents, so estimates could not be made of the representativeness of the respondents who participated in the survey. Thus, a comparison had to be made between the characteristics of the respondents and the national census data which showed that the survey under-represented the younger age groups and the healthy. This was particularly important, as the overall response rate was low (48%, n = 1,187) with 49 per cent of respondents not replying and 3 per cent refusing. Furthermore, the original sample of 2,777 was reduced to 2,489 as 288 had died or moved away. Respondents were sent three follow-up mailings in addition to the first mailing.

This study also illustrated a problem commonly found in international studies using survey methods (see Chapter 20 for a further discussion of comparative research). To enable comparison, it is important to use common core questions, although these questions must be meaningful to respondents within different countries. For example, in the English survey the two terms 'confidence' (in the doctor's competence) and 'trust' (that the doctor worked in the patient's interest) could be distinguished, but no such semantic distinction is made between the terms in Dutch or German. To deal with this difference, confidence was used as equivalent to trust in the core questions, but when undertaking the survey in England and Wales, we asked additional questions about other aspects of trust (for example, whether respondents thought the practitioner worked primarily in the interests of the patient or the organization) to see if they were associated with confidence in competence (see Figure 10.5). The statistical analysis showed that correlation between the two indicators was strong. Coupled with evidence from qualitative, informal, face-to-face interviews, this suggested that confidence was embedded in and formed part of trust (Calnan and Rowe 2008).

Using mixed methods

Postal surveys may combine various methods. For example, a survey can be preceded by a qualitative method, such as using focus groups, as an antecedent.

(Continued)

(Continued)

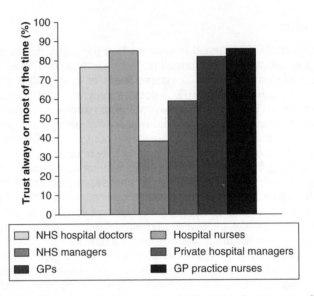

FIGURE 10.5   Public levels of trust in health services staff: putting the interests of patients above the convenience of organizations
Source: Calnan and Rowe (2008)

Focus groups may be used to identify the salient themes and help to refine the questions for a postal survey of a wider population. Alternatively, postal surveys are sometimes used as precursors to qualitative methods to identify cases for follow-up with in-depth interviews.

An example where survey methods acted as a precursor to qualitative methods may be found in a study of sufferers with upper-limb pain (Calnan et al. 2005). The study aimed to find out why people sought help and how symptoms were presented; how the problem was managed and treated; and the implications for outcome of a treatment regime. There were several design options considered, each with strengths and weaknesses. However, as the study aimed to obtain information from a broad range of informants, some of whom did not consult orthodox or unorthodox care at all, the design consisted of a community-based screening survey followed by a case-comparison study, as set out in Figure 10.6 below. The sample for the screening survey was drawn from a population of patients registered with five general practices in the local area. A postal questionnaire, which included screening questions on upper-limb pain taken from a previously validated instrument, was sent to a random sample of the working population aged 25 to 64.

Figure 10.7 shows the overall response rate (56%) and illustrates the response to the two reminders, both of which elicited around a 10 per cent response rate. The first reminder was a postcard to those who intended to take part. The second reminder was a letter, questionnaire and pre-paid envelope (identical to the first mailing) aimed at persuading the 'hard core' of non-responders to participate.

(Continued)

(Continued)

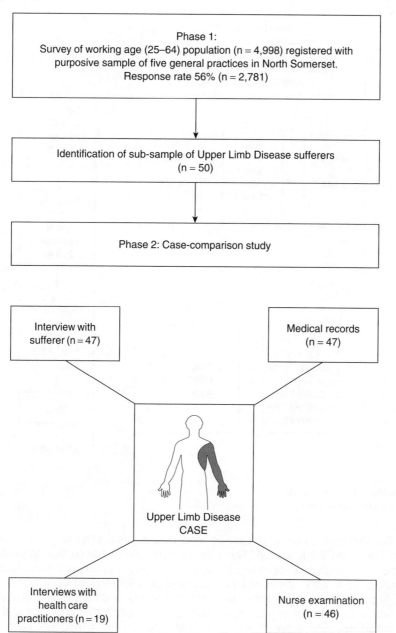

FIGURE 10.6 Study design
Source: Calnan et al. (2005)

(Continued)

(Continued)

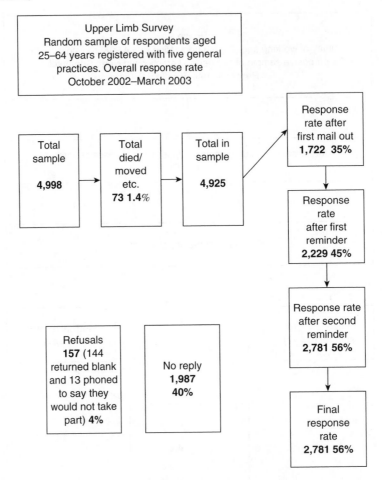

FIGURE 10.7   Response rates
Source: Calnan et al. (2005)

For this study, one of the major aims of the initial screening survey was to identify 'cases' for follow-up. These cases were selected according to predefined inclusion criteria to encompass those who had experienced arm pain during the previous 12 months; those who had had arm pain for longer than a month or not (a measure of duration); those with different levels of difficulty with undertaking activities (a measure of severity); those who had consulted a doctor and those who had not; and those who were in paid employment or not. For each group, informants were randomly selected from the survey sample. In all, 50 informants were contacted according to these criteria. It was only possible to interview 47

(Continued)

(Continued)

of the informants. Each had agreed to have their medical records examined and were invited to be examined by a nurse. Informants were asked to nominate a health care worker they had seen for their upper-limb pain. This health worker was then approached for an interview. The interview with the practitioner focused on the informant's 'case' to begin with and then expanded to general policies and practices. This example illustrates how postal surveys can be used as precursors to qualitative methods by identifying groups for follow-up.

In their study of stress in a random sample of general practices, Calnan and Wainwright (2002) used a similar two-stage methodology. A postal survey of general practices was used to identify those practices under high stress at one end of the spectrum, and, at the other end, those that had lower levels of stress. The 10 practices (five at either end) were selected according to criteria based on data collected in a survey on mental distress and job strain using the General Health Questionnaire score. Additional information about practice size and geographical location was also collected.

This was followed by in-depth interviews (n = 87) with members of the five practices who were stressed and the five who were not. Analysing this type of mixed-method database is not always straightforward, as respondents' responses to a postal questionnaire are sometimes different from their accounts in interview. The follow-up interviews showed that even among 'high-stress' practices, work stress was not the major problem it initially appeared to be. The experience of work stress in general practice was more about low morale, dissatisfaction and negative affectivity rather than severe anxiety or psychological strain.

Interview surveys

Interview surveys take at least two forms, namely face-to-face interviews and telephone interviews. A typical example of an interview survey is the British Social Attitudes Survey referred to earlier in this chapter. This survey (Park et al. 2003) began in 1983 and has been conducted annually, except for 1988 and 1992. The survey is designed to produce annual measures of attitudinal shifts. One of its main objectives is to monitor patterns of continuity and change, and the relative rates at which attitudes, in respect of a range of social issues, change over time. It is a regular survey rather than a longitudinal study as it does not follow the same sample of people (a cohort) over time, but samples from a new population each year. The interview questionnaire contains a number of core questions covering major topic areas such as defence, the economy and the welfare state. The remainder of the questionnaire is devoted to a series of questions on a range of social, economic, political and moral issues. The questions are predominantly structured and closed. Each year, the survey samples adults aged 18 and over, living in private households in Britain. It is based on a multi-stage stratified random sample. From 1993, the sample was drawn from the postcode address file, and for all years of the survey a weighting procedure is available to adjust for unequal selection probabilities. Sample sizes vary each year, and between 1983 and 2002 they ranged between 1,355 and 3,469.

A strength of the British Social Attitudes Survey is that it can be used to monitor changes in attitude over time. This is clearly illustrated by respondents' attitudes to

(Continued)

(Continued)

the NHS. A set of core questions have been included in the survey nearly every year since 1983. These have consisted of a general question:

All in all, how satisfied or dissatisfied would you say you are with the way in which the NHS runs nowadays?

There are also more specific questions:

From your own experience, or from what you have heard, please say how satisfied or dissatisfied you are with the way in which each of these parts of the NHS runs nowadays: local doctors or GPs, being in hospital as an inpatient, attending hospital as an outpatient, and NHS dentists?

It is possible from the survey to monitor changes in attitude to the NHS and specific sectors of health care over time. As Table 10.1 shows, over the last two decades there is clear evidence of a decline in satisfaction with the NHS overall. While this trend was halted in the early 1990s, possibly due to reforms in the NHS introduced at that time, the trend has continued up until the present, although there was an increase in satisfaction during the early years of the Labour administration between 1997 and 1999. The British Social Attitudes Survey data have been shown to report higher levels of dissatisfaction than other surveys, which in general record a high degree of satisfaction with health care (see Judge and Solomon 1993). This is believed to be due to the context in which the questions are asked. In the interview, the questions on satisfaction are next to questions about government priorities and public expenditure.

TABLE 10.1   Satisfaction with the NHS, 1983–2002

	1983	1986	1989	1991	1994	1997	1998	2000	2002
Very/quite satisfied	55	40	36	40	44	34	42	42	40
Neither satisfied nor dissatisfied	20	19	18	19	17	15	22	19	18
Very/quite dissatisfied	25	39	46	41	38	50	36	39	41
Net satisfaction (satisfaction minus dissatisfaction)	+20	+1	−10	−1	+6	−16	+6	+3	−1
Base	1,719	3,066	2,930	2,836	3,469	3,146	3,146	3,426	2,287

Source: Appleby and Rosete (2003)

The British Social Attitudes Survey questions may elicit a more political response, whereas other satisfaction surveys may be more firmly grounded in local knowledge. It has been suggested that general attitudes to the NHS tell us as much about government popularity as they do about the NHS per se (Appleby and Rosete 2003).

(Continued)

(Continued)

An increasingly popular method of collecting interview data is via the telephone. The high level of access to a telephone in the UK coupled with concerns about security make the telephone an increasingly acceptable medium for interview. Baeza and Calnan (1998) used telephone interviews in a national study to evaluate the new health promotion arrangements introduced into general practice in England and Wales in 1996. Once again, a mixed-method design was employed, beginning with a national survey followed by a series of in-depth case studies using qualitative methods. The objective of the survey was to explore the extent and nature of health promotion activity being undertaken through a survey of all health authorities in England.

A postal survey was not appropriate because many of the questions were semi-structured and the interviewee was the person responsible for the health promotion scheme in the health authority. This could vary depending on the health authority and could be a manager, a health promotion worker, a medical adviser or a public health consultant. A face-to-face interview survey was inappropriate due to resource constraints. In the event, the response rate to the telephone interview was high with 89 per cent (n = 85) of the 96 health authorities in England taking part. The interviews lasted, on average, an hour.

Reading Health Research Based on Quantitative Survey Methods

The appraisal of published survey research involves consideration of a number of issues, including that the research questions need to be specific and precise – particularly if a hypothesis is being tested. The key questions are:

- What types of research questions are being addressed? Are they descriptive questions: what, who, when? Or are they explanatory questions: why?
- Is the survey research design suitable for addressing these types of research questions?
- Are there causal influences imputed in the question and, if so, is there a temporal aspect to the design?
- How are concepts operationalized and how are measures or indicators selected and why?
- How reliable and valid are the indicators used in the study?
- Is there any bias in the selection of respondents?
- Are details of the response rate described and the characteristics of the non-respondents presented?
- Is there any bias in the selection of questions?
- How are the methods of data collection selected, and are they appropriate?
- How are the data analysed, and was the statistical analysis appropriate and sufficient?
- Are the conclusions derived from the evidence?
- Are the limitations in the survey methodology taken into account in the interpretation of the findings?

Conclusion

The survey is probably the most widely used and well-tested method for obtaining data from a selected population. If correct sampling techniques are used, then findings can be generalized to very large populations. As has been argued, the survey can be particularly effective when used to compare changes over time. However, surveys can also be carried out on a modest scale and telephone surveys in particular can be a useful technique for students and other researchers. Questionnaire design with critical reflection on what a question is aiming to find out and pilot testing of questions is a crucial aspect of conducting a survey. All surveys require careful planning and management and need to be underpinned by good administrative systems. If interviewers are being used, they should be properly trained and briefed prior to, and during, the course of a project. The unexpected often occurs during the course of the fieldwork or data collection phase and interviewers may require access to ongoing support and discussion with researcher leaders.

The examples set out in this chapter highlight how different survey methods have been used in practice in health research. The reader now has the opportunity to complete an exercise on translating concepts into indicators in the health field.

Exercise: Translating concepts of health into indicators

The final section of this chapter provides a problem-solving exercise which readers are invited to complete. It follows the discussion presented in an earlier section about how concepts can be operationalized into indicators by using a descending ladder of abstraction. The focus of the exercise is on translating concepts of health into indicators or questions to be used in a survey that aims to assess the health status of the adult population. Figure 10.8 provides a schema to encourage readers to break down the general abstract concept of health into various component parts. Reference back to Figure 10.1 may be helpful as a guide.

Fill in the empty boxes in Figure 10.8 which provide a ladder of abstraction by:

1 Providing a number of different definitions of health.
2 Choosing one definition on which to focus.
3 Identifying the dimensions and sub-dimensions which emerge from the chosen definition.
4 Developing questions that would act as indicators of these dimensions and sub-dimensions in the sample survey of the adult population.

Once the exercise is completed, readers might like to evaluate their indicators against a standardized instrument for measuring physical and mental health status – such as the SF-36 or the Nottingham Health Profile (Jenkinson 1994).

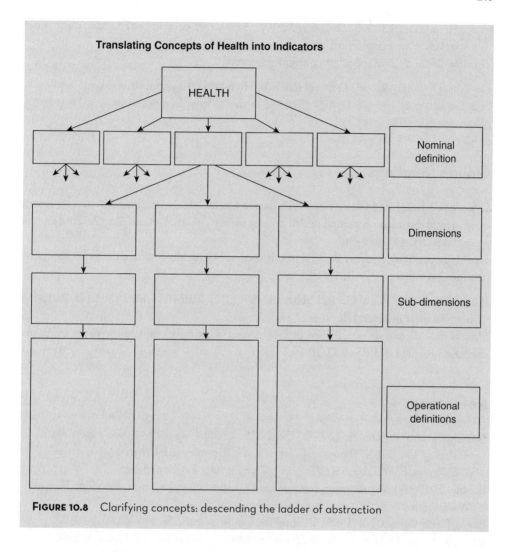

FIGURE 10.8   Clarifying concepts: descending the ladder of abstraction

Recommended Further Reading

Babbie, E. (2008) *The Basics of Social Research*, International edition. London: Thomson/ Wadsworth.
This is a very accessible introductory textbook, setting survey methods within a general context of other research methods.

Bryman, A. (2012) *Social Research Methods*, 4th edition. Oxford: Oxford University Press.
This book provides useful complementary reading to this chapter, especially in Part 2, and is strongly recommended.

Czaja, R. and Blair, J. (2005) *Designing Surveys: A Guide to Decisions and Procedures*. Thousand Oaks, CA: Pine Forge Press.
This is a detailed guide specific to designing surveys.

De Vaus, D. (2002) *Surveys in Social Research*, 5th edition. London: Routledge.
This text covers all the main issues discussed in this chapter in more detail – and is strongly recommended.

companion website ## Online Readings

O'Reilly, C., Bell, J. and Chen, T. (2010) 'Pharmacists' beliefs about treatments and outcomes of mental disorders: A mental health literacy survey', *Australian and New Zealand Journal of Psychiatry*, 44: 1089–96.
How is a quantitative survey defined in this context? Critically evaluate the paper using the checklist provided in PPS10.13/10.14.

Fitzpatrick, S. Bramley, G. and Johnsen, S. (2012) 'Pathways into multiple exclusion homelessness in seven UK cities', *Urban Studies*.
How is quantitative survey defined in this context? Critically evaluate the paper using the checklist provided in PPS10.13/10.14.

References

Appleby, J. and Rosete, A. (2003) 'The NHS: keeping up with public expectations', in A. Park., J. Curtice, K. Thomson, L. Jarvis and C. Bromley (eds), *British Social Attitudes: The 20th Report. Continuity and Change over Two Decades*. London: Sage.

Babbie, E. (2008) *The Basics of Social Research*, International edition. London: Thomson/Wadsworth.

Baeza, J. and Calnan, M. (1998) 'Beating the bands?', *Health Services Journal*, 26–7.

Bourque, L. and Fielder, E. (2003) *How to Conduct Telephone Surveys*. London: Sage.

Bryman, A. (2012) *Social Research Methods*. Oxford: Oxford University Press.

Calnan, M., Cant, S. and Gabe, J. (1993) *Going Private*. Buckingham: Open University Press.

Calnan, M. and Rowe, R. (2008) *Trust Matters in Health Care*. Buckingham: Open University Press.

Calnan, M. and Sanford, E. (2004) 'Public trust in health care: the system or the doctor?', *Quality and Safety in Health Care*, 13: 92–7.

Calnan, M. and Wainwright, D. (2002) 'Is general practice stressful?', *European Journal of General Practice*, 8(1): 5–17.

Calnan, M., Wainwright, D., O'Neill, C., Winterbottom, A. and Watkins, A. (2005) 'Lay evaluation of health care: the case of upper limb pain', *Health Expectations*, 8(2): 149–60.

Couper, M.P. (2008) *Designing Effective Web Surveys*. Cambridge: Cambridge University Press.

Czaja, R. and Blair, J. (2005) *Designing Surveys: A Guide to Decisions and Procedures*. Thousand Oaks, CA: Pine Forge Press.

De Vaus, D. (2002) *Surveys in Social Research*, 5th edition. London: Routledge.

Edwards, P.J., Roberts, I., Clarke, M.J., DiGuiseppi, C., Wentz, R., Kwan, I., Cooper, R., Felix, L.M. and Pratap, S. (2009) 'Methods to increase response to postal and electronic questionnaires', *Cochrane Database of Systematic Reviews*, Issue 3, Art. No. MR000008.

Fink, A. (2003) *The Survey Handbook*, 2nd edition. London: Sage.

Fowler, F. (2001) *Survey Research Methods*. London: Sage.

Jenkinson, C. (ed.) (1994) *Measuring Health and Medical Outcomes*. London: UCL Press.

Judge, K. and Solomon, M. (1993) 'Public opinion and the National Health Service: patterns and perspectives in consumer satisfaction', *Journal of Social and Political Studies*, 22(3): 299–322.

Litwin, M.S. (1995) *How to Measure Survey Reliability and Validity*. London: Sage.

Lozar Manfreda, K., Bosnjak, M., Berzelak, J., Haas, I., Vehovar, V. and Berzelak, N. (2007) 'Web surveys versus other survey modes: a meta-analysis comparing response rates', *International Journal of Market Research*, 50: 79–104.

Park, A., Curtice, J., Thomson, K., Jarvis, L. and Bromley, C. (eds) (2003) *British Social Attitudes: The 20th Report. Continuity and Change over Two Decades*. London: Sage.

Shih, T.H. and Fan, X. (2008) 'Comparing response rates from web and mail surveys: a meta-analysis', *Field Methods*, 20: 249–71.

Van Geest, J.B., Johnson, T.P. and Welch, V.L. (2007) 'Methodologies for improving response rates in surveys of physicians: a systematic review', *Evaluation and the Health Professions*, 30: 303–21.

Van der Schee, E., Braun, B., Calnan, M., Schnee, M. and Groenewegen, D. (2007) 'Public trust in health care: a comparison of Germany, The Netherlands, and England and Wales', *Health Policy*, 81: 56–67.

Wilson, P., Petticrew, M., Calnan, M. and Nazareth, I. (2010) 'Effects of a financial incentive on health researchers' response to an online survey: a randomized controlled trial', *Medical Internet Research*, 12(2): e13.

11

Statistical Methods for Health Data Analysis

GEORGE ARGYROUS

Introduction

- This chapter provides a basic introduction to statistics for analysing health data. Although there are a number of texts that detail the use of statistics in the health field (see, for example, Scott and Mazhindu 2009; Argyrous 2011; Dancey et al. 2012), the distinguishing feature of this chapter is its accessibility in introducing the subject of *data analysis* – what we do with quantitative research information once we have gathered it. More specifically, this chapter helps us to describe data more effectively. As such, it focuses on the first step in statistical analysis – straightforward statistical description – pointing the way to more advanced methods for those who wish to undertake further reading on the subject. For example, if we have collected measurements for the sex, age, amount of weekly exercise, smoking history and health status of patients visiting a clinic on a certain day, this chapter should help us to communicate this information more effectively, beyond simply listing the individual measurements that give the *distribution* for each of these variables.

- *Descriptive statistics* are the numerical, graphical and tabular techniques for organizing, analysing and presenting data. The major types of descriptive statistics are listed in Table 11.1.

- The great advantage of descriptive statistics is that they make a mass of research material easier to 'read' by reducing a large set of data into a few statistics, or into a graph or table.

TABLE 11.1 Types of descriptive statistics

Type	Function	Examples
Graphs	Provide a visual representation of the distribution of a variable or variables	Pie, bar, histogram, polygon (univariate) Clustered pie, clustered/stacked bar (bivariate, nominal/ordinal scales) Scatterplot (bivariate, interval/ratio scales)
Tables	Provide a frequency distribution for a variable or variables	Frequency table (univariate) Cross-tabulations (bivariate/multivariate)
Numerical measures	Mathematical operations used to quantify, in a single number, particular features of a distribution	Measures of central tendency (univariate) Measures of dispersion (univariate) Measures of association and correlation (bivariate/multivariate)

Levels of Measurement

Many considerations are involved in the decision as to which descriptive statistic most effectively summarizes a set of data. One of the most important is the level at which each variable is measured. To illustrate what is meant by *levels of measurement*, assume that the health status of the patients in our study is measured in three different ways, based on simplified measures used in the Australian Bureau of Statistics (2007–2008):

- By classifying patients according to the organ of the body affected by their disease (for example, blood and blood-forming organs, the nervous system, the respiratory system).
- By classifying patients according to whether they rate themselves as Very Unhealthy, Unhealthy, Healthy or Very Healthy.
- By counting the number of times in the previous year a patient has consulted a doctor or other health professional.

Each of these scales provides a different amount of information about the variation in health status among patients. The first scale of measurement classifies patients according to the organ system where the disease is located. This scale only allows us to say that patients are qualitatively different according to the location of the disease and, as such, is an example of a *nominal* scale: it classifies cases into categories that have no quantitative ordering.

Compare this to the second scale for measuring health status. The four categories that make up the scale have a logical order, starting with the lowest point, Very Unhealthy, and moving up to the highest point, Very Healthy. This scale allows us not only to talk about patients being different in terms of their health status, but also to say that the health status

of individual patients is better or worse than others. This ability to *rank-order* cases according to the quantity or intensity of the variable expressed by each case makes this an *ordinal*
scale. We cannot, however, measure how much healthier one person is relative to another.

The third scale for measuring health status does allow us to measure such differences. As
with nominal and ordinal scales, measuring the number of times in the past year someone
has consulted a health professional allows us to classify patients into different groups. As
with ordinal (but not nominal) scales, we can rank patients according to their respective
scores from lowest to highest. But unlike both nominal and ordinal scales, we can measure the differences – the intervals – between them. We now have a unit of measurement,
number of consultations, which allows us to quantify the difference in health status. This is
therefore an example of an *interval/ratio* scale (sometimes called a *metric* scale).

This example of measuring health status illustrates that any given variable can be measured at different levels, depending on the particular scale that is used. It is important to be
clear about the level at which a variable has been measured, since the descriptive statistics
that we calculate to express any variation across cases may be limited by this fact.

Graphs

Graphs or *charts* are the simplest, and often most striking, method for describing data, and
there are some general rules that apply to their construction. Most importantly, a graph
should be a self-contained bundle of information. In order for a graph to be a self-contained
description of the data, we need to:

- Give the graph a clear title indicating the variable displayed and the cases that make up
  the study.
- Clearly identify the categories or values of the variable.
- Indicate, for interval/ratio data, the units of measurement.
- Indicate the total number of cases.
- Explain any difference between the total in the graph and the total number of cases in
  the study.
- Indicate the source of the data.

Pie charts

The pie graph drawn for the patient survey in Figure 11.1 illustrates these rules of presentation. A *pie graph* presents the distribution of cases in the form of a circle. The relative size of
each slice of the pie is equal to the proportion of cases within the category represented by
the slice. Pie charts can be constructed for all levels of measurement and their main function is to emphasize the relative importance of a particular category to the total. They are

therefore mainly used to highlight distributions where cases are concentrated in only one or two categories. For example, the pie chart in Figure 11.1 highlights the heavy concentration of patients who have a disease of the respiratory system.

Pie graphs begin to look a bit clumsy when there are too many categories for the variable. As a rule of thumb, there should be no more than five slices to the pie. Thus, the pie chart in Figure 11.1 has grouped together a number of categories with low frequencies into an 'Other' category.

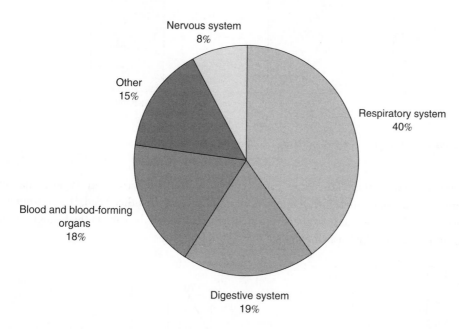

FIGURE 11.1   Pie graph: main organ affected by disease for a sample of patients (n = 200)

Bar graphs and histograms

Bar graphs and *histograms* emphasize the frequency of cases in each category relative to each other. Along one axis of these graphs are the categories or values of the scale. This axis is called the *abscissa,* and is usually the horizontal base of the graph. Along the other axis are the *frequencies,* expressed either as the raw count or as percentages of the total number of cases. This axis is known as the *ordinate.* This is usually the left, vertical axis. A rectangle is erected over each point on the abscissa, with the area of each rectangle being proportional to the frequency of the value in the overall distribution.

The difference between bar graphs and histograms is that bar graphs are constructed for discrete variables, such as the sex of patients, which are usually measured on a nominal or ordinal scale, as illustrated by Figure 11.2.

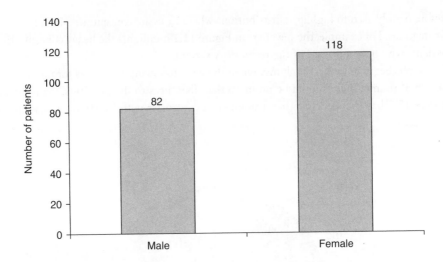

FIGURE 11.2 **FIGURE 11.2** Bar graph: sex of patients

With bar graphs, there are always gaps between each of the bars: there is no gradation between male and female, for example. A person's age, on the other hand, is a continuous variable, in the sense that it progressively increases. As a result, the bars on the histogram for age in Figure 11.3 are 'pushed together'.

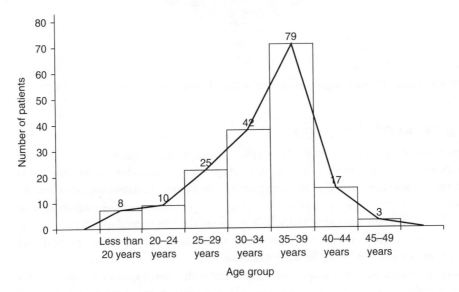

FIGURE 11.3 Histogram: age of patients

As an alternative to a histogram, Figure 11.3 also presents the distribution for age of patients in the form of a *frequency polygon*, which is a continuous line formed by plotting the values in a distribution against the frequency for each value.

Interpreting graphs

Once we have constructed the relevant graph, we then need to interpret it. When we look at a graph, we generally try to identify one or more of the following four aspects of the distribution it represents:

- The shape.
- The centre.
- The spread.
- The existence of outliers.

There are certain common *shapes* that appear in research. For example, the histogram for age in Figure 11.3 is 'bell shaped' or 'mound shaped'. For a distribution that has this 'bell shape', we also describe its *skewness*. If the curve has a long tail to the right, it is *positively skewed*, or, as is the case with the age distribution of patients, a long tail to the left indicates a *negatively skewed* distribution. If the tails on either side look reasonably similar, we describe the shape as *symmetrical*.

To gauge the *centre* of a distribution, imagine that the bars of the histogram are lead weights sitting on a balance beam. Where would we have to locate a balance point along the bottom edge of the graph to prevent it from tipping either to the left or right? This, in a loose fashion, identifies the average or typical score. In the example in Figure 11.3, we might say that the average age of patients is around 35–39 years of age.

We can also observe how tightly clustered our measurements are around the central point. Do the scores *spread* very wide across the range of possible values (that is, the distribution is *heterogeneous*) or are most similar to each other (that is, the distribution is *homogeneous*)?

Lastly, we can also note the existence of any *outliers* that are not just at the upper or lower end of the tails, but are disconnected from the rest of the group. Figure 11.4, for example, presents the annual frequency of visiting a health professional. We can immediately see an outlier with 12 visits to a health professional in the previous year. Where we identify such an outlier, we isolate the reason why it appears (data entry error or real case), and exclude it from further analysis so that it does not distort other statistics. But when we exclude an outlier from further analysis, we need to always make it clear to the reader that we have done so.

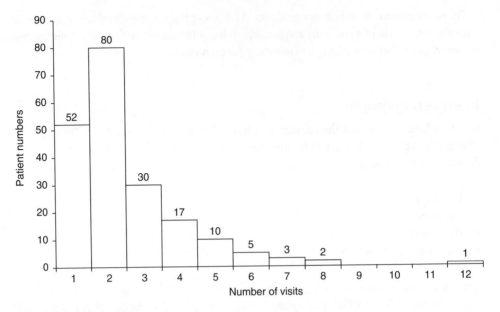

FIGURE 11.4 Number of visits to a health professional in the past year

Frequency Tables

The power of graphs is their simplicity; the visual impact of a graph can convey a message better than the most advanced statistics. The simplicity of graphs can also be their weakness. We often do want to 'dig deeper' to extract more precise understandings of the data than can be gleaned from a chart. Obtaining a more detailed breakdown of a distribution usually begins with the construction of *frequency tables*. At the very least, a frequency table tallies up the number of times (f) each value of the variable appears in a distribution. Such a table has in the first column the name of the variable displayed in the title row, followed by the categories or values of the variable down the subsequent rows of the first column. The second column then presents the frequencies for each category or value. Table 11.2 presents the same distribution as Figure 11.4, but provides much more detail about the frequency of cases across the range of scores for number of visits to the doctor.

Frequency tables follow the same rules of presentation that we listed above for graphs, with the addition of the following points:

- Arrange the values of ordinal and interval/ratio scales so that the lowest score in the distribution appears in the first row and the scale then increases down the page. Thus in Table 11.2, which presents the distribution of an interval/ratio scale, we have as the first row those who visited a health professional only once.

- Arrange the categories of nominal scales so that the category with the highest frequency (referred to below as the mode) is the first row. The category with the second highest frequency is the second row, and so on. The modal category is often of specific interest when analysing the distribution of a nominal variable, and therefore it is convenient to present it first.

TABLE 11.2   Number of visits to doctor or other health professional in the previous year

Number of visits	Frequency	Per cent*	Cumulative frequency	Cumulative per cent
1	52	26	52	26
2	80	40	132	66
3	30	15	162	81
4	17	9	172	86
5	10	5	182	95
6	5	3	187	97
7	3	2	197	99
8	2	1	199	99
More than 8	1	<1	200	100
Total	200	100		

Note: * Does not add up to 100 per cent due to rounding error.

Table 11.2 also provides the *relative frequencies*, which express the number of cases within each value of a variable as a percentage or proportion of the total number of cases. *Percentages* are statistics that standardize the total number of cases to a base value of 100, whereas *proportions* standardize the total to a base of 1. The formulae for calculating a percentage or proportion respectively are:

$$\% = \frac{f}{n} \times 100$$

$$p = \frac{f}{n}$$

where f is the frequency of cases in a particular category and n is the total number of cases.

Notice that the column of percentages in Table 11.2 should add up to 100 per cent, since all cases must fall into one classification or another. The actual percentages listed in the table, however, sum to 101 per cent, as the numbers have been 'rounded off'. Where this occurs, a footnote should be added to the table that states 'Does not sum to 100 due to rounding error', or words to that effect, as is done in Table 11.2.

With ordinal and interval/ratio data, one further extension to the simple frequency table can be made, which is also illustrated in Table 11.2. This is the addition of columns providing *cumulative frequencies* and *cumulative relative frequencies.* Since ordinal and interval/ratio scales allow us to rank-order cases from lowest to highest, it is sometimes interesting to know the number, and/or percentage, of cases that fall above or below a certain point on the scale. For example, in Table 11.2 we can see that 162 patients (81%) visited a health professional three times or less, which is the sum of the frequencies in the first three rows of the table. By implication this means that 19 per cent of patients visited a health professional more than three times in the last year. Cumulative frequencies are not appropriate where we have a nominal scale, as the ordering of the categories is not fixed, or where there are only two categories, as the simple frequencies and cumulative frequencies will be the same.

One additional point needs to be made about tabulating interval/ratio data: we often use *class intervals* rather than individual values to construct a frequency distribution. A *class interval* groups together a range of values for presentation and analysis. We use class intervals if the range of values that appears in the distribution is so large that it makes presentation and analysis difficult. For example, if we have many individual ages for the patients in our study, we may first group them into five-year intervals, such as 1–5 years, 6–10 years, and so on, before constructing the table or graph. Generally, class intervals should have the same width, although at the lower and upper end of the data range we often have open-ended intervals, such as '60 years or over'. The exception is the value of 0, which is usually listed separately. It is common for readers of tables to be specifically interested in the number of cases that have a zero value for a particular variable. The actual width of class intervals depends on the particular situation, especially the amount of information required. The wider the class intervals, the easier it is to 'read' the table, since this will reduce the number of rows. However, this increase in 'readability' comes at the cost of information, and therefore should not be undertaken if the data are already in a few, easily presented, values.

Measures of Central Tendency

We mentioned above that graphs and tables give us a quick visual sense of key features of a distribution. But we sometimes want to be more precise about the centre of a distribution. For instance, rather than stating that 'the scores tend to centre around an average of 35–39 years', we may need to be more precise about the average score. *Measures of central tendency* indicate the typical or average value for a distribution.

There are three common measures of central tendency: mode, median and mean. Each measure embodies a different notion of average and choosing the measure to calculate on a given set of data is restricted by the level at which a variable is measured.

The mode

The *mode* (M_o) is the simplest measure of central tendency, and can be calculated for all levels of measurement. The mode is the value in a distribution that has the highest frequency. The great advantage of the mode over other measures of centre is that it is very easy to calculate. A simple inspection of a frequency table is enough to determine the mode. In Table 11.2, for example, we can see that the most frequent number of times a patient visited a health professional is 2, which accounts for 80 patients. However, the mode has one major limitation that arises especially when it is used to describe interval/ratio data that have many values. Take, for example, the following scores that represent the time in seconds for a drug to take effect on a sample of patients, arranged in rank order:

36, 36, 81, 82, 84, 85, 86, 89, 91, 95, 97, 98

It is clear to the naked eye that the data are 'centred' somewhere in the range of 85–90 seconds. Yet the mode is 36 seconds since this appears twice in the distribution, whereas every other score appears only once. The mode is not really reflecting the central tendency of this distribution. We should either use other measures of central tendency, such as those we are about to discuss, or else organize the data into suitable class intervals, and report the modal class interval, rather than the individual modal score.

The mean and median

With interval/ratio data, the *mean* and *median* can be calculated as measures of central tendency rather than the mode. The mean is the sum of all scores in a distribution divided by the total number of cases. The actual formula we use to calculate the mean depends on whether we have the data in listed form or in a frequency table. If we have the raw data with each individual score listed separately, the equations for the mean of the population and the mean of a sample respectively are:

$$\mu = \frac{\sum X_i}{N}, \bar{X} = \frac{\sum X_i}{n}$$

where μ (pronounced 'mu') is the mean for an entire population, N is the size of the population, X (pronounced 'X-bar') is the mean for a sample, n is the size of the sample, and X_i is each score in a distribution. The symbol Σ (pronounced 'sigma') means 'the sum of' (or 'the total from the addition of'), so we read these equations in the following way: 'the mean equals the sum of all scores divided by the number of cases'.

Alternatively, where the scores are already grouped into a frequency table such as in Table 11.2, the relevant formula for a sample is:

$$\bar{X} = \frac{\sum fX_i}{n}$$

This formula instructs us to multiply each score by the frequency with which it appears in the table and to sum these products before dividing by the number of cases. For Table 11.2, the calculations will be:

$$\bar{X} = \frac{\sum fX_i}{n}$$
$$= \frac{(1 \times 52) + (2 \times 80) + (3 \times 30) + (4 \times 17) + (5 \times 10) + (6 \times 5) + (3 \times 7) + (2 \times 8)}{199}$$
$$= \frac{487}{199}$$
$$= 2.4 \text{ visits}$$

The mean has two major limitations, both of which derive from the fact that it is calculated using every score in the distribution. The first limitation is that it is affected by the presence of outliers, and therefore we generally exclude outliers from the calculation of the mean. Thus, when calculating the mean number of visits to a health professional, we exclude the one 'outlier' who visited a health professional more than eight times. When presenting a 'trimmed' mean as the centre of distribution, it should be noted to the reader that such 'trimming' has occurred.

The other limitation to the use of the mean as a measure of central tendency, even where outliers are excluded, is that its value is pulled away from the centre of a distribution that is skewed. For example, in Figure 11.4 we can see that the spread of scores for number of health visits is skewed to the right and this has produced a value for the mean that is higher than that we might expect from a quick visual inspection (even after we exclude outliers).

An alternative measure of central tendency to the mean, especially where a distribution is heavily skewed, is the *median* (M_d). If all the cases in a distribution are ranked from lowest to highest, the median is the score in the middle of the sequence. The actual calculation of the median will differ according to whether we have an odd or even number of scores. For an odd number of rank-ordered cases, the median is the middle score. For an even number of rank-ordered cases, the median is the mean of the two middle scores. Thus, if I lined up the 200 patients in my study according to the frequency with which they visited a doctor in the previous year, starting with patients that attended a health professional only once, the middle scores in this line-up are those for the 100th and 101st patients, both of which have a value of 2 visits. We have an even number of cases, so the median is the mean of these two middle scores, which is 2.

If a cumulative relative frequency table such as Table 11.2 has been generated, an easier way to calculate the median is to identify the value at which the cumulative per cent first passes 50 (i.e. 2 visits). We can see that the median depends solely on the value of these scores in the middle, and is not 'pulled' in one direction or another by the long tail of a skewed distribution or the presence of any outliers, factors which we have seen affect the value of the mean.

Measures of Dispersion

Measures of dispersion are descriptive statistics that indicate the spread or variety of scores in a distribution, and most of these require interval/ratio-level measurement (a measure for nominal scales, the Index of Qualitative Variation, is not covered here, but further details can be found in Argyrous 2011: 198). The simplest measure of dispersion is the *range*, which is the difference between the lowest score and highest score. This is an easily calculated measure of dispersion, because it involves a straightforward subtraction of one score from another. This advantage of the range is also its major limitation: it only uses the extreme scores, and therefore changes with the values of the two extreme scores.

The *inter-quartile range* (IQR) overcomes this problem with the simple range by ignoring the extreme scores of a distribution. The IQR is the range for the middle 50 per cent of cases in a rank-ordered series: the difference between the lower limit of the first quartile and the upper limit of the third quartile. Unlike the simple range, the IQR will not change dramatically if we add one or two cases to either end of the distribution.

The *standard deviation* is a more complex measure of spread, the value of which captures the average distance each score is away from the mean, and is calculated for a sample and population respectively by the following equations:

$$s = \sqrt{\frac{\sum\left(X_i - \bar{X}\right)^2}{n-1}} \text{ (sample)}, \sigma = \sqrt{\frac{\sum\left(X_i - \mu\right)^2}{N}} \text{ (population)}$$

where s represents the standard deviation for a sample, and σ (pronounced 'sigma') represents the standard deviation for a population.

A close look at these equations indicates how they capture the notion that the standard deviation is the average distance that each score is from the mean. The numerator is the difference between each score and the mean, and the denominator adjusts those differences by the number of cases. Unfortunately, we cannot simply add all the *positive deviations* (scores above the mean) to all the *negative deviations* (scores below the mean), since by definition these will sum to zero. This is why the equation for the standard deviation squares the differences: it thereby turns all the deviations into positive numbers, so that the larger the differences, the greater the value of the standard deviation. But the general idea is clear. Distributions that are more spread out will have many scores that are different from the mean, producing numerous large deviations and thereby a high value for the standard deviation. Another set of scores may have the same mean, but with the scores more tightly clustered around it. In this case, the deviations between each score and the mean will thereby generally be small, producing a lower value for the standard deviation.

Bivariate Descriptive Statistics: Simple Comparisons

The previous section looked at methods for describing the distribution of a single variable. This *univariate analysis* can help address simple questions such as 'what is the age distribution of patients?' or 'what is the health status of patients visiting a clinic?' This simple analysis may only be a precursor to more complex analysis that asks whether the health status of patients is related to another variable, such as their smoking history. A question that addresses the possible *relationship* between two variables requires *bivariate statistical analysis*.

Probably everyone has a common-sense notion of what it means for two variables to be 'related to' each other. We know that older children also tend to be taller: age and height are related. This example expresses a general concept for which we have an intuitive feel: as the value of one variable changes, the value of the other variable also changes. If we do believe two variables such as health status and smoking are related, we need to express this relationship in the form of a *theoretical model* before we undertake bivariate analysis to measure the relationship. A theoretical model is an abstract depiction of the possible relationships among variables. For this example, the model is easy to depict. If there is a relationship, it is because a patient's smoking history affects their health level. It is not possible for the relationship to 'run in the other direction' – a patient's smoking history will not change as a result of a change in their health level. In this instance, we say that smoking history is the *independent variable* and health status is the *dependent variable*.

Once we have specified the model that we believe underpins any relationship between two variables, we can then generate appropriate statistics to see if such a relationship does in fact appear in the data we collect. There are two ways we can assess whether a relationship exists between two variables:

- For each of the groups defined by the independent variable, calculate univariate descriptive statistics to summarize the dependent variable and compare the differences.
- Calculate measures of association and correlation.

The first method is the simpler since we generate the univariate statistics we have already discussed, but rather than doing so for the whole data set, we generate these statistics for each of the groups defined by the independent variable. For example, if I wished to see whether health status is affected by smoking history, I would calculate summary statistics for health status, but I would do so separately for smokers and for non-smokers. This is illustrated by the *stacked bar chart* in Figure 11.5. The same comparison between smokers and non-smokers is also made using the *bivariate table* in Table 11.3 (also known as a *contingency table* or *cross-tabulation*, or '*cross-tab*' for short).

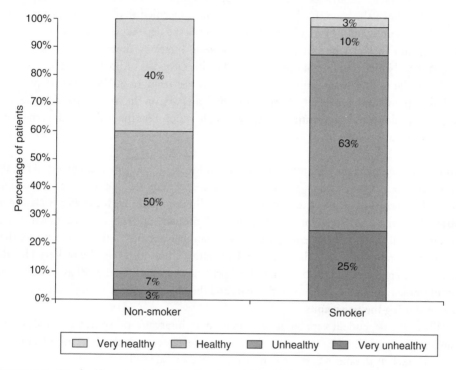

FIGURE 11.5   Stacked bar chart: health rating by smoking history of clinic patients

TABLE 11.3   Health rating by smoking history of clinic patients

Health rating	Smoking history		
	Non-smoker	Smoker	Total
Very Unhealthy	3%	25%	12%
Unhealthy	7%	63%	29%
Healthy	50%	10%	34%
Very Healthy	40%	3%	25%
Total	100%	100%	100%
	(120)	(80)	(200)

It should be noted that with cross-tabs we follow these two rules for arranging the information:

- Place the appropriate variables in the rows and columns. If there is reason to believe that one of the variables is dependent on the other, the categories of the independent variable should be arranged across the columns and the categories of the dependent variable down the rows. In this example, we have specified that smoking history is the independent (column) variable and health status is the dependent (row) variable.
- For scales that can be ranked, ensure the scale increases down the rows/across the columns. Notice that one of the variables, 'Health rating', is ordinal. Thus, the categories that make up this scale can be ordered from lowest to highest. We therefore place the lowest point on the scale, the 'Very Unhealthy' category, on the first row, so that the scale increases down the page until we reach the highest point on the scale, which is the 'Very Healthy' category.

To help us compare the difference in the health levels of smokers and non-smokers, the cross-tab presents the *column percentages*. For example, we can see that of all 120 non-smokers in the study, 3 per cent were Very Unhealthy. This compares with the 25 per cent of all 80 smokers who were Very Unhealthy. Figure 11.5 similarly presents the breakdown of each group's health status as a percentage of the total number of cases in that group, rather than the actual number of people that are Very Unhealthy, Unhealthy, Healthy or Very Healthy. In both the cross-tab and the bar chart, these percentages adjust for the different total number of smokers and non-smokers in the data, and thereby allow for a more valid comparison than just using the raw counts.

Where the dependent variable is measured on an interval/ratio scale, we can also compare the groups defined by the categories of the independent variable in terms of summary statistics such as the mean and median, as illustrated in Table 11.4.

Once we have generated graphs, tables or summary statistics such as a mean to compare the relevant groups, the task is then to interpret the differences. We must assess whether they reveal a relationship between the two variables. When comparing differences between the relevant groups, we look at the *pattern* and *strength* of any relationship that such differences reveal. For example, the cross-tab in Table 11.3 shows that the health status of smokers is lower than for non-smokers and smokers are more heavily concentrated in the

TABLE 11.4   Average annual number of visits to health professional by smoking history of clinic patients

Measure of average	Non-smoker	Smoker
Mean number of visits to health professional	1.2	3.1
Median number of visits to health professional	1	3

Unhealthy category than non-smokers. We can thus say that there is a relationship between these variables and that the relationship is negative: a higher level of smoking is associated with lower health status.

Bivariate Descriptive Statistics: Measures of Association and Correlation

In the previous section, we detected a relationship between smoking and health status by observing a difference in the set of percentages in each column of a cross-tab. The next step is to ask: what is the *strength* of this relationship? We can make an arbitrary assessment of a relationship's strength by arguing that the two sets of column percentages are very different from each other and therefore suggest a moderate-to-strong relationship. We can, alternatively, arrive at a more precise and objective measure of the strength of a relationship by calculating numerical *measures of association and correlation.* These measures are descriptive statistics that quantify a relationship between two variables. Table 11.5 lists the most common measures.

Detailing the logic of each of these measures and the methods for calculating them is beyond the scope of this chapter, but for a comprehensive guide see Liebetrau (1983). We should note here, however, that as with most other statistics, the appropriate choice is affected by the level at which the variables under analysis have been measured, as indicated in Table 11.5.

TABLE 11.5   Measures of association and correlation

Measure	Data consideration
Lambda	At least one variable nominal
Goodman and Kruskal tau	At least one variable nominal
Eta	Independent variable is nominal and dependent variable is interval/ratio
Somer's *d*	Both variables at least ordinal
Gamma	Both variables at least ordinal
Kendall's tau-*b*	Both variables at least ordinal
Kendall's tau-*c*	Both variables at least ordinal
Spearman's rho	Both variables at least ordinal with many points on the scale
Pearson's *r*	Both variables interval/ratio with many points on the scale
Kappa	Both variables at least ordinal and measured on the same scale

The general point to note about these measures is that they give a precise value on a scale from 0 to 1, indicating the *strength* of any relationship observed between two variables. We can then interpret the value according to the terminology suggested in Table 11.6. Rather than just relying on a visual impression of a cross-tab or graph, measures of association thereby provide a single figure to show the strength of association. In addition, where both variables are measured at least at the ordinal level, a + or − sign also indicates the *direction* of association: whether an increase in the quantity of one variable is associated with an increase (positive association) or decrease (negative association) in the quantity of the other variable. For instance, in the previous part of the chapter we observed that the health level decreases as the smoking level increases, and therefore we observe a negative relationship between them.

TABLE 11.6   Interpreting values for measures of association and correlation

Range (±)	Relative strength
0	No relationship
0 >−0.2	Very weak, negligible relationship
0.2–0.4	Weak, low association
0.4–0.7	Moderate association
0.7–0.9	Strong, high, marked association
0.9–<1	Very high, very strong relationship
1	Perfect association

It is important to remember that the measures only detect a *statistical association;* they do not necessarily show whether one variable causes a change in another. We may suspect theoretically that one variable causes a change in the other, but the measures listed in Table 11.5 cannot prove causation. They only provide supporting evidence for a theoretical model. For example, a relationship between the number of storks in an area and the birth rate in that area has been observed, and we may calculate a measure that quantifies this statistical relationship. However, we cannot go from this statistical regularity to a conclusion that the presence of storks determines the birth rate!

Descriptive Statistics: Advanced Methods for Analysing Many Variables

The simple statistical techniques we have discussed above can take us a long way into data analysis and help answer many of the research questions we wish to answer. However, there are many more, and more complicated, methods of analysis that are available to the researcher willing to learn and use them. One such technique readers may frequently encounter is *regression analysis*, which seeks to depict the relationship between an independent variable and one or more dependent variables in the form of a *regression equation*. For example, we may have data for the number of minutes of weekly exercise undertaken by a sample of people, along with their respective rested pulse rates. To see whether these two variables are related, we use regression analysis to yield the following equation:

Rested pulse rate = 89 − 0.3 (minutes of weekly exercise)

This equation allows us to estimate the rested pulse rate for an individual given their respective exercise level. For example, where the amount of weekly exercise is 0, we expect the rested pulse rate to be 89 beats per minute (bpm). For every minute of weekly exercise above 0, we expect the rested pulse rate to decrease by 0.3. Thus, for someone who exercises for 30 minutes per week, we predict their pulse rate to be:

Rested pulse rate = 89 − 0.3(30) = 89 − 9 = 80 bpm

Regression analysis can be extended to take into account even more complex relationships involving three or more variables. For example, the relationship between regular exercise and pulse rate may be affected by a person's sex and also their age in years, and *multiple regression analysis* produces a single equation that will measure the extent to which each of these variables affects rested pulse rate.

Table 11.7 lists the main techniques for such *multivariate analysis*. To detail these choices for undertaking multivariate analysis would take us beyond the limits of this chapter, but see Argyrous (2011) for a more detailed introduction.

TABLE 11.7 Types of multivariate analysis

Multivariate technique	Data considerations
Multiple regression	Interval/ratio independent and dependent variables. Categorical independent variables can be included as dummy variables.
Logistic regression	Dependent variable is categorical and independent variables are interval/ratio.
Loglinear analysis	All variables are categorical.

Inferential Statistics

We have discussed at some length various ways of describing our data. These data often come from a sample rather than from the whole population, so that we are faced with a problem: are the sample statistics 'representative' of the population from which the sample is drawn? The operation of *sampling error* may cause the sample to be 'off'. Sampling error occurs when random factors cause us to include in our random sample members of the population that have relatively low or high scores for the variable we are investigating. This sampling error then causes the overall sample statistics to be different from those we would have obtained if we had studied the whole population. Given that sampling error is always a possibility, on what basis can we make a valid generalization from the sample to the population?

We address this problem with *inferential statistics.* Inferential statistics are the numerical techniques for making conclusions about a population based on the information obtained from a random sample drawn from that population. The nature of inferential statistics can be illustrated by an example. Assume that we have randomly selected 200 people who perform regular weekly exercise and we find that this sample has a mean resting pulse rate of 60 bpm, and standard deviation of 10 bpm. What can we infer about the population of all people who exercise regularly?

We may have information that the general population has a mean rested pulse rate of 72 bpm. On the basis of the sample result, can we say that the *population* of all people who exercise regularly is lower than that for the general population? Maybe it is not, and our sample of 200 has produced a relatively low mean rested pulse rate as a result of sampling error. Alternatively, maybe the population of regular exercisers does have a lower mean rested pulse rate and the sample of 200 reflects this. The process of *hypothesis testing* helps us decide between these inferences by calculating the *statistical significance* of the sample result (also called the *p*-value). Statistical significance is the probability that the sample did indeed come from a population of regular exercisers whose mean rested pulse rate is the same as that for the general population, and that the low sample mean is due to sampling error alone.

Another way of making an inference from a sample result to the population is to ask from what kind of population it is reasonable to assume the sample was derived. If the sample mean is within the 'normal' bounds of sampling error, what range of values can we confidently believe includes the population mean? Answering this type of question involves the calculation of *confidence intervals.* In our example, we may calculate the confidence interval to be 60 ± 1.4 bpm. In other words, if we assume that the sample is not greatly affected by sampling error, the population from which it is drawn has a mean rested pulse rate between 58.6 and 61.4 bpm. Underlying the calculation of such a confidence interval is the simple logic that random samples will only rarely produce a result that is very different from the value for the population from which it is drawn.

This section gives some general idea about the role of inferential statistics in quantitative analysis, but the issues and calculations involved in the application of inferential statistics are far more complex than we can discuss here. The recommended further reading at the end of the chapter should be consulted as a starting point for those wishing to grapple with these issues.

Tools for Analysing Quantitative Data

It was not long ago that statistical analysis was normally undertaken 'by hand' using pen and paper (and a calculator). Since the development of affordable desktop computers, and the Internet that connects them, manual calculations are the exception rather than the rule. There are four broad classes of alternatives to calculating by hand:

- *Spreadsheet data management programs*: practically every computer has an 'office' suite of software designed to handle various tasks such as word processing and data management. Examples include Microsoft Excel, OpenOffice and Gnumeric. Such programs can generate graphs, tables and most of the statistical analysis that we require. Their advantage is their ubiquity. Their disadvantage is that they do not perform more complicated statistical analysis, or if they do it is often through the use of complicated equations that have to be precisely entered.
- *Comprehensive commercial programs*: there are many commercial programs such as SPSS, GB-Stat, InStat, JMP, Minitab, SAS and StatA. A full list of such packages is available at statpages.org. These packages often have the appearance of spreadsheet data management programs, but are specifically designed for statistical analysis, so that they have a more complete range of options, and also the type of analysis desired can be selected from a menu of options rather than by entering equations on the spreadsheet.
- *Free comprehensive programs*: an exciting development in recent years is the availability of free software, and this includes some useful statistical analysis software. A list of such software is available at freestatistics.altervista.org/stat.php and statpages.org/javasta2.html#Freebies. Of these, Epi Info developed by the US Center for Disease Control (www.cdc.gov/epiinfo) is particularly worth mentioning as a tool for health researchers. An open-source version of Epi Info, called OpenEpi, which runs on all platforms and in a web browser, is available from www.openepi.com
- *Calculation pages for specific statistical pages*: these are web pages that provide tools for conducting specific analysis. A general listing of these pages is available at the web page or statpages.org

Conclusion

The chapter has covered a wide range of tools for quantitative data analysis. A key element in determining which of these tools are appropriate is the way in which our variables of interest have been measured. In particular, we first need to determine whether our variables have been measured at the nominal, ordinal or interval/ratio levels.

We then introduced three broad classes of statistical techniques that help us describe the data that we collect, namely graphs, tables and numerical calculations, and within each of these broad groups we have further choices. For example, we saw that there are different classes of numerical calculations depending on whether we are trying to identify the central tendency of a distribution or the amount of dispersion it contains. The choices also depend on how complicated the analysis is that we wish to undertake – whether we are interested in describing the distribution of a single variable, or the relationship between two variables, or indeed the relationship among many variables.

The chapter concludes with an exercise in which the reader is invited to apply some of the statistical methods outlined to the health data set out in Table 11.8.

Reading Health Research Based on Statistics

The following is a useful checklist of questions to ask when reading statistics in the literature. When reading simple summary statistics, you should ask:

1 Which average is calculated: mean or median? (ideally both!)
2 If the mean, with or without outliers/extreme scores? If yes, note the bias this produces in the calculation of the mean.
3 If the mean, for a skewed distribution? If yes, note the bias this produces in the calculation of the mean.
4 Are measures of spread provided along with measures of average? If not, question the usefulness of averages if the data are very disperse.
5 Have the authors averaged averages or percentages? Averages should always be calculated using the raw data, rather than taken from summary statistics that have already been calculated from these data.

When reading inferential statistics, you should ask:

1 What is the practical significance of any *statistically significant* difference? A result may be statistically significant, especially when it comes from very large samples, but the measured effect in practical terms may be too small to worry about.
2 What is the confidence (alpha) level at which statistical significance is decided? Is it sufficient relative to the importance of the results or consequences of being wrong? Ideally, results should present the exact p-value for any significance test so that readers can judge for themselves whether this is statistically significant by selecting an alpha level that is appropriate to their needs.
3 What is the confidence interval around the sample result?
4 Was the sample randomly selected?
5 What is the population to which a generalization is being made?

Exercise: Statistical tests on a health data set

TABLE 11.8   Health data set

ID	Height	Weight	Age	Sex	Smokes	Exercise	Pulse
1	180	77	18	F	No	15	47
2	186	87	23	M	No	12	49
3	188	87	20	M	No	14	50
4	171	71	41	M	No	15	52
5	173	64	20	F	No	12	55
6	182	63	20	M	No	8	56
7	169	68	19	M	No	12	58
8	175	75	20	M	No	10	59
9	175	65	19	M	No	11	60
10	182	85	20	M	No	14	60
11	170	54	20	F	No	8	60
12	175	54	18	F	No	10	61
13	170	60	18	M	No	11	62
14	183	73	20	M	No	5	63
15	164	78	28	F	No	5	64
16	173	70	20	M	No	9	64
17	170	56	19	M	No	9	64
18	170	62	20	F	No	4	64
19	165	58	23	F	No	8	64
20	180	75	20	M	No	4	65
21	184	65	21	M	No	8	65
22	167	75	20	F	No	10	65
23	174	60	19	F	No	8	66
24	162	60	19	F	No	8	66
25	175	66	20	M	No	11	66
26	158	51	18	F	No	8	68
27	180	85	19	M	Yes	10	68
28	191	78	19	M	No	8	68
29	164	56	19	F	No	5	68
30	176	59	19	M	No	6	68
31	162	57	20	F	No	7	68
32	170	65	18	M	No	10	69
33	180	72	18	M	No	4	69
34	157	41	20	F	No	11	70
35	177	74	18	F	No	5	70
36	140	50	34	F	No	6	70
37	163	55	20	F	No	7	70
38	163	51	18	F	No	10	70
39	182	85	20	M	Yes	2	70
40	170	68	22	M	No	5	70
41	178	62	21	M	No	1	70
42	163	47	23	F	No	4	71

(Continued)

TABLE 11.8 (Continued)

ID	Height	Weight	Age	Sex	Smokes	Exercise	Pulse
43	195	84	18	M	No	4	71
44	169	55	18	F	No	1	71
45	175	57	20	F	No	2	72
46	172	53	20	M	No	5	72
47	167	63	28	M	No	2	72
48	164	66	23	F	No	1	74
49	168	55	24	F	No	3	74
50	180	76	21	M	No	2	74
51	189	88	45	M	No	5	74
52	178	58	19	M	No	6	74
53	160	57	19	F	No	4	75
54	185	85	19	M	No	2	75
55	194	110	25	M	No	1	75
56	170	75	20	M	No	5	76
57	166	50	19	F	Yes	2	76
58	182	98	19	M	No	3	76
59	179	80	20	M	No	2	76
60	180	102	20	M	No	1	76
61	190	82	19	M	Yes	0	76
62	171	67	18	F	No	1	76
63	171	70	26	F	No	1	76
64	178	86	21	M	Yes	4	76
65	185	110	22	M	No	0	77
66	172	59	18	F	No	5	78
67	186	96	19	M	No	6	78
68	184	74	22	M	No	2	78
69	189	60	19	M	No	1	78
70	163	55	20	F	Yes	0	78
71	155	50	19	F	No	3	78
72	187	59	18	M	No	4	78
73	185	90	18	M	No	1	80
74	180	70	18	M	No	0	80
75	160	49	19	F	No	0	80
76	192	105	21	M	No	1	80
77	182	75	26	M	Yes	1	80
78	164	54	18	F	No	0	80
79	170	60	19	F	No	2	80
80	180	80	21	M	No	2	80
81	170	59	20	M	No	2	80
82	172	60	21	F	Yes	3	81
83	179	58	19	F	No	1	82
84	155	55	20	F	No	0	82
85	166	56	21	F	Yes	0	83
86	165	48	19	F	No	2	83

ID	Height	Weight	Age	Sex	Smokes	Exercise	Pulse
87	194	95	18	M	No	1	84
88	165	63	18	F	No	1	84
89	178	63	23	M	No	3	84
90	151	42	22	F	No	4	85
91	175	79	19	M	No	0	85
92	178	56	21	F	No	1	86
93	182	60	22	M	Yes	0	86
94	173	57	18	F	No	2	86
95	165	60	19	F	Yes	3	88
96	68	63	19	M	No	4	88
97	180	65	20	M	No	0	88
98	168	60	23	M	No	1	88
99	175	60	19	M	No	2	88
100	162	50	19	F	Yes	1	90
101	170	58	21	M	Yes	1	90
102	173	64	18	F	Yes	1	90
103	161	43	19	F	No	1	90
104	170	63	20	F	No	0	92
105	167	70	22	M	Yes	0	92
106	167	62	18	F	Yes	2	96
107	155	49	18	F	No	1	104
108	164	46	18	F	Yes	0	104
109	155	65	19	F	Yes	0	119
110	179	80	20	M	Yes	2	145

The data in Table 11.8 are the results from a random sample of 110 people. The rested pulse rate of each person is measured and also their height in centimetres, weight in kilograms, age in years, sex, whether each considers themself a regular smoker, and the amount of regular exercise each undertakes in hours.

Either consider the data directly or enter them into a computer program of your choice. (The data are available from the companion website.) Then complete the following questions:

1 What is the level of measurement for each variable?
2 Produce appropriate descriptive statistics to assess the distribution of rested pulse rate. Your statistics should allow you to analyse the shape, centre and spread of the distribution, as well as the existence of any outliers. How might you explain any outliers, and how should they be handled in further analysis?
3 Compare the mean pulse rate for smokers and non-smokers. In this analysis, which variable is the independent variable and which is the dependent? What is the appropriate measure of association?

Recommended Further Reading

Argyrous, G. (2011) *Statistics for Research*. London: Sage.
This book provides reasonably comprehensive coverage of the descriptive statistics introduced in this chapter, as well as an entry point for the more advanced measures of association and inferential statistics that have only briefly been outlined here.

Liebetrau, A.M. (1983) *Measures of Association*. Beverly Hills, CA: Sage.
This is a definitive and accessible presentation of measures of association, including their calculation and respective limitations.

Sterne, J.A.C. and Smith, G.D. (2001) 'Sifting the evidence – what's wrong with significance tests?', *British Medical Journal*, 322: 226–31.
This is a short and cogent discussion of the logic and history of hypothesis testing and its limitations.

Online Readings

Aarabi, M. and Jackson, P. (2007) 'Prevention of coronary heart disease with statins in UK South Asians and Caucasians', *European Journal of Cardiovascular Prevention and Rehabilitation*, 14: 333–39.
How was the data analysed and presented?

Tettenborn, M., Prasad, S., Poole, L., Steer, C., Coghill, D., Harpin, V., Speight, N. and Myttas, N. (2008) 'The provision and nature of ADHD services for children/adolescents in the UK: Results from a nationwide survey', *Clinical Child Psychology and Psychiatry*, 13: 287–304.
How was the data analysed and presented?

References

Argyrous, G. (2011) *Statistics for Research*. London: Sage.
Australian Bureau of Statistics (2007–2008) *National Health Survey*. Cat. No. 4364.0.
Dancey, C., Reidy, J. and Rowe, R. (2012) *Statistics for the Health Sciences*. London: Sage.
Liebetrau, A.M. (1983) *Measures of Association*. Beverly Hills, CA: Sage.
Scott, I. and Mazhindu, D. (2009) *Statistics for Health Care Professionals: An Introduction*. London: Sage.

12

Randomized Controlled Trials

GEORGE LEWITH AND PAUL LITTLE

Introduction

- This chapter will focus on the underlying principles and concepts that govern all randomized controlled trials (RCTs) and will define their place within clinical research. It will also examine the different types of RCT and the practical issues that arise when carrying out a trial in a clinical setting. In the main, examples will be drawn from complementary and alternative medicine (CAM), not only because this is the first author's area of expertise, but also because some philosophical and ethical issues occur in this setting in particularly stark form.

- RCTs can be used in a number of different contexts, although they are used mostly in laboratory or clinical settings. For instance, the performance of two pieces of machinery or two devices that claim to perform the same function can be compared. A trial, holding other factors constant, can be run to compare performance on a number of criteria, such as: Which device uses the least energy? Which is the cheapest or which is the most cost-effective? Although it is much more difficult to control for variables and extraneous influences, trials can also be conducted in social care or educational settings where the outcome of an intervention can be compared with a control group to find the most appropriate solution to a particular problem. Examples have been the therapeutic benefits of 'regular good-neighbour visits' to elderly people in terms of improving their sense of well-being and the outcome of a new reading scheme compared with an existing scheme where two similar groups of 6-year-olds are studied. The fundamental principles of the RCT remain the same in whichever context they are applied. This chapter aims to outline the steps that are fundamental to setting up an RCT and meeting the requirements of a research protocol.

How to Approach Setting Up a Randomized Controlled Trial

The historical and philosophical origin of the RCT centres on the desire to find an answer to a very specific question. It sets out to evaluate the effects of a particular treatment or management strategy in a population where an intervention is introduced, by comparing the outcome with a control group where no intervention has been made. The population must be well defined and carefully selected.

A number of implicit assumptions underpin the RCT, as set out in Box 12.1 below.

Box 12.1   Assumptions underpinning RCTs

- We have an incomplete understanding of the world and knowledge evolves and develops. It is contingent and never definitive.
- Research methods evolve and change as we continue to learn about the world – thus any trial will be as good as we can make it at the time and the knowledge gained is likely to be modest and incremental.
- Logically, cause precedes effect, or, put another way, A leads to B.
- Beliefs cannot influence random events.
- In a well-designed study, the researcher's beliefs cannot influence the outcome.
- Good research aims to minimize the effects of bias, chance variation and confounding.
- Research that investigates whether treatments do more good than harm must be a priority.
- Understanding treatment and developing model validity around its delivery is vital so that the best intervention available can be evaluated.

Source: Adapted from Vickers et al. (1997)

These tenets lead to the claim that the RCT provides the 'gold standard' for research – and that it is the best means of attributing clinical real cause and effect in adding to our stock of knowledge. Not all researchers necessarily believe all of these assumptions (see, for example, Ronsenzweig 1936; Frank and Frank 1991), but they provide a sound framework for conducting an RCT.

Refining the Research Question

Setting up an RCT is a challenging task and researchers contemplating a trial must ask themselves:

- What is a good question?
- How can questions be matched to the research design?

- What is the best strategic approach to the research?
- How can an appropriate interpretation of the results be made and an inappropriate interpretation avoided?

The first prerequisite for refining a research question is to carry out a thorough literature search, as described in more detail in Chapter 3. A literature search is an iterative and developmental process that will contribute directly and indirectly to protocol development. It will help to identify whether the question one wants to ask has already been asked and also point out the strengths and weakness of previous research in addressing and answering the question.

A question is likely to be answerable if it is explicit, focused and feasible. In other words, it should be possible to link the effect of an intervention explicitly to a specific outcome. The research should be focused. There should be a very clear, simple primary question and a research method that will provide an answer – the trick is not to ask too many primary questions simultaneously even in a complex study. If there are multiple questions, then the primary research question must be given priority. The primary research question must be framed so that it is both possible and practical to answer the question. Some examples of questions are given in Table 12.1 below. The findings must be achievable within a reasonable period of time and within the bounds of the scientific and financial resources available. Factors that may allow for the misinterpretation of a study's findings, such as 'bias' and 'confounding', must be considered at an early stage and the research questions then modified, so that an appropriate trial design eventually emerges. These are considered further below.

Ways to Develop a Viable Randomized Controlled Trial

Clinical research evolves slowly, but for many therapies it is best not to try and solve too many questions simultaneously. A study's design is primarily predicated by the question it is designed to answer. The specificity and rigour of high-quality clinical trial design means that while a specific question may be asked, it is impossible to answer all the relevant questions that may surround a particular illness or a specific therapy. It is wise to recognize this at the outset when considering the details of a trial design. The study structure, rationale and design will have largely been formulated on the evidence provided in the background section of a protocol. If there is little solid RCT evidence for a particular intervention, then a feasibility or pilot study will almost certainly be required. This may be an RCT, or it may be an observational study that could be designed to evaluate recruitment and the size of the treatment effect. The study structure will need to be appropriate to the illness and the intervention. The planning stages of any clinical trial are vital – not least in terms of establishing the suitability of the research question for an RCT, as exemplified in Table 12.1.

TABLE 12.1   Different types of research question and their suitability for an RCT

Category of question	Examples	Suitable for RCT
Attributing cause and clinical effect	Does homoeopathically prepared grass pollen reduce symptoms of hay fever more than a non-active (placebo) treatment?	Y
	Is polypharmacy more effective than a single remedy approach in the homoeopathic treatment of chronic hay fever?	Y
What happens in clinical practice?	What is the cost-effectiveness of adding homoeopathic treatment to a standard care package in hay fever?	Y
	What are the patterns of cross-referral between conventional and CAM practitioners in a multidisciplinary pain clinic?	N
	How common are serious neurological complications following chiropractic cervical manipulation?	N
What do people do?	How many people visit practitioners of CAM each year?	N
	What do patients tell their primary care physician about usage of CAM?	N
	How many nurses practise CAM?	N
What do people believe and how do they explain it?	What do nurses believe about therapeutic touch? What is the patient's experience of the acupuncture consultation?	N
By what mechanisms does a therapy work?	What are the effects of needling the Hoku point on the production of endogenous opiates?	Y
Does something proposed in a therapy actually exist?	Does peppermint oil reduce histamine-induced contractions of tracheal smooth muscle?	Y
	Does homoeopathically prepared copper ameliorate the effects of copper poisoning in a plant model?	Y
	Can an acupuncture point be distinguished from non-acupuncture points by measuring the electrical resistance of the skin?	N
Is a diagnostic or prognostic test accurate?	How sensitive and specific is detection of gall bladder disease by examining photos of the iris?	N
	Is tongue diagnosis reliable?	N

Source: Vickers et al. (1997); Brien et al. (2003). Blackwell Publishing. Reprinted with permission.

Some tips for a successful project

First, based on our experience of conducting research using RCTs, we have found that working in a group with colleagues that meets on a regular basis provides an opportunity for supportive yet critical, ongoing review of projects. It helps to avoid making definitive decisions too rapidly and protects against mistakes.

Second, we believe that it is essential to carry out a thorough and ongoing literature review for each project. Data on references should be stored in a secure way, but be accessible to colleagues working on a project. Regular attendance at academic meetings, reading journals and reviewing Internet sources regularly will help to keep the researcher abreast of developments in the field.

Third, carrying out an initial pilot, or feasibility study, is often useful in testing out whether a properly constructed RCT study is worthwhile. This can help to refine the research question, develop hypotheses to be tested and check whether a project is feasible and can recruit in the specific target population. Researchers should make sure that it is or will be possible to recruit an adequate number of patients with disease X or in situation Y in the time frame they have in mind. Pilot projects allow students to test out their ideas without incurring large costs in money and time. Although the findings of small-scale studies may not be generalizable as they are likely to be underpowered (see Chapter 9), nevertheless many important questions relevant to the study can be tested. Some questions suitable for further investigation were listed in Table 12.1.

Fourth, it is essential to make sure that the volunteers or patients/clients will be able to complete the instruments that have been designed to measure outcomes. The latter should not be too burdensome for participants. Most importantly, the information sheet given to them to give their consent to the research should be written in clear and non-technical language, so it is easy for them to understand what is expected of them and makes them fully aware of any risks and costs and the time involved. They should sign the consent form and keep a copy of the information sheet.

Fifth, in relation to the technical aspects of the project, researchers should make sure that the process of randomization and blinding is feasible in the context of the study. It is particularly important to ensure that if a placebo – as a non-active treatment – is being used, it is appropriate for the control group concerned (Vincent and Lewith 1995; White et al. 2003).

Finally, the degree of variance in the main outcome measure should be calculated as this can inform decisions on the appropriate sample size for a further study.

Nowadays, for all but the most simple, small and straightforward study, clinical research is usually best conducted in teams. Given the complexity of clinical governance, ethics, requirements for trial design and protocols, trial management, data handling and statistical analysis (Mathews 2011), the sophistication of the research process is often simply too much for the lone researcher. Even for teams, advice may be needed from collaborators who are experts in particular areas and have a variety of expertise which will supplement and help develop the principal investigator's and the team's initial ideas and the development of a research protocol. However, both pilot studies and moderate-sized trials are well within the remit of undergraduate and postgraduate students working within a team and can provide an important learning opportunity.

Common Methodological Problems

A number of decisions and dilemmas must be faced by those carrying out a trial. First, while research is usually feasible and necessary, it may not be ethical. For example, it would be unethical to carry out an RCT on the benefits of antibiotics in the treatment of meningitis because the benefits of antibiotics are known and these could not therefore be withheld from a control group. Second, some research may be important but not practical. Third, research rarely provides unequivocal answers: there is often room for reasonable people to disagree about the interpretation of the findings.

Avoiding bias

Bias can occur in many stages of a trial and, unless recognized and countered, this will lead to false estimates of the effect of an intervention. There may be, as set out in Box 12.2, the following forms of bias.

Box 12.2 Forms of bias in RCTs

- *Recruitment bias:* a population may be selected for recruitment that does not represent the key population of interest – in consequence, the results of the study will only apply to the specific population recruited.
- *Selection bias:* this occurs where the intervention and control patient groups are not comparable.
- *Performance bias:* this occurs when groups within the intervention arm, for example in a multicentre study, may receive different kinds of treatment.
- *Detection bias:* this refers to systematic differences in the outcome assessment between groups.
- *Attrition bias:* this occurs when withdrawals from the study distort the symmetry of the initial selection process and therefore the results. There must be proper reporting of those who withdraw from a trial in order to avoid distortion (Feinstein 1985), as considered below.
- *Researcher/participant bias:* this occurs when the behaviour or response of those involved in a trial is affected positively or negatively by the knowledge that they are in the intervention or control group. This is sometimes referred to as the Hawthorne effect. In order to offset this, a trial may be 'blinded'. Here, the researcher does not know which group the research participant is in and whether they have been given the trial treatment or a placebo.

Assessing confounding factors

Confounding occurs when there is an association between an exposure to an intervention and the outcome as a consequence of an intervening variable – a third unknown factor. The control of confounding in the case of both known and anticipated, and unknown confounders, can be achieved through randomization, which is a major advantage of the RCT. With the randomization of those selected for trials, potential confounders can be equally distributed between groups and the effect neutralized. This is the main reason why the RCT is advocated as the best source of evidence of therapeutic benefit. An example of this is the following: a greater proportion of males over 60 die of lung cancer than males under 40. It might be incorrectly assumed that lung cancer is predominantly associated with age. However, an important intervening variable is smoking history. A history must be taken so that both age and smoking can be allowed for in interpreting trends, as they can both be measured. Randomization is discussed further below.

By definition, unknown confounders cannot be measured. An RCT that selects randomly for an appropriate size of population (statistical advice will be needed for how large that population should be for a particular trial) is a good way to attribute cause because it can allow for unknown confounding variables in, for example, attributing a therapeutic effect to a particular drug intervention. It may also be valuable in the context of a health economic evaluation. However, it is unlikely to be valuable in understanding people's activities and beliefs or the accuracy of a prognostic or diagnostic test.

Phases within a Classic Randomized Controlled Trial

The classic clinical trial process was designed to test the efficacy of drugs rather than surgical or manual interventions such as physiotherapy or osteopathy. It is essentially a prospective study. It looks forward in time. More recently, clinical trials have been divided into four main phases which represent vital progressive steps in testing the efficacy of modern pharmaceutical agents. These are pre-clinical trials and Phase I, II and III trials.

In pharmaceutical development, before a pre-clinical trial is launched, there will have been many years of very careful testing carried out both in vivo and in vitro to minimize the risk to humans of taking a particular drug and to maximize the potential therapeutic benefit. The primary aim of these studies is to assess the absorption of a drug; its distribution through the body; the effect on metabolism; and the extent of excretion – collectively known as the ADME of a drug.

In *Phase I* clinical trials, the population is not randomized into two groups and the trials are usually carried out in individuals who have a pre-existing pathology. The aim of these studies is two-fold:

- To establish the maximum tolerated dose by very cautiously increasing the dose of the medication in patients with real pathology and to look for side-effects.
- To assess whether the medication is effective.

The criteria used to define the 'maximum tolerated dose' and 'treatment efficacy' vary significantly depending on the illness. For instance, patients with terminal cancer may give consent to a trial even if there are uncomfortable side-effects because they wish to help future patients or because they believe the drug will be effective. This is less likely in the case of patients with an intermittent benign illness such as migraine.

Phase II studies are carried out in patients with a known illness and usually involve four treatment groups recruited to a prospective RCT. While a Phase I study may estimate the likely doses of a potential therapeutic agent, a Phase II study carries this work further, usually looking at three different therapeutic doses in three different arms of the trial with a placebo in the fourth arm. With most conventional pharmaceutical agents, therapeutic benefit increases with the size of the dose, but so does the potential risk of adverse reactions. The aim is to find a dose that provides the best clinical effect with the lowest level of adverse reaction. Typically, in one arm of the trial patients will receive what is thought to be the therapeutic dose; a second arm will be given half that dose and a third arm double the optimal dose, while the fourth arm receives a placebo. The specific treatment efficacy will be evaluated by comparing the balance of therapeutic benefit and adverse reaction with the active agent versus a placebo.

A *Phase III* clinical trial mirrors most closely the classic RCT. It is usually a study that involves two groups (arms) and compares the optimal dose of active treatment with a placebo over a period of time. It uses outcome measures that will allow researchers to conclude that any effects observed will be the specific effects of the drug or intervention being evaluated.

The most common trial designs used within a Phase III RCT are two armed comparative trials designed to evaluate the difference between a specific intervention and a comparative placebo or control intervention with clearly defined primary and secondary outcomes. In some instances, particularly for chronic conditions, various adaptations on this central scheme may be applied. For instance, a run-in period may be used to establish baseline symptoms prior to trial entry. This allows for the general improvement that may occur as a 'trial effect' and will become apparent as patients record their symptoms over a period of a week or month (Lewith et al. 2002a; White et al. 2004b). It may also protect against a ceiling effect as some presentation of symptoms is necessary to demonstrate that a clinical improvement has occurred as a consequence of the intervention.

The Process of Protocol Development

The process of protocol development forms the foundation of any RCT. It provides a road map or process for a trial setting out the aims and rationale, a detailed methods section covering recruitment, the process of the research over time, the end points for measurement, any risks to patients and the statistical advice received, and concludes with a patient consent form. This explains the research project in lay language and must be signed by the patient and retained by the patient. As suggested above, protocol development is generally a group activity with input required from clinicians, research methodologists, statisticians and, where appropriate, health economists, social scientists and, often, users and consumers.

Protocols are designed to clarify the researcher's thoughts but also, more importantly, to convey the scientific essence of the research proposal to others as part of a peer review process. A protocol must have clarity and focus with a logical flow that justifies the researcher's plan of investigation. It will form the basis for all relevant research applications going to ethics and governance committees as seeking external or internal funding. They will also be the basis for subsequent publications. Research protocol forms are usually obtained from the institution sponsoring the research. Forms may differ in detail, but generally cover broadly similar areas as described below.

The background section

The aim of the background section is to show that the researcher has a complete understanding of the problem they wish to investigate. It provides the argument for why a particular research question is both important and relevant within the specific field. It should be clearly and concisely written, concluding with a focused research question in the context of existing knowledge. The researcher should demonstrate an understanding of the disease process in question and its natural history, and give a clear description of issues that might impact on the disease outcome. For example, a study of one of the authors on stroke and the use of acupuncture (Hopwood et al. 2008) required an understanding of stroke and its physiological and emotional impact on functioning that might affect the outcome of the evaluation of acupuncture. A thorough review of research is required so that the research question is appropriate and logical, filling a gap in knowledge in the existing literature. The quantity of previous studies does not rule out the need for another study. For example, many studies have evaluated the use of acupuncture for back pain (White et al. 2002; White et al. 2004b; Manheimer et al. 2005). However, in some of these studies, the methodology has been flawed. Arguably, there is still a need for a large, rigorous trial.

Developing a hypothesis

The design of a research project will be influenced by the primary hypothesis, or the proposition to be tested. This can be briefly stated but must be firmly based on the research question, and is frequently a null hypothesis – that is, a proposition that suggests that statistically it is unlikely that the treatment will be shown to have an effect (see Chapter 11 on statistics). A Phase III clinical trial will inevitably have one main hypothesis, although there will almost certainly be a number of secondary research questions.

Outcomes expected and their measurement: validity and reliability

The research protocol will require a statement of how the effect of an intervention will be measured. This may be done by stating clinical measures such as blood pressure levels, air flow or exercise tests, or quality of life measures or patient questionnaires. There are advantages in using existing well-validated and reliable primary outcome measures. The concept of validity has a number of dimensions, as outlined in Box 12.3.

Box 12.3 Dimensions of the concept of validity

- *Face validity:* on the 'face' of it, the outcome measure is relevant to the study questions.
- *Content validity:* the outcome measure includes the range of issues considered important by patients and experts in the field.
- *Construct validity:* the outcome measure used in previous studies behaves in an appropriate manner which is relevant to the factors that it is measuring based on previous literature or theories – for example, a knowledge outcome should relate to training.
- *Criterion validity:* the outcome measure is congruent with an acknowledged 'gold standard' measure.

It is also important that the outcome being measured gives reliable results. The means of showing this are set out in Box 12.4.

Box 12.4 Demonstrations of reliability

- *Test–retest reliability:* measures show the same result when repeated after a short interval, such as two weeks in a stable condition.
- *Internal reliability:* this refers to the degree of rigour or consistency as a measure. For example, where questionnaire items are combined in a scale or subscale, individual questionnaire items should relate well to each other and to the scale total (Streiner and Norman 1995).
- *Outcome sensitivity:* an outcome should be sensitive to change.

New outcome measures may be developed in the context of a clinical trial, providing they are or can be compared and validated with a standard measure in the same group of patients. For example, in a study where acupuncture was used to treat neck pain, the primary outcomes used were well-validated scales measuring the quality of life perceptions of pain in a group of patients suffering from chronic, mechanical neck pain (White et al. 2004a). A further process of 'scale validation' was developed and therefore was a secondary outcome of the study. It is usual, particularly in large clinical trials, to have both primary and secondary outcomes. For instance, a study on acupuncture and pain may have a visual analogue of pain as its primary outcome, with secondary outcomes relating to quality of life and range of movement measures.

It is important to specify a primary outcome in a research study so that a Type I error, that is an error due to chance findings, can be avoided. For example, if 20 outcome measures were used in one clinical trial, it is likely that one of these would show a significant difference between an active and placebo treatment at the 5 per cent level (that is, 1:20 times), and consequently this might be considered a significant outcome. It is, in fact, likely to be simply a random event if all the other 19 outcomes show no difference between the active and the placebo treatment. The choice of primary outcome will be determined by the type of trial: thus, in a pragmatic trial where the beliefs and behaviour of the participants are as natural as possible, with minimal interference, then patient-based outcomes may be developed for use rather than objective measurement of outcomes by independent observers.

It is also important to consider, measure and control, if necessary by stratification (see below), what may predict or confound an outcome. For example, if patients are receiving either acupuncture or physiotherapy for their neck pain, then outcomes may be predicted by the attitudes and beliefs that trial participants hold about a particular intervention. If possible, these attitudes should be established in the initial part of the study (White 2003).

Ideally, outcomes should be measured independently of the investigator and, if possible, blind to the group to minimize outcome assessment bias (see 'blinding' above). Outcomes should also be measured in the same way in each group to avoid bias, as the manner and timing of a measurement may affect that measurement. For example, in the British Family Heart Study blood pressure was measured in the intervention group at the beginning and at the end, but only at the end in the control group. One finding was that a fall in blood pressure was observed in the intervention group. However, it was not possible to say whether this was due to the intervention alone or also due to the effect of a measurement that was repeated (Family Heart Study Group 1994). Poor trial design led to measurement bias. In sum, both the measurement and placebo arm of a trial should be subject to the same set of measures.

The selection of research participants: inclusion and exclusion criteria

The decision about who to include in, and who to exclude from, a trial is of key importance. An effect of an intervention is most likely to be found with a homogeneous group of patients and should include those who are most likely to benefit, if this can be predicted from previous research. If too varied a group is included, then the higher variance in the primary outcome measure will limit the ability of the treatment to show an effect, and may obscure real and important benefit. The disadvantage of using a highly selected group is that treatment effects observed in highly selected groups may not apply to a broader group generally seen in the community. If, for instance, a study is conducted involving a new intervention for chronic obstructive pulmonary disease (COPD), but excludes all patients taking oral steroids, then how relevant is such a conclusion to general practice where many patients with COPD are likely to be on long-term oral steroids? Thus, there is a continuing tension within any clinical trial between reducing variability by selecting patients with clearly defined clinical and social characteristics, and providing evidence that is generalizable to the population managed in everyday practice. Inclusion and exclusion criteria require careful thought with respect to this balance.

The recruitment process

The recruitment process used in a clinical trial will affect the generalizability of findings. For instance, a group of volunteers selected via the Web may be an entirely different population from those invited to participate in a clinical trial via a general practice. As a consequence, it is vital to keep information on the flow of patient recruitment (Moher et al. 2001; Brien et al. 2003). A good clinical trial will have a pre-specified mechanism for recording and handling the data, and it is important to track missing data from patients who drop out. The most important guiding principle is that once a patient has been entered into a clinical trial and randomized, then they must be followed up throughout the study. It is important to try and achieve a follow-up of at least 80 per cent or above, otherwise attrition bias may seriously compromise the validity of the results. If patients are rejected during a baseline recording period because they do not ultimately fulfil the entry criteria for a study (Lewith et al. 2002a) or have not otherwise entered the trial process, they do not need to be followed up throughout the study. Those who are eligible but decline to take part should be documented and reported as part of a CONSORT trial flow diagram, which is the standard mechanism for reporting the flow of patient recruitment for clinical trials.

During the development of a protocol, the sample size calculation forms the basis of the numbers that will need to be recruited to a trial in order to answer the trial's primary and secondary hypotheses. This will provide the foundation for costing and development within the context of a clinical trial.

Figure 12.1 illustrates patient recruitment in a study involving homoeopathic proving, the method used for determining which remedies are suitable for particular conditions. It records the number of people who were contacted about the study; those included in the initial baseline screening and those subsequently randomized within the study; and those who dropped out. This helps to highlight the generalizability of findings and sources of bias.

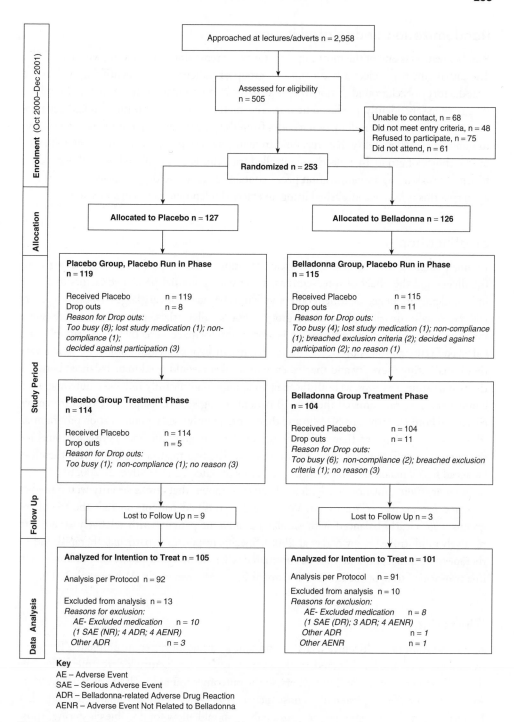

FIGURE 12.1 Patient recruitment in a study of homoeopathic proving
Source: Brien et al. (2003). Blackwell Publishing. Reprinted with permission.

Randomization and related issues

Randomization is one of the most important ways of removing confounding within an RCT. The initial aim is to select a homogeneous group of patients, while identifying within the introductory or background section to a protocol the important factors (potential confounders) that may independently predict outcome. The method of randomization should separate whoever generates the randomization codes from the person carrying out the randomization to minimize any possibility that the clinician managing the patient could have any influence on the choice of group. In a placebo-controlled trial, this is accomplished by an independent pharmacy making up randomization packs containing an active drug or placebo, and for an open trial this is best accomplished using an external telephone randomization line.

Stratification

In small single-centre clinical trials, great attention must be paid to understanding both the illness and the effect of interventions, along with potential predictive factors that may independently influence treatment outcome. This is because, for very large trials, confounders will be equally distributed between groups. For smaller trials, particularly where some variables strongly predict outcome, it is important to make sure that such variables are balanced between groups by 'stratification'. For instance, in our asthma study, we were aware that initial asthma severity and the presence of smokers would need to be balanced between the two treatment groups, as both these factors might significantly influence outcome. As a consequence, we randomized the first 10 patients using sealed opaque envelopes to receive either real homoeopathy or a placebo and then subsequently used a minimization programme. This allocates patients so that with each randomization, any difference between groups for the potential confounding variables is minimized. The two treatment groups were therefore balanced for all major known potential predictors of outcome (Lewith et al. 2002b).

In other studies, for instance with stroke, it was known that stroke severity would predict outcome irrespective of treatment. We therefore stratified patients so that the treatment groups were clearly balanced with similar numbers of patients with relatively severe and relatively mild stroke (Hopwood et al. 2008). Specific responses to particular therapies and/or therapists are important and must be considered when defining the process of randomization in a two-armed trial, or the order of treatment in a cross-over study (White et al. 2003).

Clustering

Randomization in multicentre trials can present a variety of different problems. The same treatments may not be delivered in the same way at every centre, or treatments may be delivered at some centres and not others, so the outcomes found might be centre-dependent with treatment effects 'clustered' in consequence. Every effort should be made to standardize for recruitment and sample size, and any analysis should allow for possible clustering. Those interested in multicentre trials should refer to Campbell and Machin (1999).

The statistical analysis plan

Whatever the protocol and however the study is designed, a clear plan for data analysis must be presented at the protocol stage (see Chapter 11 on statistics). An important principle in analysis is that the primary analysis should generally be an 'intention to treat' analysis – that is, where all patients, whether they complied with the intervention or not, are included in the analysis according to their original study group. This is important because, to estimate the average effect patients can expect to receive from a treatment, the results should include both patients where it has worked and those where it has not worked or who have had to stop the treatment for whatever reason. This mirrors what is likely to happen in the real world. Most studies usually also perform a so-called 'per protocol' analysis where only those patients who have complied with the intervention are assessed. This will give an estimate of the effect of the intervention in ideal circumstances.

Ethics and governance

The process of ethics and governance has changed radically with the introduction of the new European Union clinical trial directive in April 2004 and this is considered in detail in Chapter 15. It is important to recognize that ethical issues must be addressed in any research protocol, particularly with respect to data protection, obtaining fully informed consent and following good clinical practice. Researchers should inform themselves of the requirements of ethics committees. Great care should be taken in drafting the patient consent form so that the research is comprehensible in lay terms. Research ethics committees are often most critical of this aspect of a research protocol.

Methodological Issues

The replicability of research

The essence of any scientific experiment is to describe, within the methods section, an experimental procedure that can be completely duplicated by any other interested and properly trained researcher. This requires that the intervention made is described specifically and exactly. In the case of a drug trial, the exact medication used must be defined, along with its specific manufacture, dosage and delivery method. In studies involving surgical or manual intervention, such as physiotherapy, a methodological prerequisite is to describe all the interventions in all arms to a high level of specificity. A study should be capable of replication so that any other researcher would be able to carry out the same study using the same interventions and, hopefully, come to the same conclusions.

Blinding and its problems

The process of blinding is designed to remove bias and retain patient equipoise. It is used to detect the specific effects of an intervention by removing any prior 'expectation' that the researcher or participant may have of the trial results from the active or placebo treatment. It is usually possible to blind a medicinal intervention. A placebo can almost always be made to look, taste, feel and present as indistinguishable from the active treatment. However, blinding with respect to a surgical intervention or pragmatic intervention such as physiotherapy, exercise prescription or reflexology is more difficult. While it may have been ethical to blind patients as to whether they had or had not received a real surgical intervention in the mid-1950s (Beecher 1955), it is no longer thought reasonable or ethical to do so. Within the context of a clinical trial, patients must consent to receive, or not to receive, medication, surgery or spinal manipulation.

A very pragmatic definition of a double-blind trial is where neither the investigating researchers nor the trial participants (volunteers/patients) are aware of who is receiving the active or placebo treatment. Both parties are blind to the nature of the intervention, hence expectation is removed and equivalence created with respect to the treatment outcome.

A single-blind trial is where the therapist delivering the intervention knows which is the placebo and which is the active treatment, but the patient or volunteer thinks that both interventions are equally likely to be therapeutically effective. This has been achieved with some acupuncture studies (Wood and Lewith 1998). It is also the case where the primary outcome measure is achieved through, for example, a patient self-assessment questionnaire; a visual analogue scale or Short Form 36 (SF-36); or a generic quality of life measure. In this case, a patient can remain in equipoise, with an equal belief in the active and placebo treatment, although the groups receive two distinctly different treatments. Outcomes assessed either by themselves or by an entirely objective or independent source (a blood test or a blinded third party) may also mean that a study can be legitimately described as a single-blind trial.

It has been estimated that approximately 70 per cent of clinical trials fail to report the details of blinding (Schulz and Grimes 2002). Schultz argues that the removal of bias is the foundation upon which causal associations can be derived within clinical research. He points out that many conventional clinical trials fail to report the blinding and randomization process adequately and indeed a proportion of researchers may have deliberately subverted the process (Grimes and Schulz 2002). However, it is possible to minimize the effect of open (unblinded) interventions by generating a placebo effect in each group, using the therapist/physician as a placebo. For example, in an open pragmatic trial of prescribing strategies for a sore throat, the placebo effect of prescribing antibiotics was abolished by using structured advice sheets to support management in each group (Little et al. 1997).

When carrying out a trial, researchers should aim to detach themselves from preconceptions about the efficacy of a therapy. This is particularly essential during data interpretation. The Jadad score (Jadad et al. 1996) and other such scores are widely used among systematic reviewers as the basis for summarizing major sources of bias in relation to blinding, randomization and the reporting of results. However, such quality scores rarely assess generalizability to the community of individuals suffering from the illness.

Common Variations of the Randomized Controlled Trial

It has been argued above that the classic RCT is demanding on staff and resources and is often beyond the scope of the lone researcher. There are some variations that are less resource-intensive and still contribute to knowledge.

Cross-over studies

A cross-over study is a study that involves one treatment in a first phase, a washout period with no treatment and then a second randomized treatment with a control group in a further phase. Every individual takes part in both phases, but the order of treatments is randomized. The advantage of a cross-over design is that it minimizes variation. Each individual becomes their own control and so the inter-individual variation is minimized, and thus smaller numbers are needed. Cross-over designs are only appropriate for a stable disease and a therapy that has relatively short-term effects, such as the use of an H_2 blocker in the treatment of gastro-oesophageal reflux. However, it is unlikely, for example, to be the approach of choice for the treatment of mild depression in the community, largely because modern antidepressants take time to work and usually require at least a two- or three-month prescription. At the end of this period, the patient may no longer be depressed. Similarly, as interventions such as acupuncture have unpredictable long-term effects, a cross-over is not appropriate either (Lewith et al. 2002a).

Variations in control mechanisms and pragmatic studies

Some studies may attempt to control for an intervention by having an 'attention' control. This is where some patients simply spend time with a therapist, without the therapist providing a specific therapy. The methods section of the protocol may give information about the intervention, as was the case in a trial to assess the effect of exercise classes on the relief of fibromyalgia. The disadvantage of such studies is that the total effects of an intervention may involve both specific and non-specific effects, although it is often this combined effect that the patient will experience in real life. Cost-effectiveness cannot be estimated in studies which use an attention control as this would not occur in actual practice.

Pragmatic studies are defined simply as studies that look at what happens in practice. Thus, patients with chronic lower-back pain go to their conventional doctor to receive an analgesic or an anti-inflammatory and may also simultaneously visit an acupuncturist. As a consequence, a pragmatic trial of acupuncture would involve the randomization of patients to receive acupuncture plus conventional care as compared with those simply receiving the latter. Such a trial suffers from the disadvantage of being unable to define the specific effects of acupuncture, but it has the great advantage of being generalizable in a real-world context (Thomas et al. 1999, 2005).

Factorial design in the evaluation of the Alexander Technique

It is generally the case that it is preferable to answer one question at a time. However, sometimes it will be important to ask more than one question. Factorial designs provide an excellent and efficient framework for asking several questions simultaneously and, to illustrate this, a case study is provided. For instance, in a study we recently conducted which evaluates the use of the Alexander Technique in chronic back pain, we have eight groups within our clinical trial (Deyo et al. 1998). The Alexander Technique is a hands-on approach where the teacher, through both 'gentle' touch and explanation, helps pupils to release harmful muscle tensions, and improve muscle use and coordination. The questions asked in this trial were as follows:

- Primary research question: What is the effectiveness of introductory or longer courses of the Alexander Technique and of massage therapy in restoring normal activities which have been restricted by back pain?

- Then: What is the effectiveness of a general practitioner exercise prescription with a nurse follow-up appointment in restoring normal activities which have been restricted by back pain?

- What is the cost-effectiveness of these treatments compared with normal care?

We wanted to evaluate whether it was necessary to give a prolonged course (24 teaching sessions) of the Alexander Technique or whether 6 sessions could achieve the same clinical outcome. We did this as we believed that 6 sessions might be acceptable for NHS funding if the Alexander Technique proved to be cost-effective, while 24 sessions might not. However, we wished to retain the clinical assumptions prevalent among Alexander teachers and evaluate the best possible intervention, and therefore considered that our trial would be completely inadequate if one group did not receive the complete set of Alexander lessons (24 sessions).

Second, we wished to assess whether the educational element of the Alexander Technique was the key factor in improvement or whether this was simply due to a hands-on approach. For this we had one group of patients receive a massage, where there was a hands-on treatment but no education, as usually given in the Alexander Technique. The massage group was also useful to assess whether massage per se is helpful. A normal care group was required as the basic comparator for all groups. Without a normal care group, it would be difficult to estimate differences in resource use between the groups and therefore difficult to estimate cost-effectiveness.

Thus, for one 'factor' we have four groups: longer Alexander Technique (24 lessons), shorter Alexander Technique (6 lessons), massage (6 sessions) and normal care. Each of these groups was split with random assignment of subjects into two sub-groups. One of these had additional exercise and the other did not. Designing the trial with the presence or absence of exercise in all four groups allowed us to compare the Alexander Technique with standard conventional treatment plus exercise. Many recent studies suggest that this is an effective and indeed cost-effective approach to the management of chronic lower-back pain (Frost et al. 2004).

The advantage of this factorial design is that several questions may be asked simultaneously. The statistical calculations associated with this design meant that a number of questions could be asked with slightly fewer trial participants. Inevitably, multifactorial studies are complex, difficult to execute and require considerable research expertise.

Reading Health Research Based on Randomized Controlled Trials

In appraising published research on RCTs in the health field – and recognizing that there are a variety of forms of RCT – the following points arising from this chapter should be considered, among others:

- Is there a clear and important primary question in the research?
- Were there sufficient resources available to carry out the RCT?
- Is the structure of the RCT appropriate to the condition and intervention?
- Have participants been appropriately selected for the RCT?
- Have the key ethical bases been covered, including patient consent?
- How appropriate is the process of randomization and blinding?
- Have various forms of potential bias been addressed in the RCT?
- Are the outcome measures appropriate in terms of validity and reliability?
- Are the various arms of the trial subject to the same set of measures?
- Is the randomization appropriate in relation to potential confounding variables?
- Is the study described with high level specificity and capable of replication?

While the RCT is often projected as a 'gold standard', it is very important to remember that research using this method can be variable in quality.

Conclusion

This chapter describes an iterative process to enable and understand the development of RCTs. It centres on the importance of the protocol and how best to consider study development with respect to the essential issues that emerge during clinical trial development. The advent of the RCT is both a blessing and a curse. Undoubtedly, it has improved the evidence base to inform the delivery of clinical care, but inevitably any RCT is, by its nature, limited in scope. Furthermore, good science and clinical relevance do not always go hand in hand, and attempting to achieve both simultaneously requires clear thinking and the ability to work within a team. To underline the themes of this chapter, the reader is invited to engage in the short exercise set out below on evaluating the use of lavender essence as an alternative therapy.

Exercise: The evaluation of lavender essence using a randomized controlled trial

It has been suggested that *Lavandula augustifolia* (lavender essence) may be of assistance in treating insomnia. Quite a number of people just put a few drops of lavender on their pillow when they are having difficulty sleeping and say that it 'works a treat'. Insomnia affects 20 per cent of the British population, but many conventional drugs used to treat it have the potential to become addictive.

Consider the issues that you would need to take into account if you wanted to evaluate the use of *Lavandula augustifolia* using an RCT. Some of the questions you might wish to consider include:

1 How would you search the literature to find out what has already been published?
2 How would you construct a study to evaluate this?
3 If you were going to use a placebo, how might you provide a convincing one?

Recommended Further Reading

Grimes, D. and Schulz, K. (2002) A series of articles in the *Lancet* on research design (359: 57–61; 145–9; 248–52; 341–5; 515–19; 614–18; 781–5; 881–4; and 966–70).
These articles in the epidemiology series give a concise introduction to research design.

Lewith, G.T., Jonas, W. and Walach, H. (2011) *Clinical Research in Complementary Therapies*, 2nd edition. Edinburgh: Churchill Livingstone.
This book draws on the best of conventional research methods, including randomized controlled trials, and adapts them to the needs of complementary and alternative medicine.

Mathews, J.N.S. (2011) *Introduction to Randomized Controlled Clinical Trials*, 2nd edition. London: Chapman and Hall/CRC.
This text provides clear coverage of statistical concepts and medical examples for those interested in clinical trials.

 ## Online Readings

Sturkenboom, I., Graff, M., Borm, G., Veenhuizen, Y., Bloem, B., Munneke, M. and Nijhuis-van der Sanden, M. (2012) 'The impact of occupational therapy in Parkinson's disease: A randomized controlled feasibility study', *Clinical Rehabilitation*.
Critically evaluate the paper using the checklist provided in PPS12.11.

Shnayderman, I. and Katz-Leurer, M. (2012) 'An aerobic walking programme versus muscle strengthening programme for chronic low back pain: A randomized controlled trial', *Clinical Rehabilitation*.
Critically evaluate the paper using the checklist provided in PPS12.11.

References

Beecher, H. (1955) 'The powerful placebo', *Journal of the American Medical Association*, 159: 1602–6.

Brien, S., Lewith, G.T. and Bryant, T. (2003) 'Ultramolecular homoeopathy has no observable clinical effects: a randomized, double-blind, placebo-controlled proving trial of Belladonna C30', *British Journal of Clinical Pharmacology*, 56: 562–8.

Campbell, M. and Machin, D. (1999) *Medical Statistics: A Commonsense Approach.* Chichester: Wiley.

Deyo, R., Battie, M., Beurskens, A.J., Bombardier, C., Croft, P. and Koes, B. (1998) 'Outcome measures for low back pain research: a proposal for standardized use', *Spine*, 23(18): 2003–13.

Family Heart Study Group (1994) 'Randomised controlled trial evaluating cardiovascular screening and intervention in general practice: principal results of British Family Heart Study', *British Medical Journal*, 308: 313–20.

Feinstein, A.R. (1985) *Clinical Epidemiology: The Architecture of Clinical Research.* Philadelphia, PA: Saunders.

Frank, J.D. and Frank, J.B. (1991) *Persuasion and Healing: A Comparative Study of Psychotherapy.* Baltimore, MD: Johns Hopkins University Press.

Frost, H., Lamb, S.E., Doll, H.A., Taffe Carver, P. and Stewart-Brown, S. (2004) 'Randomised controlled trial of physiotherapy compared with advice for low back pain', *British Medical Journal*, 329: 708–14.

Grimes, D.A. and Schulz, K.F. (2002) 'Bias and causal associations in observational research', *Lancet*, 359: 248–52.

Hopwood, V., Lewith, G., Prescott, P. and Campbell, M.J. (2008) 'Evaluating the efficacy of acupuncture in defined aspects of stroke recovery: a randomised, placebo controlled single blind study', *Journal of Neurology*, 255(6): 858–66.

Jadad, A.R., Moore, R.A., Carroll, D., Jenkinson, C., Reynolds, D.J. and Gavaghan, D.J. (1996) 'Assessing the quality of reports of randomized clinical trials: is blinding necessary?', *Control Clinical Trials*, 17: 1–12.

Lewith, G.T., Watkins, A., Hyland, M.E., Shaw, S., Broomfield, J. and Dolan, G. (2002a) 'A double-blind, randomised, controlled clinical trial of ultramolecular potencies of house dust mite in asthmatic patients', *British Medical Journal*, 324: 520–3.

Lewith, G.T., Walach, H. and Jonas, W.B. (2002b) 'Balanced research strategies for complementary and alternative medicine', in G.T. Lewith, W.B. Jonas and H. Walach (eds), *Clinical Research in Complementary Therapies.* Edinburgh: Churchill Livingstone.

Little, P.S., Williamson, I., Warner, G., Gould, C., Gantley, M. and Kinmonth, A.L. (1997) 'An open randomised trial of prescribing strategies for sore throat', *British Medical Journal*, 314: 722–7.

Manheimer, M.S., White, A., Berman, B., Forys, K. and Ernst, E. (2005) 'Meta-analysis: acupuncture for low back pain', *Annals of Internal Medicine*, 142(8): 651–63.

Mathews, J.N.S. (2011) *Introduction to Randomized Controlled Clinical Trials*, 2nd edition. London: Chapman and Hall/CRC.

Moher, D., Schulz, K.F. and Altman, D.G. (2001) 'The CONSORT Statement: revised recommendations for improving the quality of reports of parallel-group randomized trials', *Explore*, 1: 40–5.

Ronsenzweig, S. (1936) 'Some implicit common factors in diverse methods of psychotherapy', *American Journal of Orthopsychiatry*, 6: 412–15.

Schulz, K.F. and Grimes, D.A. (2002) 'Blinding in randomised trials: hiding who got what', *Lancet*, 359: 696–700.

Streiner, D.L. and Norman, G.R. (1995) *Health Measurement Scales: A Practical Guide to their Development and Use*. Oxford: Oxford Medical Publications.

Thomas, K.J., Fitter, M., Brazier, J., MacPherson, H., Campbell, M. and Nicholl, P. (1999) 'Longer term clinical and economic benefits of offering acupuncture to patients with chronic low back pain assessed as suitable for primary care management', *Complementary Therapies in Medicine*, 7: 91–100.

Thomas, K., MacPherson, H., Thorpe, L., Brazier, J., Fitter, M., Campbell, M., Roman, M., Walters, S. and Nicholl, J. (2005) *Longer Term Clinical and Economic Benefits of Offering Acupuncture to Patients with Chronic Low Back Pain*. Final Report to NHS Health Technology Assessment Programme.

Vickers, A., Cassileth, B., Ernst, E., Fisher, P., Goldman, P., Jonas, W., Kang, S., Lewith, G., Schulz, K. and Silagy, C. (1997) 'How should we research unconventional therapies?', *International Journal of Technology Assessment in Health Care*, 13(1): 111–21.

Vincent, C. and Lewith, G.T. (1995) 'Placebo controls for acupuncture studies', *Journal of the Royal Society of Medicine*, 88: 199–202.

White, P. (2003) 'Attitude and outcome: is there a link in complementary medicine?', *American Journal of Public Health*, 93: 1038.

White, P., Lewith, G.T., Berman, B. and Birch, S. (2002) 'Reviews of acupuncture for chronic neck pain: pitfalls in conducting systematic reviews', *Rheumatology*, 41: 1224–31.

White, P., Lewith, G.T., Hopwood, V. and Prescott, P. (2003) 'The placebo needle, is it a valid and convincing placebo for use in acupuncture trials? A randomised, single blind, cross-over trial', *Pain*, 106: 401–9.

White, P., Lewith, G.T. and Prescott, P. (2004a) 'The core outcomes for neck pain: validation of a new outcome measure', *Spine*, 29: 1923–30.

White, P., Lewith, G.T., Prescott, P. and Conway, J. (2004b) 'Acupuncture versus placebo for the treatment of chronic mechanical neck pain: a randomised, controlled trial', *Annals of Internal Medicine*, 141: 911–20.

Wood, R. and Lewith, G.T. (1998) 'The credibility of placebo controls in acupuncture studies', *Complementary Therapies in Medicine*, 6: 79–82.

13

Experimental Methods in Health Research

A. NIROSHAN SIRIWARDENA

Introduction

This chapter provides an overview of non-randomized experimental and quasi-experimental methods particularly focusing on experimental techniques that provide alternatives to the randomized controlled trial (RCT) described in the previous chapter. The RCT is a particular form of experimental method, and in the double-blind controlled trial, ranks highest in the hierarchy of evidence described in Chapter 3. Randomization can control for confounding variables and double-blinding can reduce certain types of bias. However, it is not always possible to conduct an RCT for methodological, practical or ethical reasons that are discussed below. 'Experimental methods' is an umbrella term that includes a variety of techniques which aim to maintain scientific rigour in situations where it is not possible to introduce randomization, blinding or sometimes even a control. The chapter will explain the language of experimentation and discuss the advantages and disadvantages, as well as how such methods should be applied. A range of experimental research designs based on published or unpublished studies is described to illustrate the use of these methods in practice.

Non-Randomized Experimental Designs and their Rationale

Non-randomized experimental designs

The key feature of an experiment is that it assesses the effect of introducing a change where the relationship between two or more measurements is investigated by deliberately prompting a change in one of them and observing the change in the other (Robson 1994). A change based on a hypothesis of cause is introduced in one variable (the independent variable), which may lead to a corresponding change, or effect, in another (the dependent) variable. The prediction of cause and effect (A leads to B) is termed the hypothesis. Experiments test hypotheses whereas other types of quantitative study test the strength of associations between measurements (A is associated with B). Experiments, based on the scientific method of testing changes to establish a relationship between cause and effect, have advantages over other methods in their ability to test hypotheses, reduce bias and limit confounding. Arguably, they are also more robust in determining the true size of the effect of an intervention. The 'effect size' is the estimate of the magnitude of a change in a measure and may be calculated statistically.

Experimental methods should be distinguished from observational methods such as cohort, case-control or self-controlled case series studies. Case-control studies aim to compare the characteristics of a particular phenomenon in the group of interest to a control or reference group. Thus, the health of one group of people exposed to a risk, such as asbestos, or a protective factor, such as an influenza vaccination, may be compared with another group that has not been exposed in order to assess for a specific outcome – like lung cancer in the case of asbestos (Schenker et al. 1986), or a heart attack in the case of the influenza vaccine (Siriwardena et al. 2010). Cohort studies are where a selected population is studied over time to investigate the effect of a particular factor on health outcomes. Doll and Peto (1976) undertook a number of studies to assess the relationship between smoking and cancer. Self-controlled case series studies, which are a more recently introduced form of study design, aim to determine the risk of a particular outcome over time by comparing periods of exposure with non-exposure (Gwini et al. 2011). Observational methods of this type should not be confused with the participant observer or ethnographic methods used in qualitative research described in Chapter 6.

Non-randomized experimental methods include a range of study types with a single group where there is an intervention or where an intervention group is compared to a non-randomized control group. These are summarized in Figure 13.1. These methods may also be classified into pre-experimental and quasi-experimental designs on the basis that the former are not likely to provide valid evidence for effectiveness of an intervention, whereas the latter may do so in certain circumstances (Campbell and Stanley 1963; Cook and Campbell 1979).

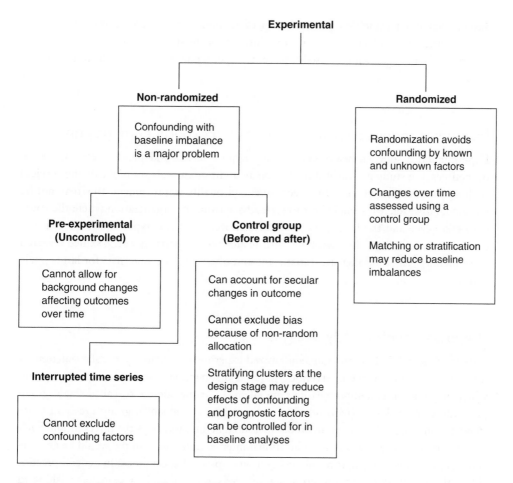

FIGURE 13.1   A classification of experimental study designs
Source: Adapted from Ukoumunne et al. (1999)

Rationale for non-randomized experimental designs

Experimental methods have a particular value in assessing the effect of innovative interventions in health care. However, health care practitioners or organizations, sometimes purposefully and sometimes inadvertently, introduce new health technologies or services. Once these are applied, they are difficult to reverse either from an ethical or practical perspective. Once a new service is introduced or an intervention is established, there are limited possibilities for more structured experimental designs to determine the effectiveness or cost-effectiveness of the changes. In this situation, non-randomized experimental designs may provide the only possibility for evaluation. For example, randomization may not be possible due to factors that are either intrinsic to the study or external to it; examples are area-wide or organization-based interventions, or a policy decision to introduce a new service.

Resources required for non-randomized experimental designs

Experimental designs in health care usually require formal independent ethical review. Sometimes, if a study is clearly shown to be an audit or an evaluation of existing services with no intervention other than a recommended quality improvement, this may not be required. However, it is usually best to seek advice from the organization where the study is to take place and the local ethics committee. Studies of this type require good access to health care settings, close working with health service partners and a skilled research team including methodologists, statisticians and often health economists for larger-scale studies.

Pre-experimental study designs

Pre-experimental designs are non-randomized experiments where a particular outcome of interest is measured in the intervention group and sometimes also in a comparison group where only post-intervention measures are taken. These include the so-called single-group post-intervention design (with or without controls) and the single-group pre- and post-intervention design when the outcome is measured before, and after, the intervention. Such designs are often used to evaluate educational interventions: an example would be an educational programme to improve the recognition of psychological illness in general practice (Hannaford et al. 1996). Pre-experimental designs are also used by researchers wishing to evaluate the impact of large-scale changes. One such study examined the effect on general practitioner (GP) workload (in terms of hours spent on general practice work per week and time spent per patient in consultations) of the introduction of a new contract for GPs in 1990 (Hannay et al. 1992).

Quasi-experimental designs

These designs include two main types of study. These are:

- non-randomized control group, before and after study
- the interrupted time series design.

The non-randomized control group before and after study method involves one or more intervention groups with one or more non-equivalent comparator groups to act as controls with measurements of outcomes taken before and after the intervention. An example of a before and after study in relation to evaluating policy innovation is a study of the impact of legislation to ban smoking in public places in the Republic of Ireland. A before and after non-randomized control group design was found to reduce passive smoking and respiratory illness in bar workers (Allwright et al. 2005). Another study, this time based in the UK, found that the introduction of legislation restricting pack sizes of analgesics led to reductions in pack sizes on pharmacy shelves. The study found that associated with this change were reductions in analgesic overdoses. It also found that the severity of the overdoses that did occur was also reduced, as were other sequelae such as the level of suicide deaths and of liver transplantation (Hawton et al. 2004).

In the second type of study using time series or interrupted time series designs, repeated measurements of the outcome of interest are taken over time from the population beginning before the intervention and continuing afterwards. The time periods used can be continuous or discontinuous, that is interrupted. Measurements are taken to assess whether there is any change over and above that which would have been expected from the secular trend prior to the intervention. Measurements for time series studies may be taken from a whole population or by sampling from a cohort of the population. Alternatively, repeated cross-sectional samples can be taken from the whole population. This method need not necessarily involve a control group but it does benefit from one in accounting for confounding external influences on the outcome to be assessed.

The Strengths and Weaknesses of Non-Randomized Experimental Designs

It is important to appreciate the advantages and disadvantages of the different types of experimental design. These are discussed firstly in relation to RCTs, then non-randomized designs in general and finally for the different non-randomized design types.

Strengths and weaknesses of randomized controlled trials

Large, well-designed and conducted RCTs ensure that intervention and control groups have a baseline of comparability. Differences in outcome can then be attributed to the intervention alone. Explanations for differences other than the intervention, or confounding factors, should be balanced equally between the intervention and control groups through randomization. The use of RCTs, despite their 'gold standard' epithet, can be hampered by a number of problems, which are illustrated in Box 13.1.

Box 13.1 Problems with the use of RCTs

- There may be such strong evidence for an intervention that a placebo group may be unethical.
- Randomization may be impossible because clinicians or organizations may advocate strongly one particular approach over another. In this situation, there is a lack of clinical equipoise, without true clinical equivalence between the intervention and control. A strong preference for either effectively prevents random allocation.
- Educational or other interventions when active participation of subjects is required for the intervention to be effective may render randomization inappropriate or impossible.
- Randomized controlled studies may be ruled out on cost terms. They are more complex and costly than non-randomized designs (Black 1996).

RCTs are also subject to a number of possible design flaws. For example, when allocation to groups is not blinded, this can lead to an inflation of effect size. Moreover, participants in RCTs are often atypical and this selection bias can affect outcomes. Only a small proportion of patients with a given condition can be included in a trial, either directly through selection and exclusion criteria or indirectly through a greater likelihood of inclusion of certain types of patient, such as those attending academic centres. Women, elderly people, children and those with other illnesses or very severe illness, are also less likely to be included in trials. This tends to increase the treatment effects and to reduce the generalizability of a study. In treatment trials, there is a bias towards the inclusion of people who are less well-off and less well educated, whereas in the case of preventive interventions, participants tend to be healthier, wealthier and better educated. The so-called 'healthy user' bias tends to increase effect size on proxy outcomes because of better compliance but conversely, to reduce effect sizes on true outcomes because of a ceiling effect. Better baseline measures have less capacity to improve.

Non-randomized experimental designs can suffer from similar problems, but as they usually tend to be less restrictive in terms of inclusion and exclusion criteria, they exhibit better external validity and generalizability. Furthermore, there is no evidence that non-randomized studies have greater effect sizes than RCTs. Potentially, trial subjects, whether individuals or organizations, tend to benefit from an intervention. For this reason, it is more critical to the internal and external validity of an experimental study to ensure that the trial group is representative of the population from which it is drawn (Britton et al. 1998). Laboratory methods often involve experimental methods too. However, these cover a variety of methods of investigation and analysis that are outside the scope of this chapter.

Strengths and weaknesses of non-randomized designs

The key advantage of a non-randomized design is that randomization need not be undertaken in situations where it would not be ethical or acceptable to clients or other stakeholders to do so. Non-randomized studies may also be the only ethical option. For example, in relation to an educational intervention versus no intervention or access to treatment versus no treatment, it can be argued that the educational intervention or the treatment may lead to some positive change. Therefore, access should not be denied to the control group. In a non-randomized educational intervention study to investigate the effect of introducing decision rules for referral for x-ray in suspected ankle and foot fractures, under the so-called Ottawa ankle rules it was decided that it was inappropriate to have a control group (Stiell et al. 1995). The results, following the educational programme, showed that the outcome led to a reduction in requests for x-ray – and, while a decrease in waiting times and costs occurred, there was no increase in the number of missed fractures. It can be assumed that, pending further research, this was due to the education effect.

Although it is widely accepted that randomization in trials reduces some types of systematic error that may interfere with the results, it has also been argued that in certain circumstances there may be an advantage in allowing patients' preferences to play a part in determining which arm of a trial they enter, even if this leads to some loss in assessing the therapeutic treatment effect. One reason for allowing patient preferences to be taken into account is that some patients may have such strong preferences that they may refuse randomization, thus leading to selection bias. In studies where there are difficulties in recruiting patients, there may be advantages in following preferences even if this motivation may skew the results.

It could equally be argued that, where it is not possible to disguise which treatment arm patients are in, the results may also be skewed by low motivation. Furthermore, certain interventions require the active engagement of participants. This is the case where self-monitoring or self-medication is required; where rehabilitation or programmes for de-institutionalization are being assessed; where behavioural or cognitive treatments for anxiety and depression are being compared with each other; and where treatments involve drug medication. In these situations, comparisons may only work if participants have no preference, which may be an unlikely scenario. One solution to this problem has been to distinguish between patients who have no preference and to apply a randomization method in their case. Thus, a trial with two interventions will have four groups: randomized to A; prefer A; randomized to B; and prefer B. An example of this type of study was conducted by Chilvers et al. (2001) on the use of antidepressant drugs and generic counselling for the treatment of major depression in primary care.

Non-randomized methods are often most useful where an innovative practice is being introduced in a single or limited number of sites for an evaluation period or to assess the effect of legislative or policy changes. An example of this type of study was where non-randomized experimental methods were used to evaluate the impact of introducing an open-access walk-in centre for people needing first-line primary care. The Department of Health favoured the introduction of open-access walk-in clinics to reduce the pressure on Accident and Emergency departments, and general practices introduced this facility in certain localities in England. In order to estimate the effect of this intervention in one locality, a study using a controlled before and after design was used to evaluate the effect of introducing an open-access clinic on the use of Accident and Emergency departments and general practices (Hsu et al. 2003). In another study, this time with a control group, a mental health facilitator was employed in six general practices to train GPs to recognize and treat postnatal depression (Holden et al. 1989). The results were compared with six control practices where there was no facilitator. In this study, there were demonstrable improvements in terms of the identification of mental illness by GPs, but not in the management or outcomes of the illness.

Strengths and weaknesses of different non-randomized design types

Pre-experimental designs suffer from a serious and often fatal flaw. It is virtually impossible to determine whether the outcomes of such studies are due to the intervention or to some other confounding factor. Such factors can include: an unpredicted external influence or the effect of changes that occur naturally over time in the process of health care, such as increased awareness of new technologies; demographic changes; or local and national influences. These are often referred to as the impact of 'secular' trends. There may also be changes in the behaviour of study participants directly as a result of being observed, termed the Hawthorne effect (see Chapter 6 and Chapter 12) or regression to the mean. There is a tendency for outlying variables to move towards mean values. Studies may also be severely compromised by selection bias as there is a tendency for researchers to select participants who are likely to benefit from the intervention.

However, such designs may have a place, particularly in quality improvement studies, where interventions are used in an attempt to improve the quality of care in a specific setting. Blenkiron (2001), for example, developed a pre-experimental design in a pilot study of the efficacy of a self-help audiocassette in coping with depression (Blenkiron 2001). The study compared the extent of patient agreement with key messages on the audiotape, before and after use. It found an improvement in attitudes and knowledge following its use. Pre-experimental studies may also be useful as a precursor to an RCT study to evaluate a complex intervention. This is where two or more interventions are combined in a single study. Many health care interventions are of this type and there is increasing evidence that multiple interventions may be more effective (Van der Wensing et al. 1998; Grimshaw et al. 2001). An example is provided in one of the case studies given at the end of the chapter.

There are a number of methodological problems with quasi-experimental studies. For instance, sometimes innovations are taken up inconsistently and comparisons can only be made between those that implement change and those that maintain the status quo. An example of this was a non-randomized control group study comparing the effect of prescribing practices of fundholding with non-fundholding general practices (Bradlow and Coulter 1993). In this case, it was only possible to compare practices that took up the initiative with those that did not. It was found that fund-holding practices were more likely to remain within their 'indicative' budget, but there may have been other intervening or confounding variables to explain the behaviour.

Other sources of bias in these types of study include external effects on outcome and secular (time-related) changes unrelated to the intervention. Although this source of bias can be minimized by having a control group, this may not be possible due to limited funding, or because a new policy is introduced. Such studies have also shown that media coverage can produce unwanted effects. For example, *Casualty*, a BBC television drama, once featured a drug overdose which led to an increase in real overdoses presenting to casualty departments (Hawton et al. 1999).

Time series designs using a particular cohort, although offering greater statistical power, are more likely over longer periods of time to lead to bias due to non-response related to the Hawthorne effect, maturation (where individual ageing is a factor) and contamination. A study can be 'contaminated' when the change that is intended for the intervention group is inadvertently introduced to the control group. This could occur, for example, due to staff moving between health facilities; an unexpected movement of patients; or the introduction of a parallel intervention, which could skew the outcomes being measured. Although a control group in a time series design may not be possible, research using this method can provide useful findings. This is exemplified by a recent study on the implementation of the National Institute of Health and Clinical Excellence (NICE) guidelines in the UK (Sheldon et al. 2004), which showed up the variable adoption of guidance.

The Medical Research Council framework for the design and evaluation of complex interventions is often used as the basis for the development of designs that may eventually lead to the classic RCT (Campbell et al. 2007). In this framework, a phased approach involving pre-clinical, theoretical modelling in Phase I and an exploratory study or studies in Phase II is the suggested approach before undertaking a definitive trial in Phase III. These initial phases could involve a qualitative study such as a case study or interviews, a before and after experimental study (with or without controls), a time series study or a combination of these.

Analysis of data, writing up and presenting the findings

Data analysis in these study designs often requires considerable statistical expertise in appropriate methods to correct for baseline imbalance, secular trends and changes over time as a result of the intervention in question. Although out of scope for this chapter, where regression models are being used, decisions need to be made about whether to analyse for variables predicting the outcome of interest in the study as fixed or random effects.

Non-Randomized Designs in Practice

Three examples of pre-experimental, non-randomized control before and after, studies and time series designs are presented below as case studies.

Increasing influenza and pneumococcal vaccination rates in high-risk groups in one primary care trust as part of a clinical governance programme

An example of a pre-experimental design was used in a study which aimed to improve influenza and pneumococcal vaccination of high-risk groups in family practices through multiple, multifaceted evidence-based interventions (Siriwardena et al. 2003). The interventions introduced to improve vaccination rates included: audit and feedback; awareness raising through various media leaflets and poster campaigns; the recommendation of vaccination by general practitioners; the use of opportunistic patient reminders and written information given during consultations; mailed reminders to patients; and advice given to practices on standardized computer coding for disease registries that included provider prompts, as well as monitoring vaccination uptake during the vaccination season.

As a result, there were significant improvements in vaccine uptake in high-risk groups in the practices participating in the study, as can be seen in Table 13.1. Practices were also able to demonstrate that they could exceed national goals for influenza vaccination rates for patients aged 65 years old and above and patients in disease risk groups. This study was undertaken to inform the design of a subsequent RCT (Siriwardena et al. 2002).

This was an uncontrolled study in a self-selected group of practices. The lack of a control group may have led to an overestimate of any effect of the intervention as it did not take into account the influence of changes over time or the Hawthorne effect. Participating practices may have been more enthusiastic about vaccination compared to those who did not participate (Siriwardena et al. 2003).

An evaluation of an educational intervention to reduce inappropriate cannulation and improve cannulation technique by paramedics

This study is an example of a non-randomized control group before and after design. It aimed to examine the effect of an educational intervention designed to improve both appropriateness and the technique used by paramedics of cannulation (Siriwardena et al. 2009). Intravenous cannulation involves the insertion of a

TABLE 13.1 Improvement in vaccination uptake of participating general practices

n = number of practices participating	Vaccination uptake		Median standard (Phase 1, Phase 2)	Mean improvement (95% CI)	Significance (p value, 2-tailed t-test)
	Phase 1 (%)	Phase 2 (%)			
Influenza vaccination uptake in CHD (n = 20)	58.3	77.5	70, 70	19.2 (14.4 to 24.0)	<0.001
Pneumococcal vaccination uptake in CHD (n = 19)	26.9	41.5	70, 70	14.6 (9.3 to 20.0)	<0.001
Influenza vaccination uptake in diabetes (n = 21)	57.6	74.5	75, 70	16.9 (10.2 to 23.6)	<0.001
Pneumococcal vaccination uptake in diabetes (n = 20)	40.2	53.5	70, 70	13.4 (4.8 to 22.0)	0.004
Influenza vaccination uptake in splenectomy patients (n = 18)	70.6	76.6	100, 100	6.1 (−2.5 to 14.7)	0.155
Pneumococcal vaccination uptake in splenectomy patients (n = 17)	81.7	83.4	100, 100	1.8 (−4.3 to 7.8)	0.546
Influenza vaccination uptake in over 65 year olds (n = 24)	48.9	73.0	60, 60	24.0 (19.7 to 28.4)	<0.001

synthetic tube into a vein using a needle and enables paramedics to administer fluids or drugs at home or in the ambulance, if patients are being transferred to hospital. When cannulae are used without good reason or inserted with inadequate infection control, there are potential risks for patients including unnecessary pain or infection.

(Continued)

(Continued)

The hypothesis of the study was that following an education session for paramedics aimed at improving their understanding of when to use cannulation and improve their technique, there would be a decrease in the use of (inappropriate) cannulation and an improvement in their cannulation technique. The primary outcome measure was the rate of appropriate cannulation, which for the purposes of the study was defined as cannulation where drugs or intravenous fluids were recorded as having been given. The secondary outcomes included the cannulation rates overall and the correct use of the cannulation technique assessed by a trained observer. The outcomes were measured two months before and two months after the educational session took place to allow time for the intervention and for a change in practice to occur.

The comparative data were analysed using logistic regression to test for both the main and interaction effects between predictor variables. The first regression model included data from the sites (intervention versus control); the timing of testing (pre-intervention versus post-intervention); and interaction between sites and the timing of testing as predictor variables. The overall cannulation rates were used as the outcome variable. The second regression model included data from the sites (intervention versus control); the timing of testing (pre-intervention versus post-intervention); and interaction between sites and the timing of testing as predictor variables – with inappropriate cannulation rates as the outcome variable.

There was a non-significant reduction in inappropriate cannulation rates, that is in the intervention area (1.0% decreasing to 0%) compared to the control area (2.5% increasing to 2.6%). There was also a significant reduction in cannulation rates in the intervention area (9.1% to 6.5%) compared with an increase in the control area (13.8% to 15.1%) (p<0.001). Finally, paramedics in the intervention area were significantly more likely to use correct hand-washing techniques post-intervention compared with paramedics in the control area (74.5% vs. 14.9%, p<0.001).

There were potential biases due to the non-equivalent group design. These included selection bias from non-random selection of intervention and control groups and confounding from possible other external influences on outcomes occurring between pre- and post-intervention phases and possible existing differences between areas in cannulation technique. Biases such as regression to the mean would have been less likely, given that the baseline rate of cannulation was greater in the control than the intervention area and baseline differences in cannulation rates were adjusted for in the analysis. The study did not account for differences in secular trends in the intervention or control areas in the analysis. The post-intervention assessment was not blinded which was another potential source of bias. Measurement of outcomes was unchanged and consistent before and after the intervention.

Investigation of the effect of a countywide protected learning time scheme on prescribing rates of ramipril – interrupted time series study

The final example is of a time series study which aimed to investigate whether an area-wide educational intervention for general practice and primary health care workers increased prescribing of the drug ramipril. This was advocated for reducing cardiovascular risk and preventing heart attacks (Siriwardena et al. 2007).

As a result of the benefits of specific drugs called angiotensin converting enzyme (ACE) inhibitors in improving clinical outcomes for patients at risk of heart disease, including those with diabetes, we used prescribing rates for ramipril, an ACE inhibitor widely used for prevention at the time, as an outcome measure. This was based on the Heart Outcomes Prevention Evaluation (HOPE) trial, which provided evidence that patients with coexisting diabetes and hypertension or other cardiovascular risk factors, if treated with ramipril, had lower rates of cardiovascular disease and death.

A time series design was used to analyse prescribing data in 101 practices in one county in England. Data were collected in one year, before and after the educational session to assess changes in the rate of prescribing ramipril.

The time study showed a significant change in the rate of ramipril prescribing at a therapeutic dosage following the educational intervention (OR: 1.50, 95%; CI: 1.07 to 1.93), despite a background of secular change. Within this overall change, there were a number of patterns of change in prescribing. There were, for instance, practices in which prescribing rates rose either a little or a lot after the intervention. There were practices that delayed prescribing the drug, in contrast to those where the rate of prescribing continued to rise.

The time series design was chosen for the study because it would have been inappropriate to randomize practices as all were invited to the educational session. It was difficult to provide an unbiased control group because of potential contamination. The study took into account secular trends and assessed whether the intervention had a significantly greater effect than the underlying secular trend. A change occurred, but this was partly related to increased ramipril prescribing for diabetes and probably also for heart failure and hypertension.

The data collection was retrospective to reduce the likelihood of the Hawthorne effect biasing the results. The design did not preclude effects other than the chosen intervention affecting the particular outcome.

Reading Health Research Based on Experimental Methods

Despite their value, the reader needs to be able to critically appraise published health research based on experimental methods that are not RCTs, including non-randomized experimental and quasi-experimental methods. Key questions to ask include the following:

- Are such experimental methods most suited to the research in question?
- Are there good reasons for not directly conducting an RCT?
- Are the limitations of non-randomized experimental methods appreciated?
- How are these limitations addressed in the research design?
- What approach is taken to potentially confounding variables?
- What arrangements are made for internal and external validity?
- Are there plans for an RCT to follow in a phased approach?
- Has the study been appropriately ethically reviewed?

The reader should also see the comments on reading health research based on RCTs in Chapter 12, given that the RCT is a specific form of experimental method.

Conclusion

In this chapter, it has been shown why and how experimental designs in health research extend beyond the traditional RCT. A number of pre-experimental, quasi-experimental and experimental designs have important potential applications for assessing and evaluating health technologies, interventions and services, and for modelling prior to RCTs, particularly of complex interventions. Finally, an exercise is set out for the reader to complete. It asks which experimental methods can be applied to the ambulance service, and in what way.

Exercise: Non-randomized experimental designs

In 2004, the UK Healthcare Commission report on ambulance services noted that a majority of patients, four out of five, said they had suffered pain from their presenting condition while in the ambulance. Although 81 per cent felt that the ambulance crew did everything they could to control pain, one in five wanted more pain relief; 14 per cent said the crew did this to some extent; and 5 per cent said that the crew did not do everything they could to control their pain.

As a result of this report, you are asked to design and implement a quality improvement protocol for improving the assessment and control of pain in an ambulance service in which you are working. Pain control is assessed in adults (aged 16 and over) using a verbal pain rating scale from 0 (no pain) to 10 (the most severe pain) and should be recorded for all patients. The NHS Trust board is keen to see improvements across the service and both you and they consider an RCT study to be neither ethical nor feasible.

In your report, address the following questions:

1 Which patients or patient groups would you study in relation to pain? Who would you exclude, and why?
2 What outcomes measures could you use for your evaluation?
3 What methods could you use to improve pain control and why?
4 Consider what other experimental methods could be used in this situation.
5 Which of these would you prefer to use and why?
6 Where would you find a control group for your study?
7 Describe any sources of bias and confounding factors in your preferred study design. How might you address these?

Recommended Further Reading

Shadish, W.R., Cook, T.D. and Campbell, D.T. (2002) *Experimental and Quasi-experimental Designs for Generalized Causal Inference.* Boston, MA: Houghton-Mifflin.
This is an updated version of a classic text, in which experts in the field of quasi-experimentation discuss in comprehensive fashion key issues relating to the theory and practice of experimental and quasi-experimental designs.

Trochim, W.M. (2006) *Research Methods Knowledge Base*, 2nd edition. Available at: www.socialresearchmethods.net/kb/
For a very readable and accessible account of quasi-experimental methods, this is an excellent site to look at. It is written by an expert in quasi-experimental research methods from Cornell University.

Ukoumunne, O.C., Gulliford, M.C., Chinn, S., Sterne, J.A.C. and Burney, P.G.J. (1999) 'Methods for evaluating area-wide and organisation-based interventions in health and healthcare: a systematic review', *Health Technology Assessment*, 3(5): 9.
This HTA monograph is a systematic review comparing randomized and non-randomized designs and supporting the use of well-designed quasi-experimental designs to answer particular types of research question.

Online Readings

Korwanich, K., Sheiham, A., Srisuphan, W. and Srisilapanan, P. (2008) 'Promoting healthy eating in nursery schoolchildren: A quasi-experimental intervention study', *Health Education Journal*, 67: 16–30.
How is experimental design defined in this context? Critically evaluate the paper using the check-list provided in PPS13.11.

Taylor, L., Poland, F., Harrison, P. and Stephenson, R. (2011) 'A quasi-experimental feasibility study to determine the effect of a systematic treatment programme on the scores of the Nottingham Adjustment Scale of individuals with visual field deficits following stroke', *Clinical Rehabilitation*, 25: 43–50.
How is experimental design defined in this context? Critically evaluate the paper using the checklist provided in PPS13.11.

References

Allwright, S., Paul, G., Greiner, B., Mullally, B.J., Pursell, L., Kelly, A., et al. (2005) 'Legislation for smoke-free workplaces and health of bar workers in Ireland: before and after study', *British Medical Journal*, 331: 1117.

Black, N. (1996) 'Why we need observational studies to evaluate the effectiveness of health care', *British Medical Journal*, 312: 1215–18.

Blenkiron, P. (2001) 'Coping with depression: a pilot study to assess the efficacy of a self-help audio cassette', *British Journal of General Practice*, 51: 366–70.

Bradlow, J. and Coulter, A. (1993) 'Effect of fundholding and indicative prescribing schemes on general practitioners' prescribing costs', *British Medical Journal*, 307: 1186–9.

Britton, A., McKee, M., Black, N., McPherson, K., Sanderson, C. and Bain, C. (1998) 'Choosing between randomised and non-randomised studies: a systematic review', *Health Technology Assessment*, 2(13): 3.

Campbell, D.T. and Stanley, J.C. (1963) *Experimental and Quasi-Experimental Designs for Research*. Chicago, IL: Rand McNally College Publishing.

Campbell, N.C., Murray, E., Darbyshire, J., Emery, J., Farmer, A., Griffiths, F., Guthrie, B., Lester, H., Wilson, P. and Kinmouth, A.L. (2007) 'Designing and evaluating complex interventions to improve health care', *British Medical Journal*, 334: 455–9.

Chilvers, C., Dewey, M., Fielding, K., Gretton, V., Miller, P., Palmer, B., Weller, D., Churchill, R., Williams, I., Bedi, N., Duggan, C., Lee, A. and Harrison, G. (2001) 'Antidepressant drugs and generic counselling for treatment of major depression in primary care: randomized trial with patient preference arms', *British Medical Journal*, 322: 772–5.

Cook, T.D. and Campbell, D.T. (1979) *Quasi-experimentation: Design and Analysis Issues for Field Settings*. Chicago, IL: Rand McNally College Publishing.

Doll, R. and Peto, R. (1976) 'Mortality in relation to smoking: 20 years' observations on male British doctors', *British Medical Journal*, 2: 1525–36.

Grimshaw, J.M., Shirran, L., Thomas, R., Mowatt, G., Fraser, C., Bero, L., Grilli, R., Harvey, E., Oxman, A. and O'Brien, M.A. (2001) 'Changing provider behavior: an overview of systematic reviews of interventions', *Medical Care*, 39(8): 112–45.

Gwini, S.M., Coupland, C.A. and Siriwardena, A.N. (2011) 'The effect of influenza vaccination on risk of acute myocardial infarction: self-controlled case-series study', *Vaccine*, 29(6): 1145–9.

Hannaford, P.C., Thompson, C. and Simpson, M. (1996) 'Evaluation of an educational programme to improve the recognition of psychological illness by general practitioners', *British Journal of General Practice*, 46: 333–7.

Hannay, D., Usherwood, T. and Platts, M. (1992) 'Workload of general practitioners before and after the new contract', *British Medical Journal*, 304: 615–18.

Hawton, K., Simkin, S., Deeks, J., Cooper, J., Johnston, A., Waters, K., Arundel, M., Bernal, W., Gunson, B., Hudson, M., Suri, D. and Simpson, K. (2004) 'UK legislation on analgesic packs: before and after study of long term effect on poisonings', *British Medical Journal*, 329: 1076.

Hawton, K., Simkin, S., Deeks, J.J., O'Connor, S., Keen, A., Altman, D.G., Philo, G. and Bulstrode, C. (1999) 'Effects of a drug overdose in a television drama on presentations to hospital for self poisoning: time series and questionnaire study', *British Medical Journal*, 318: 972–7.

Holden, J.M., Sagovsky, R. and Cox, J.L. (1989) 'Counselling in a general practice setting: controlled study of health visitor intervention in treatment of postnatal depression', *British Medical Journal*, 298: 223–6.

Hsu, R.T., Lambert, P.C., Woods, M. and Kurinczuk, J.J. (2003) 'Effect of NHS walk-in centre on local primary healthcare services: before and after observational study', *British Medical Journal*, 326: 530.

Robson, C. (1994) *Design and Statistics in Psychology*, 3rd edition. Harmondsworth: Penguin.

Schenker, M.B., Garshick, E., Munoz, A., Woskie, S.R. and Speizer, F.E. (1986) 'A population-based case-control study of mesothelioma deaths among US railroad workers', *American Review of Respiratory Disease*, 134(3): 461–5.

Sheldon, T.A., Cullum, N., Dawson, D., Lankshear, A., Lowson, K., Watt, I., West, P., Wright, D. and Wright, J. (2004) 'What's the evidence that NICE guidance has been implemented? Results from a national evaluation using time series analysis, audit of patients' notes, and interviews', *British Medical Journal*, 329: 999.

Siriwardena, A.N., Fairchild, P., Gibson, S., Sach, T. and Dewey, M. (2007) 'Investigation of the effect of a countywide protected learning time scheme on prescribing rates of ramipril: interrupted time series study', *Family Practice*, 24(1): 26–33.

Siriwardena, A.N., Gwini, S.M. and Coupland, C.A. (2010) 'Influenza vaccination, pneumococcal vaccination and risk of acute myocardial infarction: matched case-control study', *Canadian Medical Association Journal*, 182(15): 1617–23.

Siriwardena, A.N., Iqbal, M., Banerjee, S., Spaight, A. and Stephenson, J. (2009) 'An evaluation of an educational intervention to reduce inappropriate cannulation technique by paramedics', *Emergency Medical Journal*, 26(11): 831–6.

Siriwardena, A.N., Rashid, A., Johnson, M.R.D. and Dewey, M.E. (2002) 'Cluster randomised controlled trial of an educational outreach visit to improve influenza and pneumococcal immunisation rates in primary care', *British Journal of General Practice*, 52: 735–40.

Siriwardena, A.N., Wilburn, T. and Hazelwood, L. (2003) 'Increasing influenza and pneumococcal vaccination rates in high risk groups in one primary care trust', *Clinical Governance: An International Journal*, 8(3): 200–7.

Stiell, I., Wells, G., Laupacis, A., Brison, R., Verbeek, R., Vandemheen, K. and Naylor, C.D. (1995) 'Multicentre trial to introduce the Ottawa ankle rules for use of radiography in acute ankle injuries: Multicentre Ankle Rule Study Group', *British Medical Journal*, 311: 594–7.

Ukoumunne, O.C., Gulliford, M.C., Chinn, S., Sterne, J.A.C. and Burney, P.G.J. (1999) 'Methods for evaluating area-wide and organisation-based interventions in health and healthcare: a systematic review', *Health Technology Assessment*, 3(5): 9.

Van der Wensing, M., Van der Weijden, T. and Grol, R. (1998) 'Implementing guidelines and innovations in general practice: which interventions are effective?', *British Journal of General Practice*, 48: 991–7.

14

The Use of Economics in Health Research

ALAN MAYNARD

Introduction

All societies face the twin problems of the inevitability of death and the scarcity of resources. These problems impose difficult choices on decision makers, whether they are prime ministers, nurses, doctors or patients. Every choice has an opportunity cost: a value forgone. A decision to use the drug Herceptin to treat primary breast cancers consumes scarce resources that could be used to replace diseased and painful hips or treat patients with Alzheimer's disease. Every diagnostic or treatment choice made by a doctor or nurse uses resources and deprives other patients of care from which they could benefit. The scarcity of resources makes rationing in health care inevitable. The issue is what principles should determine who will receive care and who will be deprived of care and be left in avoidable pain and discomfort, and perhaps to die? The policy issue is not whether to ration but how to do so. A number of economic techniques have been used to develop principles and to evaluate the costs and benefits of different treatments. In this chapter, the rationale for economic evaluation is considered; the techniques for economic evaluation to prioritize treatments are described and their limitations discussed; the different types of economic evaluation are outlined; and a case study is provided to illustrate the process in practice.

The Rationale for Economic Evaluation

In the NHS and other publicly funded health care systems around the world, society has rejected the use of the price mechanism and the willingness and ability of people to pay as the means by which access to health care is determined. In these systems, the dominant access criterion is 'need' but this concept has to be carefully defined.

Rationing access to health care in the face of scarcity involves depriving some patients of care from which they could benefit and wish to have. Given that the demand for care usually exceeds supply, some argue that we should deliver those interventions that 'work', but this raises another definitional problem – how should this clinical effectiveness be defined? For instance, with a hip replacement, the major benefits are the removal of pain and improved mobility. With some cancer care, the focus of doctors is on survival rates of perhaps months or years, often with little attention being paid to the quality of life during this period. Identifying and agreeing the 'end point', that is what outcomes should be evaluated and how should they be measured in clinical trials, is never easy and makes economic evaluation challenging, as we will see later.

Dilemmas of Economic Assessment

However, the crucial issue at this juncture is whether determining clinical effectiveness as the criterion for access to care is necessary and sufficient. The economic argument is that clinical effectiveness is a necessary characteristic for rationing access to care, but is not sufficient. As argued in Maynard (1997), what is clinically effective may not be cost-effective but what is cost-effective is always clinically effective. Economists have developed a measure for clinical effectiveness in terms of the number of Quality Adjusted Life Years (QALYs) that can be expected from a particular treatment (Williams 1985). All these words require definition but, put briefly, a QALY is one added year of perfect health. This measure must be set against the costs of treatment to assess clinical cost-effectiveness. QALYs provide the basis for comparing one treatment with another, as described in the example in Box 14.1.

Box 14.1 An example of the dilemmas of economic assessment

Let us assume that there is a limited budget of £70,000 and that the costs of the alternative procedures, X and Y, for the particular disease that you will treat are known. Furthermore, let us assume that the benefits of each procedure are known and measured in QALYs, where a QALY is one year of perfect health.

(Continued)

(Continued)

If therapy X produces 5 QALYs and therapy Y produces 10 QALYs, on the basis of clinical effectiveness, Y is superior and will be preferred by the patient and their physician who, motivated by the individualistic Hippocratic Oath, wishes to do the best for the patient.

But what if therapy X costs £1,500 and therapy Y costs £7,000? Therapy X produces a QALY at an average cost of £300, while therapy Y produces a QALY for £700. Therapy Y produces an additional 5 QALYs for an additional cost of £5,500 (£7,000 minus £1,500). The marginal cost of producing a QALY using Y is £1,100 (£5,500 divided by 5).

Therapy X is superior in terms of cost-effectiveness as it produces health QALYs at least cost, while therapy Y is clinically superior as it produces more QALYs. From the individualistic perspective of the patient and their agent, the doctor, therapy Y is preferred. However, from the social perspective of the economist and public health physician, therapy X is preferred as it produces the greatest health gain from a fixed budget. Thus, if a clinic had a fixed budget of £70,000, using therapy Y would produce 100 QALYs of health gain, but if it uses therapy X it will produce more than twice as many QALYs.

This example highlights that society's goal is to get the maximum health gain from its finite health care budget. Indeed, the necessary and sufficient condition for resource allocation and determining access to health care is the relative cost-effectiveness of competing interventions. Those interventions that are cost-effective give the 'biggest health care bang for the NHS buck'. Decision makers at the National Institute for Health and Clinical Excellence (NICE) use this criterion to determine access to the new technologies they evaluate (www.nice.org.uk). Internationally, this approach is gradually challenging and eroding the narrow clinical perspective and the individualistic ethic reflected in the Hippocratic Oath.

While techniques of economic evaluation are increasingly used to prioritize interventions competing for funding in the NHS, the actual practice of both clinical and economic evaluation could be said to be flawed as many studies are inadequately designed. Despite this, studies with basic methodological and design faults are often reported and published in highly prestigious journals (Freemantle and Maynard 1994). Consequently, it is important for practitioners of the 'dark arts' of economic evaluation and the patients and carers who use services to be able to deconstruct and appraise studies using QALYs. To facilitate this, there are checklists of good practice and these provide a useful way of elaborating the component parts of an economic evaluation. An economic evaluation checklist developed by Williams (1976) and given in Box 14.2 is very pragmatic, but provides an extremely useful start from which to explore any study.

Box 14.2 Economic evaluation checklist

To evaluate the costs and benefits of treatments, consider the following questions:

- What precisely is the question which the study is trying to answer?
- What is the question that it has actually answered?
- What are the assumed objectives of the activity studied?
- By what measures are these represented?
- How are they weighted?
- Do they enable us to tell whether the objectives are being attained?
- What range of options was considered?
- What other options might there have been?
- Were the other options rejected, or not considered, for good reasons?
- Would the inclusion of other options have been likely to change the results?
- Is anyone likely to be affected who has not been considered in the analysis?
- If so, why are they excluded?
- Does the cost go wider or deeper than the expenditure of the agency concerned?
- If not, is it clear that these expenditures cover all the resources used and accurately represent their value if released for other uses?
- If so, is the line drawn so as to include all potential beneficiaries and losers, and are resources costed at their value in their best alternative use?
- Is the differential timing of the items in the streams of benefits and costs suitably taken care of (for example, by discounting, and, if so, at what rate)?
- Where there is uncertainty, or there are known margins of error, is it made clear how sensitive the outcome is to these elements?
- Are the results, on balance, good enough for the job at hand?
- Has anyone else done better?

Source: Williams (1976)

Over the three decades since the Williams questions were posed, guidelines have been refined and differentiated by a range of authors – for example, by Maynard (1990), Drummond and the British Medical Journal Economic Evaluation Working Party (1996) and Drummond et al. (2005).

The list in Box 14.2 can be divided into a number of categories that raise particular questions and are elaborated below.

Technical questions

What is the role of the particular service or treatment intervention and what would be the consequence of doing nothing? In all evaluations, the option of 'doing nothing' may be the one that is the most cost-effective!

What is the comparator? Any new service has to be compared with an alternative. The study description should not only define the alternatives being compared but also explain the choice of alternatives. Sometimes in drug evaluations a placebo or dummy drug is used. This is usually insufficient as we need to know not just whether the new treatment has an effect compared with using a dummy tablet, but whether it is better than the accepted 'best available' treatment being used now. Whatever the alternative, its selection should be explicit and explained.

Identifying costs

Are all the costs of the new service or treatment identified, measured and valued? The range of costs that are evaluated has to be clearly stated and defended. These should include operating or current costs, as well as capital costs. There should also be consideration of system costs (for example, the opportunity cost of resources denied to others) and the cost to patients (for instance, in travel time) and other agencies such as local authority social services.

Identifying benefits

Are all the benefits identified, measured and valued? There are a number of important issues to be considered here: in particular, the nature of the clinical trial method; the measurement of the 'end point' or benefit; and the valuation of the benefit or end point.

First, the randomized controlled trial (RCT) is generally regarded as the best way of measuring clinical effectiveness. The Cochrane Collaboration (www.cochrane.org) is an international collaboration that has established good practice in the evaluation of 'what works' in clinical practice, and is discussed further in relation to involving health care users in Chapter 20. Its website and related sites such as the National Electronic Library for Health (www.nelh.nhs.uk) and the NHS Centre for Reviews and Dissemination (www.york.ac.uk/inst/crd) provide a starting place for identifying previous work, showing not only what works, but also what is in use yet unproven. The Cochrane criteria of validity and robustness should be used to guide you through these minefields. This is facilitated by systematic reviews that collect data from trials and then filter out those of poor quality to give an unbiased view of what works (NHS Centre for Reviews and Dissemination 2001).

Second, any review of a clinical area will immediately highlight the issue of selection of the end point, or benefit, from trial interventions. The health economist prefers to use direct evidence of improvement in the length and quality of life. However, trials often use intermediate or incomplete 'end points'. For instance, in cancer the principle focus is often on survival or additional months or years of life, with the quality of survival being ignored. An end point such as a myocardial infarction (heart attack) avoided, begs the question: for how long is survival enhanced and with what quality of life? Economic evaluations build on the clinical evidence base. If practitioners are not cautious, their work can be undermined by poor practice in clinical trials.

The final complex issue in outcome measurement and evaluation is the assignment of preferences and the valuation given to them. Ideally, we would like a benefit indicator that incorporates increased length and quality of life in a composite measure. However, patients themselves experience many health attributes, including things such as physical and mental functioning and pain. Such attributes of the health effects of interventions can be explored by generic quality of life measures using, for example, Short Form 36. This asks patients to self-assess their health state before and after treatment. While SF-36 can provide a patient profile of quality of life over time, it provides no insight into how a particular patient would trade off different health attributes. Consequently, for economic evaluation, efforts are made to measure the utility or value of particular combinations of health outcomes.

This is done using either 'the standard gamble' or 'time trade-off' approach. The former is regarded as the best option and involves an individual being asked to choose between the certainty of one health state and a gamble between the probability (p) of surviving for the same period with no disability or a probability $(1 - p)$ of immediate death. The value of p is changed until the individual is indifferent between the certain option and the gamble. This probability measure defines the utility for that particular person of the health state being considered, on a scale of 0 (death) to 1 (perfect health). The method and the simpler alternative, the time trade-off approach, are detailed in texts such as Drummond et al. (2005).

This preference-based, multi-attribute, health status measurement is epitomized by the EQ5D (EuroQol Group 1991). EQ5D has five dimensions (mobility, self-care, usual activities, pain/discomfort and anxiety/depression – see www.euroqol.org). The scores from EQ5D can be used as a 'weighted health index' that gives a numerical value for quality of life in a given health state. Such scores can be used in the calculation of QALYs, which are discussed below in the cost-utility evaluation section of this chapter (for further explanation, see also Jefferson et al. 2000; Drummond et al. 2005).

The Timings of Costs and Benefits

In terms of health benefits, an investment now may produce health benefits over decades. An example is that if you are persuaded to stop smoking, this will add years to your life and quality to those years in the future as you avoid premature heart disease, cancer and other ailments. For an individual, the treatment of hypertension involves costs for the rest of that person's life. So the question can be asked, what is the opportunity cost of a pound spent now compared with a pound spent in 10 years' time on this treatment? In these cases, it is expected that you will prefer gain now and loss in the future. To cope with the time preferences of individuals and of a society, streams of benefits and costs are adjusted in a process called discounting. Good economic evaluations should include this process (Drummond and the British Medical Journal Economic Evaluation Working Party 1996).

Sensitivity analysis

Inevitably, there will be uncertainty about both the estimated stream of benefits and that of costs. A good study will carry out sensitivity analysis and this will involve, for instance, re-estimating the results if costs are 5 and 10 per cent higher and benefits are 5 and 10 per cent less. Sensitivity analysis using such variations in assumptions tests the robustness of results in a world where estimates of clinical effectiveness and cost-effectiveness are inevitably somewhat imprecise.

Decision analysis

Increasingly, the uncertainty surrounding cost and benefit data is leading to the use of decision analysis. Decision analysis is a clearly defined, systematic approach to decision making when there is uncertainty. Uncertainty is common in medicine as diagnostic tests may generate false positives and false negatives. Patients vary, and treatments are never certain in their effects and may generate differing side-effects. Furthermore, the cost of treatment alters over time. Such uncertainty can be dealt with by quantifying it in terms of probabilities. For example, if an antibiotic has a 0.80 probability of removing a bacterial infection, there is a 0.20 probability that it will not. In this case, probability represents the strength of the belief an individual has, as a result of their knowledge and experience. Thus, data from clinical trials can be supplemented or even supplanted by eliciting expert opinions. Decision trees can be constructed that make the alternative costs and benefits explicit and assign probabilities to them. A checklist for such analysis has been published in Philips et al. (2004) and this approach is also discussed in Drummond et al. (2005).

When scrutinizing economic evaluations, the issues discussed above need to be studied with care. While such checklists have been available for three decades, practice continues to disappoint. Studies to evaluate the costs and benefits of particular treatments continue to fall short in terms of rigour and quality. The aim of research studies should be to inform the clinical evidence base in an unbiased fashion.

Types of Economic Evaluation

The terms 'economic evaluation' and 'cost-benefit analysis' can be confusing if they are used loosely and without precision. In effect, there are several types of economic evaluation, of which the cost-benefit analysis discussed so far is just one. The following five types of economic evaluation can be found in the literature and are explored further below:

- Costing studies.
- Cost minimization analysis.
- Cost-effectiveness analysis.
- Cost-utility analysis.
- Cost-benefit analysis.

Costing studies

The first study type listed is costing studies (CS). These are common, but are not economic evaluations, as alternatives are not compared. They are useless for deciding on how to invest resources in competing interventions in the health care sector. However, they are common because they are used by, for instance, the pharmaceutical industry, to draw attention to the costs of a disease. CS are used for marketing by the sponsoring company just about to launch a product. Such studies tell us that, for example, diabetes costs many billions and heart disease even more.

Such disease costings reveal nothing about how a disease can be treated efficiently with treatments that minimize costs and maximize benefits. They are discussed here to empha-size that they are not a form of economic evaluation as there is no comparison with alterna-tive interventions, but they are a common element of the marketing armoury of commercial companies seeking NHS funding.

Cost minimization analysis

Cost minimization analysis (CMA) involves the identification, measurement and valuation of the costs of competing therapies. In such a study, it is assumed that the outcome of the alternatives is identical. Thus, the focus of the analysis is partial. It seeks to identify which of two alternatives is cheapest.

One of the early examples of the CMA approach was an analysis of alternative methods for treating varicose veins. Piachaud and Weddell (1972) identified two interventions: surgery and injection-compression therapy in an outpatient clinic. They measured the cost of health service resource use and the individual cost to patients in terms of the time and cost of entering treatment. The authors also examined the wage cost losses of those treated but made no attempt to value unpaid activity such as the services of carers.

The study was based on an RCT that showed that after three years of follow-up the results for patients under 60 were equally good. The authors concluded that as the cost of injection was less than a third of surgery, and the loss of earnings was much less than in the non-surgical arm of the trial, injection therapy was to be preferred as it was less costly.

However, subsequent follow-up of the patients in the trial showed that at five years the assumption of equivalence of outcome was valid only for patients aged less than 35, among whom there were no signs of venous insufficiency. For the majority of patients, the outcomes of surgery were superior and thus decision makers faced the choice of whether to fund an intervention that was more expensive but gave better results.

Cost-effectiveness analysis

Cost-effectiveness analysis (CEA) is an approach devised by the US military during the Korean War. Their problem was to identify the cheapest way of killing enemy soldiers. For instance, what were the relative costs of bombing the enemy, napalming them, using tanks and using infantry, and how successful were these methods as measured by 'body count'?

This grim example demonstrates the essence of CEA. The method involves the costing of alternatives and the use of an intervention-specific measure of success. In health care where our interest is in improving the length and quality of patients' lives, the CEA approach involves costing alternatives and using outcome measures such as reductions in blood pressure or lives saved.

It is obvious that CEA has a particular use. It can identify which alternative intervention in a particular clinical area is best. However, CEA does not enable us to make evaluative comparisons across specialities. The measurement of reductions in blood pressure provides information about whether drugs, exercise and diet alone, or in combination, have a beneficial effect and hence reduce the risk of heart attack and stroke. Using dialysis or transplantation to treat chronic renal failure produces additional years of life. However, these two areas of study do not inform us as to which of treating renal failure or reducing blood pressure is the better area for investment.

A good example of the use of CEA addresses this issue of treating chronic renal failure with hospital dialysis, or transplantation (Klarman et al. 1968). This study was incomplete in some aspects. In analysing the mix of treatments, such as dialysis before transplant (which is usual) and hospital dialysis before home dialysis (which is community based and used to train recipients for home treatment), the study showed that transplantation is the cheapest way of producing additional years of life for such patients. This option also produces the best quality of life for survivors. The great problem is insufficient supply of spare parts available to meet patient demand.

Cost-utility analysis

The absence of a generic benefit measure that informs choices between interventions among therapeutic areas in CEA has led to the development of cost-utility analysis (CUA). Initially devised by the USA Office of Technology Assessment in the late 1970s, it was developed in the UK by Williams (1985) and is now a core element in the appraisal process for new technologies used by NICE. The goal of CUA is to identify the cost of producing an additional unit of benefit, the QALY. A QALY combines estimated increases in survival with health status valuations using quality of life measures such as EQ5D. One QALY is one year of perfect health and because it is measured on an interval scale, two half QALYs can be summed to one QALY. Thus, if treatment A for hypertension is valued at 0.85 QALYs and treatment B is valued at 0.60 QALYs, the incremental difference in utility is 0.25 QALYs or 250 QALYs per 1,000 patients per year.

In using QALYs, a major issue is whose valuation of quality of life should be used. Doctors and nurses are better informed about health states and interventions. However, patients are informed about the health states they experience, but not about those that they have not experienced. Typically, patients rate health states higher than health care professionals. An alternative source of evaluation is the wider society, which mixes informed and uninformed views, and typically gives values lower than patients.

There continues to be considerable argument about the validity of QALY estimates. Typical challenges include: Do they really measure what they claim to measure? Are they reliable (that is, reproducible and consistent)? Are they sensitive to small health state changes? Are they stable over time and independent of the duration of time in a health state? One pragmatic response of QALY adherents is that they may be imperfect, but they are the best approach available.

Cost-benefit analysis

Cost-benefit analysis (CBA) involves the identification, measurement and valuing of both the monetary costs of each alternative treatment considered in an evaluation and the monetary value of the benefits. This is an ambitious enterprise requiring the analyst to elicit values in terms of how much is given up (the opportunity cost) and how much is gained (that is, the value of reduced pain and increased length and quality of life).

Translating the stream of benefits from any intervention into monetary equivalents is done by contingent valuation (CV) or willingness to pay (WTP) studies whose purpose is to elicit a monetary valuation for common or societal goods, such as pollution and services, or, for example, the value patients place on control over their symptoms. These goods are not traded in markets. CV seeks measures to value all health factors such as the length and quality of life outcomes and non-health factors such as privacy and politeness in the treatment process.

This type of study involves investigating how much individuals are willing to pay to avoid ill health or to improve their health. For instance, let us assume that you are in pain. There are two treatments: drug X and drug Y. You are informed that drugs X and Y are equally effective in controlling your pain. However, drug X gives 1 patient in 100 stomach bleeds, while drug Y gives bleeds to 3 in 100 patients. How much would you be willing to pay, to get drug X? How much will you pay to reduce the risk of a stomach bleed from 3 to 1 per cent?

This approach is burgeoning in both health economics and environmental economics. However, it poses some difficulties. For instance, there is evidence that the method used to elicit valuations affects the values given. There is also a risk that respondents may state high values for their preferred alternative as in the NHS they do not actually have to pay. The principal concern about this method is that the values are hypothetical. Despite these concerns, work in this field progresses with practitioners seeking to devise methods to test for bias.

What follows, now, though, is a case study that illustrates some of the key areas and concepts in health economics so far considered.

CASE STUDY

Coronary artery bypass grafting – an overview of types of economic evaluation

Conjoint analysis (willingness to pay) studies, cost-effectiveness work and cost-utility analyses increasingly fill not only the pages of specialist health economics journals (such as *Health Economics*), but also medical journals. Clinicians increasingly recognize that the development and use of new technologies is not now determined on the basis of clinical effectiveness alone, but also on economic efficiency. In reviewing data or in carrying out your own studies, it is important to adopt the appropriate approach for the task in hand and to use a checklist to ensure that the design of the study is robust and comprehensive. This will now be explored through questions raised about coronary artery bypass grafting, as set out in Box 14.3.

Box 14.3   Questions relating to coronary artery bypass grafting

Should the number of coronary artery bypass grafting interventions be increased, decreased or maintained at the current level? Elaborating on this:

- Which groups gain least and most per unit of cost from this procedure?
- Which groups gain more per unit cost from related cardiac procedures such as pacemaker insertion, transplantation, angioplasty and valve insertion?
- Which groups gain more per unit of cost from other procedures outside heart disease (for instance, renal dialysis and transplantation)?

Source: Williams (1985)

In this respect, the following comments may be made:

The author, Williams (1985), took the Rosser matrix valuations of different combinations of health state, in particular disability and distress, where 1 was healthy and 0 was

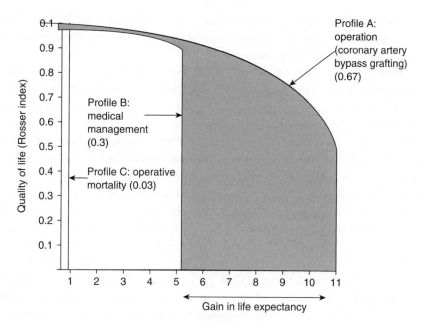

FIGURE 14.1   Severe angina and left main vessel disease
Source: Williams (1985) Reproduced with permission from BMJ Publishing Group

dead (Rosser et al. 1982). At the time, there was no clinical data that gave information on quality of life, so Williams used (only) three cardiologists to give him their judgements on the health profiles of patients with angina who had, or did not have, coronary artery bypass grafting (CABG). With this information, the author derived Figure 14.1 above, which gives the expected length and quality of life gained for patients with severe angina and left main vessel disease. The judgement was that, for 67 per cent of patients with CABG, it would give considerable health gains, while 30 per cent would get no advantage and 3 per cent would die. The author derived different results for patients depending on the level of angina, disease spread and location. The benefits were discounted at 5 per cent.

The author also used available cost data from the Department of Health and international data to adjust the figures. Costs were also discounted at 5 per cent. A range of results was computed. For instance, the cost per QALY of treating a patient with severe angina and left main vessel disease was just over £1,000 in 1985 prices, whereas a pacemaker for atrioventricular heart disease produced a QALY for £700. A heart transplant and a kidney transplant were estimated as producing a QALY for £5,000 and £3,000 respectively.

This is shown in Figure 14.1 where quality of life based on the Rosser values is indicated on the vertical axis and the duration of survival is shown on the horizontal axis. Three curves on this quality duration of life space depict three outcomes: the outcome with CABG, the outcome with medical management of angina and the operative mortality rate. The gain from the CABG is the difference between the first and second curves, minus the area under the curve reflecting the mortality outcome.

The valuation of benefits has developed substantially since this study with the development of generic quality of life measures such as EQ5D. It is instruments such as this that are now required in technology appraisals by regulatory agencies such as NICE. The study was a major development as it switched attention away from benefit measurement merely in terms of survival, and towards quality of survival, which is a major attribute of CABG. The valuation of costs has improved, but further development is needed. NHS data are improving but remain crude and the creation of private cost data remains challenging.

The use of ranked-cost QALY data in 'league tables' that rank technologies has been criticized because, inter alia, such estimates have been developed using differing methods (Maynard 1991). This approach illustrates how increasingly the relative ranking of technologies can determine regulatory sanction or rejection (see Maynard et al. 2004).

Typically, the system of ranking reflects the CUA characteristics of the technology – that is, their costs and benefits in terms of QALYs. Some argue that the value of a QALY for different groups might be weighted to reflect equity concerns: for example, whether an additional QALY for a poor recipient as opposed to a rich one is of greater value to a society interested in decreasing health inequalities. Williams (1997) proposed the concept of a 'fair innings', whereby elderly citizens could give up use of efficient interventions to fund the inefficient treatment of young people who would otherwise die prematurely after a short life span. Technology assessments typically do not use weights based on social class or age, but there continues to be a vigorous academic debate about such issues.

Efficiency, Ethics and Equity

Is economic evaluation ethical? From the economic perspective, waste or the inefficient use of society's scarce resources is unethical as it deprives potential patients of care, from which the only ethical way of allocating resources seems to be by drawing lots – that is, a lottery (Harris 1997). Such contentious views challenge the notion that the social goal to be adopted is that all should benefit. However, the economic paradigm is contentious. Harris takes this as maximizing the health of the community. Moreover, the application of techniques of economic evaluation assumes that the policy maker's objective is efficiency – namely, maximizing health gains (QALYs) from a finite budget. Nonetheless, society often chooses to act inefficiently, for example by intervening to save the lives of very low birthweight babies. This is inefficient because of the incidence of disability, but it is funded as society values young lives highly.

Other social values may override the pursuit of efficiency. For instance, QALYs are weighted equally in routine economic evaluations but if your objective is to reduce health inequality, perhaps QALYs accruing to the poor should be weighted higher than QALYs accruing to the rich? As noted earlier Williams (1997), when considering the health care costs of elderly people, advocated the 'fair innings' argument. He claimed that life beyond the allocated 'three score and ten' was a bonus that should be discriminated against, such that the efficient treatment of elderly people should be foregone and resources shifted to the inefficient treatment of the young who might not have a fair innings due to, for example, disability. Equity arguments such as these are generally ignored by health technology agencies such as the National Institute for Clinical Excellence (NICE) in the UK and parallel bodies in Europe, Canada and Australasia. Their concern, perhaps contentiously, remains the maximization of society's overall health status.

Reading Health Research Based on Economics

Much advice has already been given in this chapter on critically assessing the role of economics in health research, especially in the evaluation of service or treatment interventions. In this respect, the following high-level questions, among others, are worth reiterating:

- Is the research question and associated objectives clearly identified?
- What is the role of the particular service or treatment intervention?
- What would be the consequence of doing nothing?
- What is the comparator service or treatment intervention?
- Are all the costs of the new service or treatment identified?
- Have these costs been measured and valued against comparators?
- Are all the benefits identified, measured and valued?
- What are the political/ethical implications of the analysis?

Of course, health economists are not only concerned with the cost-effectiveness and cost benefits associated with service or treatment interventions, but this is a very important part of their work as regards health research methods.

Conclusion

The influence of economic evaluation has grown considerably in recent decades due to the influence of Alan Williams and his students such as Michael Drummond. This has been the product of increasing recognition that the rationing of health care should not be based on the advocacy of those who shout loudest, but on the evidence base of clinical and cost effectiveness. The battle continues, with patients often urgently seeking potentially life-saving care and their clinicians anxious to provide such care, but with the NHS having to assign priority between competing medical interventions and patients.

Economic evaluation techniques offer an explicit framework into which evidence of cost and effect can be inserted, often as probabilistic statements. This facilitates the critical analysis of data and helps to inform those charged with making the difficult rationing choices facing society. The chapter has made a distinction between different types of economic evaluation and what they aim to do. It has also drawn attention to the weaknesses of many studies. The reader should look for rigour and objectivity in the research that underpins economic assessments. An exercise now follows in which the reader can apply some of the principles covered in this chapter.

Exercise: Which treatment alternative in implant surgery should be funded?

Implant A has the lowest rate of complications. Implant B produces a quality adjusted life year at least cost. Implant C is the least expensive, and therefore its adoption facilitates the treatment of the largest number of patients from a given budget. Answer the following questions:

1 Which of the following questions might be regarded as 'equitable'?

- Which of these choices is most clinically effective?
- Which of these choices is efficient?

Choices and consequences: there are 500 patients requiring treatment and the NHS Primary Care Trust (PCT) has a budget of £500,000 for implants. Implant A costs £2,500 per patient and produces a QALY at a cost of £425. Implant B costs £1,500 and produces a QALY at a cost of £415. Implant C costs £1,000 and produces a QALY at a cost of £700.

2 Considering the options:

- With implant A, how many patients can be treated and what is the total number of QALYs produced?
- With implant B, how many patients can be treated and what is the total number of QALYs produced?
- With implant C, how many patients can be treated and what is the total number of QALYs produced?

3 Addressing the issues:

- If this PCT is maximizing improvements in health (as proxied by the level of QALY production), as it should in the NHS, how many patients will be left untreated?
- What information would you seek as the Chief Executive of the PCT to provide a case for increasing the budget allocation for these implants?
- What are the costs and benefits of adopting implants?

Recommended Further Reading

Drummond, M., Sculpher, M.J., Torrance, G.W., O'Brien, B. and Stoddart, G.L. (2005) *Methods of Economic Evaluation of Health Care Programmes*, 3rd edition. Oxford: Oxford University Press.
This book is an essential guidebook for practitioners on the issues raised in this chapter.

Jefferson, T., Demicheli, V. and Mugford, A. (2000) *Elementary Evaluation in Health Care.* Oxford: Oxford University Press.
This is more of an elementary and introductory guide to the use of economics in health research.

 ## Online Readings

Farnham, P. G., Sansom, S. L. and Hutchinson, A. B. (2012) 'How much should we pay for a new HIV diagnosis? A mathematical model of HIV screening in US clinical settings', *Medical Decision Making*, 32: 459–69.
How is economic evaluation defined in this context? What are the advantages of the approach adopted?

Modayil, M. V., Consolacion, T. B., Isler, J., Soria, S. and Stevens, C. (2011) 'Cost-effective smoke-free multi-unit housing media campaigns: Connecting with local communities', *Health Promotion Practice*, 12: 173S–185S.
How is economic evaluation defined in this context? Critically evaluate the paper using the checklist provided in PPS14.8.

References

Drummond, M. and the British Medical Journal Economic Evaluation Working Party (1996) 'Guidelines for authors and peer reviewers of economic submissions to the BMJ', *British Medical Journal*, 313: 275–83.
Drummond, M., Sculpher, M.J., Torrance, G.W., O'Brien, B. and Stoddart, G.L. (2005) *Methods of Economic Evaluation of Health Care Programmes*, 3rd edition. Oxford: Oxford University Press.
EuroQol Group (1991) 'EuroQol: a new facility for the measurement of health related quality of life', *Health Policy*, 16: 199–208.
Freemantle, N. and Maynard, A. (1994) 'Something rotten in the state of clinical and economic evaluations?', *Health Economics*, 3(2): 63–7.

Harris, J. (1997) 'Maximising the health of the community: the case against', *British Medical Journal*, 314: 669.

Jefferson, T., Demicheli, V. and Mugford, A. (2000) *Elementary Evaluation in Health Care.* Oxford: Oxford University Press.

Klarman, H.E., Frances, J.O. and Rosenthal, G.D. (1968) 'Cost effectiveness analysis applied to the treatment of chronic renal failure', *Medical Care*, 6: 48–54.

Maynard, A. (1990) 'The design of future cost-benefit studies', *American Heart Journal*, 119(3): 761–5.

Maynard, A. (1991) 'Developing the health care market', *Economic Journal*, 101: 1277–86.

Maynard, A. (1997) 'Evidence based medicine: an incomplete method for informing treatment choices', *Lancet*, 349: 126–8.

Maynard, A., Bloor, K. and Freemantle, N. (2004) 'Challenges for the National Institute for Clinical Excellence', *British Medical Journal*, 329: 227–9.

NHS Centre for Reviews and Dissemination (CRD) (2001) *Undertaking Systematic Reviews.* Report No. 4. York: University of York.

Philips, Z., Ginnelly, L., Sculpher, M., Claxton, K., Golder, S., Riemsma, R., Woolacoot, N. and Glanville, J. (2004) 'A review of guidelines for good practice in decision analytic modelling in health technology assessment', *Health Technology Assessment*, 8(36): 1–158.

Piachaud, D. and Weddell, J.M. (1972) 'The economics of treating varicose veins', *International Journal of Epidemiology*, 1: 287–94.

Rosser, R., Kind, P. and Williams, A. (1982) 'Valuation of quality of life: some psychometric evidence', in M. Jones-Lee (ed.), *The Value of Life and Society.* Amsterdam: Elsevier.

Williams, A. (1976) 'The cost benefit approach', *British Medical Bulletin*, 30(3): 252–6.

Williams, A. (1985) 'Economics of coronary artery by-pass grafting', *British Medical Journal*, 291: 326–9.

Williams, A. (1997) 'The rationing debate: rationing health care by age – the case for', *British Medical Journal*, 314: 820–5.

PART IV

Contemporary Issues in Researching Health

15

Governance and Ethics in Health Research

PRISCILLA ALDERSON

Introduction

- This chapter considers formal and informal approaches to ethics review and governance, their gradual development in the past and how ethics is addressed in health research today. The final part of the chapter discusses the broader politics of research ethics and governance.
- To begin with some definitions, 'participants' is the current term used for people taking part in research. This implies an active involvement and a shared control of the research process between researchers and participants. In practice, this does not always occur as people may have little or no awareness about why they are being researched and what the process involves. In such cases, people are being treated as the subjects, or even the objects, of the research rather than as participants. Therefore, the term 'subjects/participants' is used here. The term 'medical' is used to refer to clinical scientific research on the body and body parts, and the term 'social' includes all the disciplines that research people's views and their experiences of health and illness. At present, a spectrum of views about research ethics and governance is found among social researchers, ranging from active interest and support through resignation to and unwilling compliance with ethics committees' requirements to direct criticism of the lack of political and socio-economic concern in abstract bioethics.

The Changing Context of Health and Medical Research Ethics

Medical research ethics in the past

The history of medical ethics records doctors' gradual movement from rejection, for example see Tobias and Souhami (1993), to general support for research ethics and governance. Before 1950, there were few formal ethics guidelines and committees. During the 1930s to 1940s, formal guidelines in Germany did little to prevent harmful research, which was also widely conducted in the USA, Europe and the Far East (Proctor 1988; McNeill 1993). Unethical medical research has continued into this century (see Sharav 2003; Save the Children 2007; Slesser and Qureshi 2009; Boseley 2010; Kolch et al. 2010). Recently, a leading British paediatric journal published a report of unethical research without comment. The paper reported 'non-therapeutic' research on newborn babies with severe cardiac defects. This included 60–90 minutes of extra anaesthesia with administration of carbon dioxide before surgery (Hoehn et al. 2005).

From the 1970s and 1980s, research ethics committees and, in the USA, institutional review boards for medical research, began to be introduced widely. In the 1980s and 1990s, philosophy departments at risk of closure set up flourishing health care ethics centres and courses and there are now numerous health care ethics journals and conferences. However, as the neonatal cardiac example above illustrates, some research ethics committees still allow high-risk research that contravenes the guidelines set by the World Medical Association (1964, 2008) and the Royal College of Paediatrics and Child Health (2000) to take place.

In general, sociologists have only recently begun to consider formal ethics governance seriously within their own discipline. Burgess (1989) identified three main areas for attention to ethics: sponsorship in terms of how sponsors may assist with research or impede it; research relationships that involve access, power, deception, harm and secrecy; and the dissemination of research findings. Recently, Petersen (2011) is among many who have pointed out the inescapably ethical, normative and value-laden nature of social research. Gouldner (1971: 50–1) considered that research methodology is 'infused with ideologically resonant assumptions about what the social world is' (see Chapter 2 for further discussion). According to this view, ethics is not a matter of adding a paragraph or veneer of respect for rules, but involves thinking about ethics in every aspect of the research project.

The influences that stimulated interest in social research governance are outlined in Box 15.1 which follows.

Box 15.1   Influences stimulating interest in social research governance

- Risk, cost and the threat of litigation
- The institutionalized increase and formal management of risk and mistrust (see Beck 1992)
- A few highly publicized cases of the death of a clinical research subject
- The exponential growth of other governance and legalistic bureaucracy in research institutions
- Institutions' desire for standards to promote and protect profits from research and development
- The aim to reassure the public and sustain their support, donations and willingness to take part in research
- The many recent Acts and Conventions on human rights and data protection.

In consequence during the past decade, research agencies and funders and professional academic associations have revised their ethics guidelines, and British universities now have ethics committees intended to safeguard research subjects/participants, researchers themselves and the standards and reputation of research. Social and health care research ethics committees have reorganized their national institutions and websites. The context of this chapter is continuing change and debate on the pros and cons of health research ethics and governance; on whether the relevant disciplines require different forms of ethics governance; and on how the various disciplines concerned with health can work together.

Developing a Framework for Medical Ethics

In 1981, I joined a group which met monthly over three years to discuss and write a book on the law and ethics of medical research on children (Nicholson 1985). Modelled on the USA National Commission for the Protection of Human Subjects in Medical and Behavioral Research (1977, 1978), the group in London included doctors, lawyers, a nurse, lay people, philosophers and psychologists. Given the history of unregulated medical research on children, we were critical of existing arrangements. We aimed to identify and agree on principled, but flexible, standards to protect both child research subjects and the interests of all future patients who might benefit from research findings. We were influenced by three main frameworks for medical ethics relating to the principles, rights and outcomes set out in Box 15.2.

Box 15.2   Frameworks for medical ethics

- *Principles of ethics* that centre on a respect for autonomy, justice, doing no harm and using resources fairly and efficiently.
- *Rights* that provide for basic needs with the best available health care; protect people from harm, abuse, neglect and discrimination; respect their freedom of information, expression, thought and conscience; and promote social inclusion and self-determination.
- *Outcomes* that aim to avoid or reduce harm and costs and to promote benefits.

Sources: USA National Commission for the Protection of Human Subjects in Medical and Behavioral Research (1978); United Nations (1989); Beauchamp and Childress (2001)

These principles, rights and outcomes, alongside other ethical frameworks such as virtue ethics, all have strengths but leave gaps, which are widely analysed and debated (see, for example, Gillon 2003; Council of Europe 2005; Halliwell et al. 2005; Royal College of Physicians 2007; Fox and Swazey 2008; UK Research Integrity Office 2009; General Medical Council 2010; Hedgecoe 2010; and Petersen 2011). Moral questions about power, honesty and respecting or abusing people, arise throughout the research process and, formally or less consciously, researchers tend to resolve questions by thinking about principles. They are concerned with the right thing to do; about human rights in respecting and protecting people; and about outcomes. What might be the benefits to promote and the harms to avoid? Many researchers combine these approaches. Although the frameworks do not provide easy answers to ethical problems, they can help to identify and clarify problems and possible ways to solve or reduce them.

Key Questions in Health Research Ethics and Governance

The key questions for those concerned with research ethics and governance are set out in Box 15.3 below.

Box 15.3   Key questions for research ethics and governance

- How can we prevent poor standards and promote high standards of research?
- How can ethics and governance be efficient and effective?
- What ethical questions arise throughout projects in the choice of research questions, theories and methods to apply?
- How can the many disciplines and lay people involved in research and governance work well together?

In the UK, the *Research Governance Framework for Health and Social Care* (Department of Health 2004) defines governance as: setting standards; defining ways to deliver standards; monitoring and assessing the arrangements; improving research quality; safeguarding the public by promoting good practice; reducing and preventing poor practice and misconduct; and ensuring that lessons are learnt from adverse incidents. These standards apply to all research conducted in British health or social services and relate to other areas of research. Increasingly, funding bodies also require reports on ethical standards.

Concerns about Ethics Guidelines

A central question is whether guidelines are useful and effective. They have been central to greater understanding and practical implementation of high standards in research. However, some common confusion arises in the guidance, particularly on covert research, therapeutic research and harm–benefit equations.

Consent and covert research

In 1947, the first international guidance on research ethics, the *Nuremberg Code* (1947), began: '1. The voluntary consent of the human subject is absolutely essential'. The code assumed that people could base their consent or refusal on an 'enlightened' decision. This emphasis on voluntary consent was lost later in the far more widely used *Declaration of Helsinki* (World Medical Association 1964) which emphasized the doctor's duty to relieve suffering, advance progress through research and protect human beings' 'health and rights' (World Medical Association 2008). Consent is not mentioned until clause 9 in 1964, and not until clause 22 in the 2008 version is free agreement mentioned. Although later clauses enlarge on consent, power has shifted from the voluntary subject to the responsible medical researcher. *The Declaration of Helsinki* also does not mention covert research – that is, research carried out without the subject/participant's knowledge and consent – but appears to veto it by repeatedly stating that consent must always be sought.

Within social science, the British Psychological Society (2009) aims to 'protect the dignity of participants', but – as is the case with the British Sociological Association (2004) – covert research, that is research without people's knowledge or consent, is allowed. The central principle to be determined is: 'the reaction of participants when deception was revealed. If this led to [their] discomfort, anger or objections ... then the deception was inappropriate.' Yet an accurate prediction of people's reaction after an event is often not possible to determine, particularly when the judgement is being made by researchers who have decided to deceive them.

Therapeutic research

Until 2000, *The Declaration of Helsinki* used the somewhat misleading phrase 'therapeutic research'. This implied research that was directly beneficial research and required lower ethical standards than for 'non-therapeutic research', which had no direct benefit to patients. However, all research concerns collecting and analysing data rather than providing care or directly benefiting people. Researchers might do so coincidentally, if they provide care/treatment that they are also researching or evaluating, but the main purpose of research is systematic enquiry. The term 'therapeutic' implies benefits that the researcher cannot ensure. Indeed, many people have been classed as being in 'therapeutic research' and the treatment was later shown to be unhelpful or harmful. If they were in a placebo control group, they would, by definition, be receiving a non-treatment. Research ethics committees may still evaluate potentially dangerous drug trials as 'therapeutic', and therefore permissible, while at the same time criticizing 'non-therapeutic' data collection. This might later prove to be far more useful in understanding the aetiology or process of disease or the social and emotional needs of patients.

For decades, the care-based concept of 'therapeutic research' has tended to confuse discussions of medical ethics as it is used to excuse risks that might be accepted in treatment, but not in research. This confusion is also found in social research, when researchers justify intrusive interviews by claiming that people like to talk, or find relief in relating their experiences. They may do, but that is not the aim or purpose of the encounter and cannot be guaranteed. The claim blurs the reality that subjects/participants are helping the researcher by providing data. To recognize that the research encounter is essentially a meeting between strangers can help to promote protection and respect. Some guidelines for health and social care workers may blur the roles of researcher and service provider. Butler (2002: 245) comments:

> Both the process of social work/care research, including the choice of methodology, and the use to which any findings might be put, should be congruent with the aims and values of social work practice and, where possible, seek to empower service users, promote their welfare and improve their access to economic and social capital on equal terms with other citizens.

The statement does not explain how the process of collecting and reporting data can either meet the aims of social work/care to provide a service or directly benefit and empower a client. Promises directly to help subjects/participants can undermine the key principle of respect for consent (or refusal) that is freely given. Such promises have the potential to mislead researchers, subjects/participants and gatekeepers into believing that there is a direct benefit of taking part in research and that permission should not be refused.

Turning to other research areas, some clinical trialists claim that patients do better simply by being in a trial, although the evidence for this is inconclusive (Vist et al. 2005). Feminist research ethics also tend to emphasize the ethic of care in research (Edwards and Mauthner 2001). This can imply a direct benefit of care from the researcher or from being in a research project. It risks over-conceptualizing the subject/participant as dependent and needy. In contrast, codes of medical ethics have placed an emphasis on respect for the person's independence from the researcher. It is seen as being crucial to the research process. In sum, there are vital distinctions between treatment and research and between both the relationship of practitioner–patient/client and of researcher–subject/participant. As Cooter (1992) records, well-meant 'caring' intentions have on occasion cloaked and excused extremely harmful 'welfare', dietary and medical practices in research.

The harm–benefit analysis

Another longstanding confusion in the guidelines relates to the harm–benefit analysis. Too often, likely risks, harms, costs and inconvenience to subjects/participants were weighed against the supposed direct benefits to them of taking part in research and/or of receiving the treatment being tested. Participants might also have received the treatment outside the research. Alternatively, if a treatment were only available within trials, then its efficacy would be likely to be too questionable to count as a definite assured benefit. *The Declaration of Helsinki* (World Medical Association 2008: 18) still makes this error in mentioning 'the foreseeable benefits' to subjects, but does add 'and to other individuals or communities affected by the condition under investigation'. The real balance is between possible harm to subjects versus possible benefit to future people, and this should be explained to each potential participant so that they can make a decision on the basis of a personal harm–benefit assessment.

Ethics guidelines can be vague, confusing and contradictory and it has been argued that practice cannot be made to fit written codes, however well they are devised. For instance, two or more values can have 'different, even conflicting implications' (Lindsay 2000: 18). Nevertheless, ethics guidelines do address complex questions of justice, respect, harm and benefit that have been debated, though not conclusively, for many centuries. Moreover, they raise vital questions that science and research methods do not deal with directly and so they can help to promote reflection and debate that contribute to the gradual rise in ethical standards in research.

Governance Through Research Ethics Committees

The role of research ethics committees

The uncertainty about interpreting ethical guidelines is arguably one reason for having formal reviews and discussion to help to clarify complex arguments, instead of leaving decisions to individual researchers alone. The various potential roles of research ethics committees are set out in Box 15.4.

Box 15.4 The role of research committees

Research committees:

- Act as a protective barrier between researchers and potential subjects/participants.
- Raise awareness about ethics within the research community.
- Review whether the anticipated benefits justify any risks to subjects/participants.
- Veto unethical research early and warn and advise about potential ethical problems that might be avoided or prevented.
- Check that potential participants receive clear written information and have an opportunity for discussion so that they can give informed consent or refusal.
- Check that certain groups are not over-researched, that particular needs are met, such as for interpreters, and that the protocol is not too onerous.
- Collect data on best research ethics practice and disseminate ideas.

The priority during an ethics review is that subjects/participants have clear written information, and know that consent should be adequately informed and freely given or withheld. The review of basic science raises such questions as: Is the research worth doing? Do the hoped-for benefits justify the risks and costs? Will the research duplicate previous work? Are the methods likely to answer the research questions? Is the sample size large enough? How original and useful might the research findings be?

It may be claimed that only relevant specialists can be competent reviewers. However, if research is to be ethical, it can be explained and justified clearly enough to enable 'ordinary' people to give or withhold informed consent. Research ethics committees that include members with a range of expertise, including 'lay' people, aim to review proposals from the point of view of potential participants rather than of informed specialists (West and Butler 2003).

The websites of the Association of Research Ethics Committees (AREC) (www.arec.org.uk) and the National Research Ethics Service (NRES) (www.nres.nhs.uk) under the Health Research Authority, with email lists such as the Center for Genetics and Society (cgs@geneticsandsociety.org), BioEdge (bioedge@bioedge.org) and GeneWatch UK (www.genewatch.org), give frequently updated news on ethical problems, guidelines and debates about rights, privacy, data protection, consent, low and high standards in research, patenting and related matters. AREC gives advice on writing patient/participant information sheets.

Common Criticisms of Research Ethics Committees

It is often suggested by researchers that health care ethics committees lack interest in, and knowledge about, social research (Christensen and Prout 2002; Lewis 2002; Glendenning and McKie 2003; Iphofen 2004; and Brindle 2005). Yet having to explain social research theories and methods convincingly to ethics committees can prepare researchers to give skilful explanations to potential subjects/participants in order to obtain their informed consent. Explaining and justifying qualitative methods, with clear protocols and information leaflets, can also help to increase public understanding and gain support for social research. Increasingly, health research ethics committees understand and support social research and have social researchers as members.

Some social researchers argue that while medical research can cause harm and distress, social research does not, and, indeed, people enjoy and benefit from taking part in social research. However, the parents who protested after their deceased children's organs were removed between 1988 and 1995 for research at Alder Hey Hospital said they supported scientific/medical research on the children's organs. Their objection was a social concern – they were not informed or asked for their consent. Similarly in the 1980s, women who enrolled into covert breast cancer trials without their consent said that they felt wronged primarily because they had not been respected, rather than physically harmed. Even the seemingly innocuous social research question 'Tell me about who you live with at home' can distress people who may be going through domestic turmoil. In practice, it is impossible to predict when a subject/participant might feel harmed, distressed, humiliated, anxious, wronged or betrayed if, say, their identity is revealed or they are misquoted. An ethics committee review and form-filling can offer time to consider such potential problems, to prevent them or prepare a researcher in how to respond to them if they arise.

Ethics committees are said to be against open-ended ethnography and grounded theory that raise new questions, as well as being critical of opportunistic and informal research. However, research funders – and not only research ethics committees – require detailed plans, justifications and safeguards for subjects/participants. In practice, ethnographic and other unfolding research methods may be approved by health care ethics committees as long as their objectives and methods are clearly described and justified. If questions and methods alter or emerge during a project in major ways, then research ethics committees and subjects/participants can be informed. Indeed, in such projects participants may share in planning the initial approaches and subsequent changes (see also Chapters 8, 17 and 20).

A critical analysis of research ethics, its complexity as well as its use and misuse, can be extremely valuable. However, social researchers should be accountable for their practice. They could reflect on how far they themselves would trust other professions, such as police or journalists, bankers or doctors, on whose services they sometimes rely, if these professionals claimed to need little or no regulation of ethics or accountability. In recent years, self-regulation in many professions has been found to be inadequate (see, for instance, Allsop and Saks 2002). It is therefore questionable why 'lay' subjects/participants should trust unaccountable social researchers.

Completing forms and reports is part of efficient research, but there are concerns about the time spent on form-filling and delays during ethics reviews. This can severely disrupt timetables and staff employment contracts. The NRES now coordinates all the committees into a rapid response national review process. Sylvester and Green (2003) and others are concerned about delays to students' limited time for completing dissertations, and they give the example of research with people having palliative terminal care. They warn that their Masters students might have to undertake literature reviews instead of research. Yet it can be argued that a literature review may be preferable to exposing very ill, vulnerable 'participants' to hurried and therefore potentially unethical research by inexperienced Masters students.

Informally, social researchers may discuss how research ethics committees approve poor and harmful protocols, reject good ones and probe trivial points. It is the case that committee members may have too little time to do their (unpaid) work properly and certainly they need training and support. Some committees are dominated, and possibly misled, by assertive individuals. Yet they do invite researchers to respond to their queries and criticisms and to attend a meeting if they wish. Another criticism is that the lay members are neither 'representative', nor democratically elected. However, professional members are not 'representative' either, as they too may be appointed for their personal qualities, expertise and willingness to join the committee. Research ethics committees are part of public service and decision making. Like juries, they may look unsatisfactory until the alternatives are considered.

The Politics of Research Ethics and Governance

Research ethics governance is a contentious arena, with researchers from different disciplines often aiming to protect their own interests, while they compete for research opportunities and funding, power and influence. Doctors dominate health research in access to resources and in the management of research processes, and they are usually the leaders of interdisciplinary teams. A further complication for ethics is that some medical staff and ethicists have lucrative contracts and research prospects with the companies that sponsor research and manufacture products, opportunities that social scientists, perhaps fortunately, seldom have.

Whereas medical research ethics guidelines and international networks are well established, paradoxically social science research ethics is less socially and collectively developed. Many social researchers prefer the private, informal ethics of 'self-regulation' and personal conscience (British Sociological Association 2004). Social science ethics committees are less likely to have independent and lay members, even though it is arguably easier for lay people to understand social than, say, biochemical research, although they routinely sit on health care ethics committees. Social scientists seem to be less aware of the British Sociological Association (2004) code, than their medical and nursing colleagues are about their codes (Nursing and Midwifery Council 2007 and World Medical Association 2008). This is partly because those professions have to be registered in order to practise and can be struck off for breaking ethical rules. By contrast, Lewis et al. (2003: 4) state that: 'It was unexpected to find that a considerable number [of sociological researchers] reported the absence of [consent] procedures.' However, a year later Webster et al. (2004) and Boulton et al. (2004) reported growing support among social researchers for research ethics committees and for ethics training.

Some authors criticize ethics rules and formal guidelines/review for the reasons given in Box 15.5 which follows.

Box 15.5 Criticisms of ethics rules and formal guidelines/review

Ethics rules and guidelines are held by some to be:

- Too inflexible.
- Unable to deal with unforeseen situations.
- Too easily becoming a routine or a fig leaf.
- No substitute for the active engagement of individual researchers and the whole social science community with ethics (Christensen and Prout 2002).

Indeed, it has been observed that formal guidelines and review might unethically 'invite the individual to surrender the moral conscience to a professional consensus' (Homan 1992: 331).

Of course, there are dangers in bureaucratic ethics (Bauman 1993) of 'ethical inflation' and imposed 'external drivers' that could 'restrict the conduct of important, high quality, social science research' (Lewis et al. 2003: 1–4). Lewis et al. warn that overly prescriptive, imposed, 'highly formalised or bureaucratic ways of securing consent' could undermine the desirable ethics 'embedded' in everyday research. They suggest that formal review is 'marginal to fostering relationships in which a process of ongoing ethical regard for participants could be sustained', and that it conflicts with what 'constitutes good (necessary, relevant) practice'. They add that 'ethical vigilance' should be 'proportionate to the risks borne by research participants'.

Consultations on social research guidelines (for example, Boulton et al. 2004 and ESRC 2005) have partly addressed criticisms of research ethics review systems. They have helped to develop higher standards of research ethics 'literacy' and governance that benefit researchers and subjects/participants and aim to treat social research ethics as public and negotiated. Yet many urgent questions remain such as: How can personal privacy be respected in national surveys of disease or in family genome research? How can longitudinal researchers obtain subjects'/participants' informed consent when secondary research teams will use their databanks for as-yet-unknown purposes? Health care research ethics committees and guidance from the Department of Health in the UK only partly address such problems. How can health research effectively help to raise standards of health?

To dismiss ethics as yet another discourse of power ignores how researchers themselves can be seen to have a vested interest in maximizing their autonomy and power. The critics of the ethics governance cited above claim that this will either force researchers to observe higher standards or force them to lower their standards. Perhaps they should accept that the first point is reasonable and the second unlikely and still each researcher's personal choice? The opposition to review also denies the value of formal and group means of critically improving research designs and overlooks how morality in research is neither a private nor collective concern, but a complicated combination of the two.

Learning from Social Research Ethics

While medical ethics has tended to construct policies and systems, social research can also contribute to health care ethics, which has long been seen as too abstract and impersonal. When one abstract philosopher claimed that it was necessary to clear away the contingent 'rubbish' of social experience in order to see ethical problems clearly (Raphael 1976), a practical feminist philosopher replied that ethical problems are constituted in this everyday 'rubbish' (Grimshaw 1986). Grounded in practical everyday experiences, social research ethics can introduce the practical, realistic insights too often ignored in abstract ethics. Social scientists may contribute to the development of practical research ethics by:

- Learning from feelings and emotions during the research process.
- Acknowledging practical problems throughout the research process.
- Explicitly acknowledging ethics in the social, political and economic contexts of research.

Learning from emotions

Researchers develop insights through learning from their emotions by looking inwards at their hopes and fears about their work: their anxiety about mistakes and dealing with stress from lack of time and resources. Researchers gain from sharing their satisfaction about new data and theories, as well as responding to the hopes and fears of subjects/participants. Although emotions can mislead and cloud judgement, there are grave dangers if researchers lose empathy and pity. Macintyre (1966) analysed how overly rational Kantian ethics, which dismissed emotions, contingencies and empathy, ended by validating Nazism, notorious for its inhumane research. Researchers can become detached from their 'moral self constituted by responsibility' and become blindly obedient to rules, instead of carefully negotiating a way forward through unpredictable and ambiguous interactions (Bauman 1993). During stressful and often sensitive research in health care, ethics can contribute to supporting and debriefing researchers during shared research analysis sessions.

Acknowledging practical problems

On the numerous practical and unpredictable problems that arise during research projects, solutions can be found. Halliwell et al. (2005: 142) review these rarely reported problems and contend that social research 'is first and foremost a moral activity'. It is about negotiating human relationships and achieving a complicated balance between many opposing options. They conclude that at every stage, ethical research relies on codes, research ethics committees and researchers' good intentions. It also relies on their skills and their respect for participants, as well as their reflections on their work and their efforts to raise practical standards in an open and transparent way.

Explicitly acknowledging ethics in the social world

The greatest contribution that social researchers can make to ethical practice is to expand the economic and political dimensions of health care ethics. Some doctors, lawyers and philosophers regard the social sciences as younger disciplines with less tried-and-tested methods, theories and body of knowledge. Yet the dominant methods of the medical case study or the statistical survey both tend to atomize individuals and use variables in ways that exclude the social context. This works against a more integrated social science that connects private troubles to public issues (Mills 1959). Conventional bioethics tends to take justice to mean enforcing present rules, not working towards redistribution and equity. It avoids explicitly examining power differences, both between researchers and subjects/participants and within research teams. Power has greatest force when it is least obvious, visible or acknowledged, and when it is exerted through subtle persuasion and knowledge withheld. Power is weaker when it is overt and can be countered by open resistance (Lukes 2005). It is therefore important to be aware of power in research in several ways, as set out in Box 15.6.

Box 15.6 Dimensions of awareness of power in research

Awareness of power in research can be found in:

- Methods of researcher–participant relations, such as watching for cues that subjects/participants might feel too intimidated to refuse to take part or to say they wish to withdraw.
- Fair relations within interdisciplinary research teams, fostered by clear foresight and written agreements from the start about responsibility, authorship, freedom to publish and other potentially contentious matters, which are then discussed during regular, well-chaired team meetings.
- Choosing research topics and methods of analysis that take due account of political power in, for example, connections between social inequalities, morbidity and mortality.

Research reports can greatly affect research subjects/participants and also, potentially, everyone in the group associated with them, as is the case with research involving people affected by HIV/AIDS. The media and policy makers are liable to cite research in ways that can increase prejudice, discrimination and the further social exclusion of these disadvantaged groups. Although the social inclusion and health of many groups (such as women and black, disabled and gay people) has improved over the past 50 years – particularly for those group members with higher incomes – poor health and social exclusion can occur among members of groups who are low paid or unpaid. Such groups include children and young people (one third of the world's population), immigrants, Roma and homeless people. Despite researchers' attention to the social and health status of disadvantaged groups, many of these groups are not significantly healthier in the 2010s than they were in the 1960s. Rates of obesity, diabetes, cancer, asthma and dementia are rising, as is ill health associated with growing inequalities (Wilkinson and Pickett 2009). This raises questions about the purpose and effectiveness of public health research and policy. Researchers may therefore wish to make efforts to prevent policy makers and the mass media from using their work in ways that increase prejudice, discrimination and inequality.

Bioethics can be censured for endorsing biomedical research uncritically. Through abstract, universal, mechanistic over-use of the four principles (respect for autonomy, beneficence, non-maleficence and justice), bioethics tends to concentrate on detailed, personal consent to research and treatment, rather than on broader social contexts, the uncertainties, risks and political economies relating, for example, to genomics, biobanks, cloning, stem cells, nanotechnology and synthetic organs. Research in these areas can be seen to produce costly medical and surgical interventions for those who can afford them – potentially overlooking the dangers these technologies pose to civil liberties. Currently, the main use of DNA knowledge is to maintain banks for the police while neuro-scanning might one day be able to 'read thoughts'. Bioethics could more strongly challenge large-scale investment in biotechnology research, instead of concentrating on micro-ethics questions related to personal risk and consent, abstracted from political questions about the 'environment', social and economic influences on health and illness and research (Fox and Swazey 2008; Hedgecoe 2010; Petersen 2011). In this vein, bioethicists and scientists may be seen to collude with the mass media and commercial interests in raising false hopes of miracle medical discoveries as this serves to sustain public support and funding for their research (Evans et al. 2011).

Ethnography, the sociological critics contend, could help to 'save' bioethics by enriching its social and political dimensions and analysing how science is socially co-constructed and does not simply produce facts. At present, however, sociologists have tended to concentrate on areas already defined and dominated by bioethics and scientists, rather than considering future, long-term, population-related possibilities. On this view, social researchers can be seen to be restricted by major funders' biomedical-technical-bioethical programmes – as illustrated by the operation of the Research Councils and Wellcome Trust in the UK. These organizations may be seen to grant funds to bioethics research to 'resolve ethical dilemmas' through bureaucratic, neo-liberal analyses of cost-effectiveness validating the new biotechnologies and their seemingly inevitable emergence, rather than taking a more challenging view of ethics (Fox and Swazey 2008; Hedgecoe 2010; Petersen 2011). They may therefore side-step questions such as: how research commodifies bodies; how commercial companies privatize and then sell knowledge gained from state-funded research; the relative lack of democratic consultation about research plans and processes; and public misinformation.

There is therefore criticism of some of the approaches to research ethics highlighted in this chapter. It has been argued that questions of human rights and informed consent are too narrow to encompass unknown future research on biobanks (Fox and Swazey 2008). Social researchers may be well advised to attend more to ethical dilemmas such as: 'Is the research worth doing?' (see Alderson and Morrow 2011), and 'Who is likely to gain or lose by the findings?' From this perspective, health care ethics should move beyond informed consent, which is stretched to tenuous extremes over questions concerning longitudinal research. There should perhaps be more concern with democratic public engagement with biotechnical research and questioning of who has the power to set international research agendas.

Yet instead of criticizing 'principilism', as the sociological critics do, we need to recognize how principles of respect for autonomy, to do no harm and achieve justice, in fact underlie arguments for human rights and sociologists' criticisms of bioethics and their proposed alternatives. The valuable standards developed in bioethics for specific, personal, short-term decisions about health care research and treatment should be retained, but we also need to expand on and politicize the principles of respect and justice that bioethics has made unduly narrow and abstract.

Conclusion

During debates about research ethics, opinions are sharply divided between beliefs that formal regulations and reviews inhibit research, and the belief that ethics is essential to protect research subjects/participants and high standards in research. This chapter has aimed to highlight the nature of these arguments. The practical implication for researchers is to take care at every stage of the research process, from initial plans to final dissemination. They should aim for ethical standards throughout, working with subjects/participants as far as possible, from the initial planning and selection of topics, questions, methods and samples. Participants or their representatives can advise on and encourage respectful approaches, and provide a deeper understanding of research subjects' motives and values during data collection and analysis, report writing and dissemination – as further discussed in Chapter 20. However, ethics governance can be seen to be unduly shaped by an abstract, apolitical philosophy, which serves the commercial research programmes of governments and industry. Sociology and the other social sciences could contribute more critical and wide-ranging socio-economic-political analyses that would raise standards of justice and human rights at all levels of health care research and governance.

Exercise: Writing a leaflet for participants in health research

Health Research Authority-based ethics committees require researchers to write a leaflet for potential participants to accompany the project application form. The leaflet has to include the following:

A short project title

Researcher's name, institution and contact details

Information on:

- The nature, timing and purpose of the research.
- The key questions and methods.
- The potential harms/risks.
- The hoped-for benefits that any findings might yield.
- Participants' rights:

  o to withdraw from the project, or to refuse to take part.
  o to have their data protected.
  o to anonymity in reports.

Write a clear and respectful leaflet of up to two A4 sides about one of your own projects. Assume that the people reading it will have a reading age of about 10 years, and use short words and sentences. See www.arec.org.uk for further practical details.

Recommended Further Reading

Alderson, P. and Morrow, V. (2011) *The Ethics of Research with Children and Young People: A Practical Handbook*, revised 3rd edition. London: Sage.
This book breaks research projects into 10 stages and discusses the many ethical questions that can arise for researchers at each stage. It is relevant to all age groups with extra questions relating to children.

Petersen, A. (2011) 'Can and should sociology save bioethics?', *Medical Sociology News*, 6(1): 2–14. Available at: www.medicalsociologyonline.org
Petersen summarizes sociological criticisms of bioethics and proposes broader, more sociological approaches to research ethics.

World Medical Association (2008) *The Declaration of Helsinki*. Fernay-Voltaire: WMA.
The basic international guide to health care research ethics has been regularly updated since it was originally agreed in 1964 and is relevant to all health researchers.

Online Readings

Griffiths, P. (2008) 'Ethical conduct and the nurse ethnographer: Consideration of an ethic of care', *Journal of Research in Nursing*, 13: 350–61.

What are the key issues relating to ethical research conduct identified by the author? What solutions are proposed? How effective do you think they will be in this context?

Morrisey, B. (2012) 'Ethics: Ethics and research among persons with disabilities in long-term care, *Qualitative Health Research*, 22: 1284–97.

What are the key issues relating to ethical research conduct identified by the author? What solutions are proposed? How effective do you think they will be in this context?

References

Alderson, P. and Morrow, V. (2011) *The Ethics of Research with Children and Young People: A Practical Handbook*, revised 3rd edition. London: Sage.

Allsop, J. and Saks, M. (eds) (2002) *Regulating the Health Professions*. London: Sage.

Bauman, Z. (1993) *Postmodern Ethics*. Oxford: Blackman.

Beauchamp, T. and Childress, J. (2001) *Principles of Biomedical Ethics*. New York: Oxford University Press.

Beck, U. (1992) *Risk Society*. London: Sage.

Boseley, S. (2010) 'Nigeria: drug trial tale of "dirty tricks"', *Guardian Weekly*, 17 December.

Boulton, M., Brown, N., Lewis, G. and Webster, A. (2004) *Implementing the ESRC Research Ethics Framework: The Case for Research Ethics Committees*. York: SATSU, University of York and School of Social Sciences and Law, Oxford Brookes University.

Brindle, D. (2005) 'Getting permission for social research is now a nightmare', *The Guardian*, 5 February.

British Psychological Society (2009) *A Code of Conduct for Psychologists*. Leicester: BPS.

British Sociological Association (2004) *Statement of Ethical Practice*. Durham: BSA.

Burgess, R. (1989) *The Ethics of Social Research*. London: Falmer.

Butler, I. (2002) 'Critical commentary: a code of ethics for social work and social care research', *British Journal of Social Work*, 32: 239–48.

Christensen, P. and Prout, A. (2002) 'Working with ethical symmetry in social research with children', *Childhood*, 9(4): 477–97.

Cooter, R. (ed.) (1992) *In the Name of the Child: Health and Welfare 1880–1940*. London: Routledge.

Council of Europe (CE) (2005) *Additional Protocol to the Convention on Human Rights and Biomedicine, Concerning Biomedical Research*. Brussels: CE.

Department of Health (2004) *Research Governance Framework for Health and Social Care: Implementation Plan for Social Care*. London: HMSO.

Economic and Social Research Council (ESRC) (2005) *Framework for Research Ethics*. Swindon: ESRC.

Edwards, R. and Mauthner, M. (2001) 'Ethics and feminist research: theory and practice', in M. Mauthner, M. Birch, J. Jessop and T. Miller (eds), *Ethics in Qualitative Research*. London: Sage.

Evans, J., Meslin, E., Marteau, T. and Caulfield, T. (2011) 'Deflating the genomic bubble', *Science*, 331: 861–2.

Fox, R. and Swazey, J. (2008) *Observing Bioethics*. Oxford: Oxford University Press.

General Medical Council (2010) *Consent to Research*. London: General Medical Council.

Gillon, R. (ed.) (2003) *Principles of Healthcare Ethics*. Chichester: Wiley.

Glendenning, C. and McKie, L. (2003) 'BSA working in partnership with SPA: ethics in social research', *BSA Network*, Summer: 15–16.

Gouldner, A. (1971) *The Coming Crisis of Western Sociology*. London: Routledge.

Grimshaw, J. (1986) *Feminism and Philosophy*. Brighton: Wheatsheaf.

Halliwell, N., Lawton, J. and Gregory, S. (2005) *Reflections on Research: The Realities of Doing Research in the Social Sciences*. Buckingham: Open University Press.

Hedgecoe, A. (2010) 'Bioethics and the reinforcement of socio-technical expectations', *Social Studies of Science*, 40(2): 163–86.

Hoehn, K., Wernovsky, G., Rychik, J., Gaynor, J., Spray, T., Feudtner, C. and Nelson, R. (2005) 'What factors are important to parents making decisions about neonatal research?', *Archives of Disease in Childhood*, 90: 267–9.

Homan, R. (1992) 'The ethics of open methods', *British Journal of Sociology*, 42(3): 321–32.

Iphofen, R. (2004) 'A code to keep away judges, juries and MPs', *Times Higher Education Supplement*, 16 January: 24.

Kolch, M., Ludolph, A., Plener, P., Fangerau, H., Vitiello, B. and Fegert, J. (2010) 'Safeguarding children's rights in psychopharmacological research: ethical and legal issues', *Current Pharmacological Design*, June.

Lewis, J. (2002) 'Research and development in social care: governance and good practice', *Research Policy and Planning*, 20(1): 3–9.

Lewis, G., Brown, N., Holland, S. and Webster, A. (2003) *A Review of Ethics and Social Science Research for the Strategic Forum for the Social Sciences, Commissioned by the ESRC: Summary*. York: SATSU.

Lindsay, G. (2000) 'Researching children's perspectives: ethical issues', in A. Lewis and G. Lindsay (eds), *Researching Children's Perspectives*. Buckingham: Open University Press.

Lukes, S. (2005) *Power: A Radical View*. Basingstoke: Palgrave Macmillan.

Macintyre, A. (1966) *A Short History of Ethics*. New York: Macmillan.

McNeill, P. (1993) *The Ethics and Politics of Human Experimentation*. Cambridge: Cambridge University Press.

Mills, C. Wright (1959) *The Sociological Imagination*. Oxford: Oxford University Press.

Nicholson, R. (1985) *Medical Research with Children: Ethics, Law and Practice*. Oxford: Oxford University Press.

Nuremberg Code (1947) Available at: ohsr.od.nih.gov/guidelines/nuremberg.html

Nursing and Midwifery Council (2007) *The Code: Standards of Conduct, Performance and Ethics for Nurses and Midwives*. London: NMC.

Petersen, A. (2011) 'Can and should sociology save bioethics?', *Medical Sociology News*, 6(1): 2–14. Available at: www.medicalsociologyonline.org

Proctor, R. (1988) *Racial Hygiene: Medicine under the Nazis*. Cambridge, MA: Harvard University Press.

Raphael, D. (1976) *Problems of Politics and Philosophy*. London: Macmillan.

Royal College of Paediatrics and Child Health (2000) 'Ethics Advisory Committee: guidelines on the ethical conduct of medical research involving children', *Archives of Disease in Childhood*, 82: 177–82.

Royal College of Physicians (2007) *Guidelines on the Practice of Ethics Committees in Medical Research on Human Participants*. London: Royal College of Physicians.

Save the Children (2007) *Why Social Corporate Responsibility is Failing Children*. London: Save the Children Fund.

Sharav, V. (2003) 'Children in clinical research: a conflict of moral values', *American Journal of Bioethics*, 3(1): 1–99.

Slesser, A. and Qureshi, Y. (2009) 'The implications of fraud in medical and scientific research', *World Journal of Surgery*, 33(11): 2355–9.

Sylvester, S. and Green, J. (2003) 'An excess of governance? Social research and Local Research Ethics Committees', *Medical Sociology News*, 29(3): 39–44.

Tobias, J. and Souhami, R. (1993) 'Fully informed consent can be needlessly cruel', *British Medical Journal*, 307: 1199–2001.

UK Research Integrity Office (2009) *Code of Practice for Research*. London: UKIR. Available at: http://ukrio.org

United Nations (1989) *Convention on the Rights of the Child*. New York: United Nations.

USA National Commission for the Protection of Human Subjects in Medical and Behavioral Research (1977) *Research Involving Children: Report and Recommendations*. Washington, DC: DHEW.

USA National Commission for the Protection of Human Subjects in Medical and Behavioral Research (1978) *The Belmont Report: Ethical Principles and Guidelines for the Protection of Human Subjects of Research*. Washington, DC: DHEW.

Vist, E.G., Hagen, K., Devereaux, P., Bryant, D., Kristoffersen, D. and Oxman, A. (2005) 'Systematic review to determine whether participation in a trial influences outcome', *British Medical Journal*, 330: 1175.

Webster, A., Lewis, G., Brown, N. and Boulton, M. (2004) *Developing a Framework for Social Science Research Ethics: Project Update for ESRC*. York and Oxford: SATSU, York and Oxford Brookes University.

West, E. and Butler, J. (2003) 'An applied and qualitative LREC reflects on its practice', *Bulletin of Medical Ethics*, 185: 13–20.

Wilkinson, R. and Pickett, K. (2009) *The Spirit Level*. London: Penguin.

World Medical Association (1964) *The Declaration of Helsinki*. Fernay-Voltaire: WMA.

World Medical Association (2008) *The Declaration of Helsinki*. Fernay-Voltaire: WMA.

16

Researching Complementary and Alternative Medicine

JANET RICHARDSON AND MIKE SAKS

Introduction

- This chapter addresses a controversial area – that of researching complementary and alternative medicine (CAM), at a time when CAM has come under heavy attack by orthodox scientists on both sides of the Atlantic for lacking research evidence and being tantamount to quackery (see, for example, McHale 2011). In the context of rising public interest in CAM (Saks 2008), it particularly focuses on the challenges of researching health beyond the boundaries of orthodox medicine – arguing that there is a strong case for adopting a more eclectic approach centred on both quantitative and qualitative approaches. The chapter includes a discussion of the evidence base of CAM and orthodox medicine, as well as some of the specific challenges to researching the former, linked to the politics of health – with suggestions as to how these may be overcome. The key themes of the chapter are illustrated by a case study involving the Lewisham Complementary Therapy Centre, in which one of the authors was centrally involved.

- In this context, orthodox medicine and CAM are both defined politically in terms of how far at any point in time they are formally underwritten by the state – as regards, for example, the level of research funding and their inclusion in the undergraduate medical curriculum (Saks 2003). The current Western medical orthodoxy is usually seen as being based on the biomedical model outlined in Chapter 2 and is heavily state-supported. This tends to place emphasis on objective indicators of health and to focus on specialized surgical and other procedures involving specific areas of the body in cases of disease pathology (Stacey 1988). In this biomedical approach, the randomized controlled trial (RCT) described in Chapter 12 has been proclaimed as the definitive standard in research evaluations. However, this chapter highlights the difficulties inherent in applying this model to health care interventions other than those involving drug trials – even within orthodox biomedicine.

Outside the bounds of biomedicine, such difficulties are most strongly exemplified in the case of CAM, on which this chapter is centred. CAM consists of a diverse range of therapies outside the political mainstream, from aromatherapy and crystal therapy to acupuncture and homoeopathy. These do not share a common philosophy, but tend to be ideologically positioned more towards the holistic end of the spectrum – in which the subjective views of clients and mind–body links are usually regarded by their proponents as more central to treatment than in orthodox medicine (Saks 2000). This can be illustrated with reference to classical acupuncture where clients are treated holistically according to their individual characteristics through the insertion and manipulation of complexes of needles in prescribed points – to adjust the energy flow along a system of channels called meridians that are held to run through the body (Saks 2005b). The key question, however, is whether the RCT is applicable to this area and, if not, how such therapies are to be assessed. A number of possible solutions to this research dilemma will be set out in this chapter using examples from research practice. Ultimately, it will be proposed that health care research in CAM – and indeed in orthodox medicine – requires a multidisciplinary approach and the use of mixed research methods to address the wide range of issues that arise.

The Development of Evidence-Based Orthodox Medicine

Historically, the purpose of orthodox medical research has been to understand the mechanisms of disease, produce new treatments and use them pragmatically, not to test for effectiveness using a rigorous scientific method (Smith 1995). Despite their introduction in the mid-twentieth century, many conventional treatments have not been subjected to RCTs and, as a result, new interventions have been introduced on a wide scale on the basis of opinion rather than evidence (Smith and Rennie 1995). Many have also been employed widely before being shown to be harmful and of little benefit – as, for example, in the use of insulin coma therapy, leucotomy and regressive electro-convulsive therapy (ECT) for the treatment of schizophrenia (Andrews 1989). Innovations in health service delivery have also been unregulated and unevaluated, and few decisions have been made on the basis of sound evidence regarding their efficiency and safety in pragmatic settings (Fitzpatrick 1994).

In this respect, a lack of evidence has inhibited the effective use of resources and led to wide variations in clinical practice in diagnostic procedures and health care interventions in orthodox biomedicine, centred largely on drugs and surgery. However, this is not to deny some of the dramatic advances in medicine, from the use of antibiotics to hip surgery, which have been evidence-based and have brought about substantial patient benefit (Le Fanu 2011). The very thin and patchy application of rigorous evaluative approaches in orthodox medicine in the UK eventually gave rise to a systematic NHS research and development programme to create an NHS where decisions are evidence-based (Department of Health 1993), the basic principles of which have since been restated and embellished (see, for example, Department of Health 2006, 2010). This has placed the RCT even more centrally at the heart of the NHS. Nevertheless, some clinicians have feared that 'scientific' evidence-based medicine threatens the 'art' of patient care, and will lead to the neglect of good clinical skills and experience (see, for example, Grahame-Smith 1995).

Debates about 'Evidence' in Orthodox and Complementary and Alternative Medicine

The question as to what constitutes 'evidence' in orthodox medicine remains. The strongest type of evidence in biomedicine is thought to be provided by systematic reviews of well-designed RCTs, as outlined in Chapter 12. Here, the overall approach is 'reductionist', which emphasizes the generation of objective 'hard data' to establish particular cause–effect relationships for generically defined diseases (Brown et al. 2003). The experimental methodology in RCTs, where strenuous efforts are made to isolate independent and dependent variables and eliminate 'non-specific' variables, has fitted closely with the theoretical assumptions contained in the orthodox biomedical model (Pocock 1983). This approach, however, can exclude the role of social, psychological and cultural factors in the development and resolution of health problems, and the experience of health problems of different individuals. These issues have been central to the more individualistically tailored approach in CAM.

Although CAM has seen a dramatic recent rise in popularity with the public in the UK and most of the developed world, there remains a lack of credible evidence for the effectiveness of CAM therapies. Despite queries raised about the efficacy and safety of some CAM therapies (Ernst et al. 2008), the main problem has been, with a few notable exceptions, the lack of methodologically rigorous studies that might convince, or otherwise, the sceptics (Saks 2006). The debate on the most relevant methodological approaches to evaluating alternative therapies pivots on the apparent contrast and conflict between two different and diverse world views or paradigms (Richardson 2000), as discussed in Chapter 2. It is frequently asserted by practitioners of CAM that research methods developed in the orthodox biomedical frame of reference are not transferable to the evaluation of more holistic CAM therapies – particularly in relation to the application of RCTs (see, for instance, the debate over their appropriateness in cancer care in Block et al. 2004).

This is in part because those practising CAM therapies typically claim to treat the individual client specifically rather than providing a standard treatment for a given condition, as in orthodox biomedicine. This makes organizing subjects into control and experimental groups in a randomized trial – with the administration of a placebo treatment alongside the therapy being evaluated – more problematic in the case of CAM than in drug assessment (Saks 2006). In this regard, blinding procedures also raise considerable difficulties in the evaluation of CAM as compared with trials of pharmaceuticals. The purpose of blinding is to exclude non-specific factors or placebo effects which may produce a desirable outcome, but which are not due directly to the active intervention. Yet even for many orthodox health care interventions, it may be extremely difficult to arrange a double-blind trial with a credible placebo (Pocock 1983). Anthony (1993) also suggests that blind designs may be impossible in CAM as the therapist is usually regarded as an integral part of the intervention.

This critique fails to acknowledge adequately that, despite the ideology of holism, some CAM therapies, like osteopathy for bad backs, can be as mechanistic and reductionist as many of those in orthodox biomedicine (Saks 1997). In the case of acupuncture, this is well illustrated by the formula, as opposed to the classical, variant which involves needling the same points for a given condition, irrespective of the individual patient (Saks 1992). Even in relation to more holistic therapies, moreover, RCTs may be conducted in which both patients and practitioners are not blind to the procedure, as has been the case in evaluating the effects of psychotherapeutic techniques, healing and prayer (Vickers 1996). Nonetheless, Black (1996) has argued that in such instances, the artificiality of the trial may reduce the placebo element of any intervention. This may limit the extent to which the researcher can capitalize on the non-specific treatment effects, and, as in the case of more mechanistic CAM therapies, the outcome of the trial may reflect the minimum rather than the maximum level of benefit that can be expected.

It can be argued therefore that it is important to evaluate care as it is normally delivered in clinical practice. Who then decides which evidence is important? Reilly and Taylor (1993) used a survey method to produce a profile of the evidence required by general practitioner trainees for CAM and orthodox medicine. The same profiles for both were demanded by 59 per cent of responders. However, 44 per cent placed greater emphasis on the patient experience for CAM than clinical trials for orthodox medicine.

Nonetheless, purchasers of health care are in a different position. They are accountable and driven by limited resources. They must therefore ensure the greatest cost benefit and value for money. Although CAM is increasingly provided in the NHS, especially in primary care through either direct provision or subcontracting relationships (Thomas et al. 2003), cost constraints have undoubtedly led to short-term 'quick-fix' planning. This may have worked to the prejudice of CAM, especially as there is relatively little state funding for research as compared with orthodox medicine (Saks 2005a). This is despite government capacity-building initiatives following the field-breaking report on CAM by the House of Lords

Select Committee on Science and Technology (2000) which favoured greater investment in research into CAM.

Patients, however, may be looking for different health benefits than those indicated by the results of conventional RCTs based on a biomedical model, particularly when they have long-term chronic disease. Increasingly, lay people place importance on such factors as how far treatment enhances or sustains emotional well-being, a healthier lifestyle and more satisfying relationships. This may lead to very different perceptions by patients of what constitutes relevant evidence in evaluating the efficacy of CAM and other therapies as compared with orthodox practitioners and researchers (Mercer et al. 1995). Furthermore, studies suggest that patients frequently choose CAM due to the adverse effects of conventional treatments and perceive CAM to be lower risk (Vincent and Furnham 1996). Although this may be regarded as a rather blunt instrument for gauging the efficacy of therapeutic interventions in clinical circles, subjective levels of consumer satisfaction with CAM have been consistently high whatever their objective deficiencies or merits (Saks 2003). In this sense, patients may have been disempowered by RCTs with their emphasis on objective rather than subjective outcome measures (Brown et al. 2003).

Orthodox Medicine and the Politics of Research in Complementary and Alternative Medicine

In terms of the 'politics' of research, it is important to note that doctors who are the prime beneficiaries of state research funding in health care in the UK have an interest in restricting their research to areas where they are recognized as competent, which may operate to the detriment of CAM research. This may explain, for example, the long history of the rejection of acupuncture as a therapy in modern times. It may also explain why, following public pressure in the 1960s and 1970s, doctors have been keener to examine acupuncture from a neurophysiological perspective with reference to the production of endorphins, rather than the traditional focus on balancing yin and yang along meridians (Saks 1992). The effect of this has been to limit research in acupuncture to pain and the treatment of addictions, rather than looking at a wider application based on classical Oriental theories. These tend to lie outside the knowledge and experience of Western medical researchers. Nevertheless, from the viewpoint of medical interests, acupuncture has opened up new areas for doctors to colonize while at the same time avoiding legitimating the growing numbers of traditional acupuncturists operating in private practice. In turn, this has helped to maintain the status, income and power of the medical profession (Saks 2005b).

From this standpoint, it can be seen that research into health care, and the choice of research methodologies, is not simply a technical operation, but is also related to maintaining dominant medical interests (Mulkay 1991). The influence of such interests may also extend to the powerful multinational pharmaceutical companies which have generally seen CAM as a threat (Walker 1994), even if it could be argued that they themselves are now being colonized through the range of CAM preparations for standard conditions now available in chemists' shops and supermarkets. This raises serious questions about the main drivers for state and privately funded research in CAM and other areas of health care – and the extent of tolerance towards more eclectic approaches to research, as well as how far the policies adopted are synonymous with the wider public interest (Saks 2006).

A good example of research into CAM that showed that the medical establishment does not always live up to high 'scientific' standards was a study based on a trial by Bagenal and colleagues (1990) which led to an attack on the Bristol Cancer Help Centre. This study suggested that women with breast cancer attending the centre – which offered a range of alternative health provision – were more likely to die earlier than those receiving orthodox medical treatment. Unfortunately, though, there were a variety of flaws in the methodology of this study, such as poorly matched subjects in the trial and the control group (Stacey 1991). This meant that the research findings were not supported by the data. The effects of the publication of the study findings were devastating for the women concerned. This led to suggestions that the study was part of a politically inspired medical campaign to demonize CAM.

Challenges to Research in Orthodox and Complementary and Alternative Medicine

The example of the Bristol Cancer Help Centre highlights that the RCT is itself socially constructed and is not a neutral approach, as it inevitably rests on certain paradigmatic assumptions (see, for instance, Richardson 2003, as well as Chapter 2 of this volume). As ever, the decision to use RCTs depends on the nature of the research question being asked (Dyson and Brown 2006). There are also further criticisms of the RCT when used in either CAM or orthodox medicine (Kelner et al. 2003). One key instance of these is the contentious methodological assumption underlying the use of the RCT that patients have no treatment preferences (Fitter and Thomas 1997). While the issues that this raises can be overcome by using patient selection criteria (Brewin and Bradley 1989), critics like Heron and Reason (1984) go further in seeing clinical trials as a source of alienation, as they separate individuals from what is going on in their body and deprive them of the opportunity to participate in decisions about their treatment. In order to help to resolve such dilemmas about assessing efficacy, a number of alternative and complementary approaches to health research are now considered in turn.

The role of pragmatic and explanatory studies

One approach that addresses some of the problems concerned with RCTs is that of making a distinction between pragmatic trials and explanatory trials. In a pragmatic trial, the intention is to study the policy context in which a therapy will be used and ask whether the therapy will work in everyday practice. The explanatory trial, on the other hand, tries to separate the policy into its constituent parts – for example, time, active intervention and therapeutic setting – to discover which specific component of an intervention produces the outcome (Schwartz and Lellouch 1967).

The main difference between pragmatic and explanatory studies is the extent to which protocol violations, such as patient non-compliance, are considered in the interpretation of results. The explanatory approach confines the analysis to only those patients who receive therapy according to the protocol. Pocock (1983), however, suggests that all eligible patients, regardless of compliance, should be included in the analysis where possible. In the pragmatic trial all patients, including those who withdraw from therapy, need to be accounted for, and all protocol violations and major deviations should be recorded. Withdrawals and deviations are considered in the analysis to avoid distorting treatment comparisons. This is particularly important if patients are withdrawn because of side-effects, as they will otherwise not be reported. This may therefore create uncertainty about the results of the trial, even if a lack of response data from those who withdraw may sometimes mean that they have to be excluded from the analysis (Pocock and Abdalla 1998). In relation to assessing the efficacy of CAM in particular, the term 'pragmatic' refers to a research design that allows practitioners to treat patients individually in clinical practice, in a manner that capitalizes on, rather than restricts, non-specific placebo effects. Meade and Frank (1993) illustrate how such a pragmatic approach using individualized treatments compared the policies for outpatient management with chiropractic for the treatment of low-back pain. Knipschild (1993) also advocates the use of pragmatic trials in comparing the best orthodox and CAM therapy for patients.

Two major problems exist for patient selection to CAM research trials. The first problem also relates to trials in orthodox medicine and originates from the premise that patients play an active part in the outcome of their treatment. In this model, the patient's motivation to follow treatment regimens is held to be influenced by preferences before treatment is started. In general, the greater the need for participation (for example, by following a special diet) and the greater the motivation, the more likely it is to influence outcome. In pragmatic trials, the objective is to discover the effect and outcome of 'packages' of management, even though most treatments are complex, mixing supposedly active components with contextual factors – including the way treatment is given. In explanatory, as opposed to pragmatic, trials, the contextual factors are 'equalized' by randomization and artificial constraints which do not allow the role of expectation in treatment outcome to be evaluated. Brewin and Bradley (1989) therefore suggest that the alternative is to optimize motivation by ascertaining patients' preferences prior to randomization to a treatment or control group and allocating them to their preferred treatment choice.

The second problem relates to patient selection, which can be based on diagnosis by orthodox medical or CAM system criteria. Wiegant et al. (1991) propose that there are four possible ways of dealing with this dilemma:

- Following selection criteria based on orthodox diagnosis.
- Basing selection on orthodox criteria, but allowing the practitioner to treat the patient on an individual basis according to the therapy they are practising.
- Conducting an initial trawl based on orthodox diagnosis, then creating subdivisions according to the appropriate CAM diagnosis.
- Defining selection criteria by following the CAM diagnosis alone.

Whatever means is chosen, it should be consistently employed. Combining this precept with a pragmatic trial that takes into account in some way patient preference, allows practitioners to treat patients on an individual basis and goes some way to addressing the criticisms of using RCTs in CAM. In this frame of reference, blinding should be included in the design where possible, and every effort made to identify and control for potential bias in order to ensure that the outcome is due to the intervention.

The use of appropriate outcome measures

A health care intervention is intended to maintain or improve functioning and well-being, and subsequently to improve the quality of life. It is therefore very important to measure patients' subjective experiences of illness and the care that they receive in CAM research if trials are to be employed, especially given the significance that is accorded to this in the CAM field (Kelner et al. 2003). Yet the biomedical model of disease is rooted in the belief that well-being is an objective and measurable state – a philosophy that has often been enshrined in RCTs. Attempts to evaluate interventions purely in terms of this model have been contested due to limited success in producing objective standards of assessment that reflect different perceptions of health and illness (Turner 2003). One of the anomalies in contemporary practice is that patients' subjective perception of personal well-being may be discordant with their 'objective' health status. For example, a person can feel ill without medical science being able to detect disease and many people live with pathologies of which they are unaware (Bowling 2004).

It is therefore important to employ appropriate outcome measures. Dixon and colleagues (1994) found that most health outcome assessments in use were multidimensional, the main indices being included in the Short Form 36 (SF-36). This has the merit of being well validated and used frequently as a generic quality of life measure in outcome assessment, as well as having been employed to evaluate CAM therapies (see, for instance, Fitter and MacPherson 1995). Outcome measures such as the SF-36 ask specific questions about physical, social and emotional functioning. However, it is also important to define and measure what is significant to the patient. In this respect, the Measure Yourself Medical Outcome Profile (MYMOP) is a very helpful patient-generated, individualized, outcome questionnaire (Paterson 1996). It is problem-specific, but includes general well-being and is also suitable for assessing a range of symptoms, which can be physical, emotional or social. This is illustrated by a recent study of acupuncture (Paterson et al. 2011). In addition, MYMOP is brief, with only seven items, simple to administer and sensitive to change. Prior to commencing a clinical research trial or outcome assessment, the nature of the research questions about CAM needs to be clearly defined. The selected outcome measures should be appropriate, valid and reliable.

Qualitative approaches

It is also vital to note that using such quality of life measures and trials in orthodox medicine or in CAM studies does not facilitate a deeper understanding of the experience of health and illness. In order to address this question, qualitative research methods can usefully be deployed. They are particularly appropriate to new fields of study where experiences of individuals are of concern – providing rich descriptions of what it is like to experience illness and suffering. Pope and Mays (1995) suggest that qualitative approaches should be an essential component of health service research, as they allow access to areas not amenable to quantitative research, such as by providing a fuller understanding of lay and professional beliefs. Various dimensions of such research methods and the specific balance of benefits and costs are explored in the chapters contained in Part III of this volume. These are reinforced by the general criteria for the evaluation of qualitative research set out in Box 16.1.

Box 16.1 Criteria for the evaluation of qualitative research

Four general criteria can be given for the evaluation of qualitative research:

- *Truth value:* this is subject-oriented and not defined by the researcher in advance. Here, the researcher recognizes that there are multiple realities and attempts to report the perspectives of informants as clearly as possible.
- *Applicability:* this is the criterion used to determine whether findings can be applied in other contexts or settings.
- *Consistency:* this is whether the findings would be consistent if the enquiry were replicated without the same subjects or in a similar context.
- *Neutrality:* this is freedom from bias in the research procedure and results.

Source: Lincoln and Guba (1985)

Such approaches to ensuring validity and reliability are fundamental to challenging the criticisms of qualitative methods as 'quick', 'dirty' and 'at the bottom of the hierarchy of evidence' (Greenhalgh 1998). This is particularly the case when they are used in the CAM area, which is already marginalized compared with orthodox medicine.

A systematic review and thematic analysis of qualitative studies in CAM specifically found that qualitative methods enabled an assessment of the integrity and feasibility of interventions and study design, if undertaken prior to large-scale clinical trials (Richardson et al. 2004). Qualitative studies provide an understanding of the complexity of the patient experience, including how the experience of the intervention impacts on patients' self-knowledge, and important self-directed changes in behaviour and lifestyle. A common finding in a number of studies is that the experience of an intervention allowed patients to explore meaning, which brought about a desire for inner change.

While strenuous efforts to control 'extraneous variables' are desirable in controlled clinical trials, it should also be recognized that, in reality, the world is not best conceptualized by being polarized into 'objective' quantitative and 'subjective' qualitative studies. This is highlighted by the fact that the therapeutic effect of any intervention will be at least partly due to the way that intervention is delivered (Helman 2007). Researchers have therefore attempted in various ways to evaluate the benefits of CAM therapies from chiropractic to homoeopathy using pragmatic trials that assess therapies in the context in which they are practised in individualized treatments (Meade et al. 1990; De Lange de Klerk et al. 1994). In such trials, the intervention is often compared with an alternative or standard treatment or the use of a waiting list control group. This chapter concludes by indicating how the challenges that this poses can be addressed using a case study from the field – drawing heavily on the recent practical experience of one of the authors, Janet Richardson, in a CAM therapy centre in Lewisham.

The Lewisham Complementary Therapy Centre

The Lewisham Complementary Therapy Centre, on which this case study focuses, was recognized as a 'good model' of service delivery and evaluation that maintained the integrity of CAM therapies by basing its evaluation of effectiveness on pragmatic trials using sensitive approaches (Fulder 1996). It originated in June 1994 when an innovative new project was launched in Lewisham Hospital NHS Trust in South East London. The project introduced a number of CAM therapies into the NHS – acupuncture, homoeopathy and osteopathy – alongside an evaluation programme (Richardson 1995). The launch followed approximately four years of working towards raising the profile of CAM therapies within the hospital through study days, workshops, and establishing a massage and osteopathic service for staff within the hospital.

Janet Richardson established a steering group to draw together a proposal for funding the service. This was followed by setting up, organizing and managing the service once it was funded, and evaluating the outcome of the care it provided (Richardson 1996). The development of the service was based on a survey of local general practitioners to assess the level of support, followed by the generation of referral guidelines using a modified Delphi technique – a survey method for establishing consensus views (Richardson 2001a). The initial intention to conduct RCTs was hampered by lack of funding from medical research charities which considered

(Continued)

CASE STUDY

(Continued)

funding the researcher but not the practitioners. A contract to provide the service was therefore sought and awarded by the relevant health authority. As agreed with the health authority, the evaluation took the form of an outcome assessment based on the SF-36 and open-ended questions about expectations and experience, using the waiting list as a control group.

Patients attending the clinic for acupuncture, osteopathy and homoeopathy over a nine-month period were evaluated and their SF-36 scores, measuring eight dimensions of health, were compared with the waiting list controls. There were statistically significant differences in outcome between the treatment group (N = 179) and the control group (N = 151) on all dimensions of the SF-36 questionnaire with the exception of 'physical functioning'. Here, the treatment group still had higher health status than the controls. As a result of a large non-response rate in the control group, sensitivity analysis was carried out in line with an 'intention to treat' approach. Based on the assumption that non-responders in the control group experienced a moderate clinical/social improvement, this demonstrated that the differences at outcome between the treatment and control group remained significant, except for mental health (Richardson 2001b, 2004).

The evaluation of patient expectations prior to the intervention found that patients anticipated the relief of symptoms; a therapeutic/holistic approach; improvement in quality of life; provision of information; reduction of the risks of allopathic treatments; the need for self-help advice; and greater accessibility of such treatments on the NHS (Richardson 2004). A qualitative evaluation of the patient experience showed that patients reported additional positive benefits such as relaxation and feelings of increased well-being; experienced a therapeutic and 'holistic' approach; were helped to develop coping strategies; and had appreciated being listened to by practitioners.

This service evaluation illustrates how a pragmatic approach can maximize the therapeutic effect, maintain the integrity of the intervention and benefit from both quantitative and qualitative research. It also provides an example of a systematic approach to service development. Fulder (1996) suggests that the Lewisham complementary therapy project was successful as a result of the specific referral guidelines that were established through intensive dialogue between doctors and the CAM therapists. The issue of dialogue was extremely important as the service was based on three 'complete' systems of treatment, two of which were grounded in world views very different from conventional medical science. Crucially, the focus of the dialogue was not inhibited by the different paradigms within which the CAM practitioners were working. For the local general practitioners, the issue was moving towards a collective agreement about the kind of patients who might be helped by these treatments. This was achieved by the CAM practitioners translating their respective paradigms into a conventional diagnostic system.

Unfortunately, the Lewisham Complementary Therapy Centre had its funding withdrawn, in spite of achieving positive therapeutic outcomes. This is a clear example of 'moving goal posts', and reinforces again how 'evidence' cannot be divorced from the politics of health care (Richardson 2003) – a theme which is very apparent in contemporary debates over orthodox medicine and CAM in Britain and other countries, which have been highly politically charged (Saks 2011).

Conclusion

In summary, then, there are many questions to ask in research, and diverse questions require a range of approaches in researching CAM – and more orthodox forms of medicine. Even very sophisticated RCTs can fail to detect the complexity that lies beneath the swampy lowlands in research linked to therapeutic outcomes (Richardson 2002). Researchers should therefore think very carefully about the nature of their questions, as well as their own motivation, and consider the possibility of a more eclectic approach to research methods in general and RCTs in particular, in line with the support given for mixed methods and multidisciplinary research in Chapter 22 of this book. By the same token, in areas like CAM where there is less conventional evidence of the efficacy of the therapies concerned, there also needs to be a sensitivity to the ethical issues involved – not least for health professionals offering advice to clients (Snyder 2007). The chapter has, nonetheless, suggested how research can be moved forward in relation to CAM as well as orthodox medicine by going beyond the straightforward application of an RCT. It now winds up with an exercise for the reader that brings some of the themes the chapter has covered more sharply into focus.

Exercise: Researching the effects of massage on patients with cancer

With the question in mind of what is to count as evidence, and in light of the issues raised in this chapter about research questions and methodologies in relation to CAM, and indeed orthodox medicine, consider the example below.

You are asked to design a study to evaluate the effects of massage on patients with cancer who are receiving supportive (palliative) care. Address the following questions:

1 What kind of study would you design and what method(s) would you use?

2 How would you recruit study participants and how many would you require?

3 What would you measure?

4 Who would you involve in the study – in terms of both researchers and practitioners?

5 Where would you apply for funding?

Finally, you may wish to consider what political issues arise from the study.

Recommended Further Reading

Ernst, E., Pittler, M.H., Wider, B. and Boddy, K. (2008) *Oxford Handbook of Complementary Medicine*. Oxford: Oxford University Press.

This book provides an accessible, critical overview of research issues and evidence for CAM which is helpful for health professionals in advising patients.

Richardson, J. (2004) 'Developing complementary therapy services: a systematic approach', *Health Psychology Update*, 13(3): 23–33.
This article discusses further the establishment and evaluation of the CAM service established within an NHS setting in Britain, which is considered as a case study in this chapter.

Saks, M. (2003) *Orthodox and Alternative Medicine: Politics, Professionalization and Health Care.* London: Sage.
This book aids our understanding of how orthodox medicine and alternative medicine have developed in Britain and the USA, and the significance of politics in the struggle for legitimacy in research and other areas.

Online Readings

Segar, J. (2012) 'Complementary and alternative medicine: Exploring the gap between evidence and usage', *Health: An Interdisciplinary Journal*, 16: 366–381.
What are the barriers to identifying an evidence base for CAM? How far is the adoption of CAM within the NHS driven by the power of the medical profession in the UK?

Golden, I. (2012) 'Beyond randomized controlled trials: Evidence in complementary medicine', *Journal of Evidence-based Complementary and Alternative Medicine*, 17: 72–75.
What does the author argue are the key flaws in the RCT model? How appropriate is the RCT model for researching CAM?

References

Andrews, G. (1989) 'Evaluating treatment effectiveness', *Australian and New Zealand Journal of Psychiatry*, 23: 181–6.

Anthony, H.M. (1993) 'Clinical research: questions to ask and the benefits of asking them', in G.T. Lewith and D. Aldridge (eds), *Clinical Research Methodology for Complementary Therapies.* London: Hodder & Stoughton.

Bagenal, F.S., Easton, D.F., Harris, E., Chilvers, C.E.D. and McElwain, T.J. (1990) 'Survival of patients with breast cancer attending the Bristol Cancer Help Centre', *Lancet*, 336: 606–10.

Black, N. (1996) 'Why we need observational studies to evaluate the effectiveness of health care', *British Medical Journal*, 312: 1215–18.

Block, K.I., Cohen, A.J., Dobs, A.S., Ornish, D. and Tripathy, D. (2004) 'The challenges of randomized trials in integrative cancer care', *Integrative Cancer Therapies*, 3(2): 112–27.

Bowling, A. (2004) *Measuring Health: A Review of Quality of Life Measurement Scales*, 3rd edition. Buckingham: Open University Press.

Brewin, C.R. and Bradley, C. (1989) 'Patient preferences and randomised clinical trials', *British Medical Journal*, 299: 313–15.

Brown, B., Crawford, P. and Hicks, C. (2003) *Evidence-based Research: Dilemmas and Debates in Health Care*. Maidenhead: Open University Press.

De Lange de Klerk, E.S.M., Blommers, J., Kuik, D.J., Bezemer, P.D. and Feenstra, L. (1994) 'Effect of homoeopathic medicines on daily burden of symptoms in children with recurrent upper respiratory tract infections', *British Medical Journal*, 309: 1329–32.

Department of Health (1993) *Research for Health*. London: Department of Health.

Department of Health (2006) *Better Research for Better Health*. London: Department of Health.

Department of Health (2010) *Equity and Excellence: Liberating the NHS*. London: Department of Health.

Dixon, P., Heaton, J., Long, A. and Warburton, A. (1994) 'Reviewing and applying the SF-36', in *Outcomes Briefing*. Leeds: UK Clearing House on Health Outcomes – Nuffield Institute for Health, 4: 3–25.

Dyson, S. and Brown, B. (2006) *Social Theory and Applied Health Research*. Maidenhead: Open University Press.

Ernst, E., Pittler, M. H., Wider, B. and Boddy, K. (2008) *Oxford Handbook of Complementary Medicine*. Oxford: Oxford University Press.

Fitter, M. and MacPherson, H. (1995) 'An audit of case studies of low back pain: a feasibility study for a controlled trial', *European Journal of Oriental Medicine*, 1(5): 46–51.

Fitter, M.J. and Thomas, K.J. (1997) 'Evaluating complementary therapies for use in the National Health Service: "Horses for Courses". Part 1: The design challenge', *Complementary Therapies in Medicine*, 5: 90–3.

Fitzpatrick, R. (1994) 'Applications of health status measures', in C. Jenkinson (ed.), *Measuring Heath and Medical Outcomes*. London: UCL Press.

Fulder, S. (1996) *The Handbook of Alternative and Complementary Medicine*. Oxford: Oxford University Press.

Grahame-Smith, D. (1995) 'Evidence based medicine: Socratic dissent', *British Medical Journal*, 310: 1126–7.

Greenhalgh, T. (1998) 'Qualitative research', *British Journal of General Practice*, September: 1626–7.

Helman, C. (2007) *Culture, Health and Illness*, 5th edition. London: Hodder Arnold.

Heron, J. and Reason, P. (1984) 'New paradigm research and holistic medicine', *British Journal of Holistic Medicine*, 1: 86–91.

House of Lords Select Committee on Science and Technology (2000) *Report on Complementary and Alternative Medicine*. London: The Stationery Office.

Kelner, M., Wellman, B., Pescosolido, B. and Saks, M. (eds) (2003) *Complementary and Alternative Medicine: Challenge and Change*. London: Routledge.

Knipschild, P. (1993) 'Trials and errors', *British Medical Journal*, 309: 1706–7.

Le Fanu, J. (2011) *The Rise and Fall of Modern Medicine*, 2nd edition. London: Abacus.

Lincoln, Y.S. and Guba, E. (1985) *Naturalistic Inquiry*. Beverly Hills, CA: Sage.

McHale, K. (2011) *Homoeopathy: The Basics, History and Debate over the Effectiveness of Using Natural Treatments in Medicine*. Webster's Digital Services.

Meade, T.W. and Frank, A.O. (1993) 'Manipulation and low back pain: an example of principles and practice', in G.T. Lewith and D. Aldridge (eds), *Clinical Research Methodology for Complementary Therapies*. London: Hodder & Stoughton.

Meade, T.W., Dyer, S., Browne, W., Townsend, J. and Frank, A.O. (1990) 'Low back pain of mechanical origin: randomised comparison of chiropractic and hospital outpatient treatment', *British Medical Journal*, 300: 1431–7.

Mercer, G., Long, A.F. and Smith, I.J. (1995) *Researching and Evaluating Complementary Therapies: The State of the Debate*. Leeds: Collaborating Centre for Health Service Research, Nuffield Institute for Health.

Mulkay, M. (1991) *Sociology of Science: A Sociological Pilgrimage*. Milton Keynes: Open University Press.

Paterson, C. (1996) 'Measuring outcomes in primary care: a patient generated measure, MYMOP, compared with the SF-36 health survey', *British Medical Journal*, 312: 1016–20.

Paterson, C., Taylor, R.S., Griffiths, P., Britten, N., Rugg, S., Bridges, J., McCallum, B. and Kite, G. (2011) 'Acupuncture for "frequent attenders" with medically unexplained symptoms: a randomised controlled trial (CACTUS study)', *British Journal of General Practice*, 61: 295–305.

Pocock, S.J. (1983) *Clinical Trials: A Practical Approach*. Chichester: Wiley.

Pocock, S.J. and Abdalla, M. (1998) 'The hope and the hazard of using compliance data in randomized controlled trials', *Statistics in Medicine*, 17: 303–17.

Pope, C. and Mays, N. (1995) 'Reaching the parts other methodologies cannot reach: an introduction to qualitative methods in health and health services research', *British Medical Journal*, 311: 42–5.

Reilly, D. and Taylor, M. (1993) 'Developing integrated medicine: Report of the RCCM Research Fellowship in Complementary Medicine, The University of Glasgow 1987–1990', *Complementary Therapies in Medicine*, 1 (Suppl. 1): 1–50.

Richardson, J. (1995) 'Complementary therapies on the NHS: the experience of a new service', *Complementary Therapies in Medicine*, 3: 153–7.

Richardson, J. (1996) 'Non-conventional therapy in the NHS: can it work?', *International Journal of Alternative and Complementary Medicine*, July: 20–1.

Richardson, J. (2000) 'The use of randomized control trials in complementary therapy: exploring the methodological issues', *Journal of Advanced Nursing*, 32(2): 398–406.

Richardson, J. (2001a) 'Developing and evaluating complementary therapy services. Part 1. Establishing service provision through the use of evidence and consensus development',

The Journal of Alternative and Complementary Medicine: Research on Paradigm, Practice, and Policy, 7(3): 253–60.

Richardson, J. (2001b) 'Developing and evaluating complementary therapy services. Part 2. Examining the effect of treatment on health status', *The Journal of Alternative and Complementary Medicine: Research on Paradigm, Practice, and Policy*, 7(4): 315–28.

Richardson, J. (2002) 'Evidence-based complementary medicine: rigour, relevance and the swampy lowlands', Editorial, *Journal of Alternative and Complementary Medicine*, 8(3): 221–3.

Richardson, J. (2003) 'Complementary and alternative medicine: socially constructed or evidence-based?', *Healthcare Papers*, 3(5): 30–6.

Richardson, J. (2004) 'Developing complementary therapy services: a systematic approach', *Health Psychology Update*, 13(3): 23–33.

Richardson, J., Smith, J. and Pilkington, K. (2004) 'Qualitative research in complementary therapies: is it of any value?', *FACT (Focus on Alternative and Complementary Therapies)*, 9(1): 43.

Saks, M. (1992) 'The paradox of incorporation: acupuncture and the medical profession in modern Britain', in M. Saks (ed.), *Alternative Medicine in Britain*. Oxford: Clarendon Press.

Saks, M. (1997) 'Alternative therapies: are they holistic?', *Complementary Therapies in Nursing and Midwifery*, 3: 4–8.

Saks, M. (2000) 'Medicine and the counter culture', in R. Cooter and J. Pickstone (eds), *Medicine in the Twentieth Century*. Amsterdam: Harwood Academic.

Saks, M. (2003) *Orthodox and Alternative Medicine: Politics, Professionalization and Health Care*. London: Sage.

Saks, M. (2005a) 'Improving the research base of complementary and alternative medicine', Editorial, *Complementary Therapies in Clinical Practice*, 11: 1–3.

Saks, M. (2005b) 'Regulating complementary and alternative medicine: the case of acupuncture', in G. Lee-Treweek, T. Heller, S. Spurr, H. MacQueen and J. Katz (eds), *Perspectives on Complementary and Alternative Medicine: A Reader*. London: Routledge/Open University.

Saks, M. (2006) 'The alternatives to medicine', in J. Gabe., D. Kelleher and G. Williams (eds), *Challenging Medicine*, 2nd edition. London: Routledge.

Saks, M. (2008) 'Plural medicine and East–West dialogue', in D. Wujastyk and F.M. Smith (eds), *Modern and Global Ayurveda: Pluralism and Paradigms*. Albany, NY: SUNY Press.

Saks, M. (2011) 'Power and professionalization in CAM: historical and contemporary perspectives'. Paper presented at the conference on Regulation and Professionalization in Complementary and Alternative Medicine, University of Birmingham, UK, May.

Schwartz, D. and Lellouch, J. (1967) 'Explanatory and pragmatic attitudes in therapeutic trials', *Journal of Chronic Disease*, 20: 637–48.

Smith, R. (1995) 'The scientific basis of health services', *British Medical Journal*, 311: 961–2.

Smith, R. and Rennie, D. (1995) 'And now, evidence based editing', *British Medical Journal*, 311: 826.

Snyder, L. (ed.) (2007) *Complementary and Alternative Medicine: Ethics, the Patient, and the Physician*. Totowa: Humana Press.

Stacey, M. (1988) *The Sociology of Health and Healing*. London: Unwin Hyman.

Stacey, M. (1991) 'The potential of social science for complementary medicine', *Complementary Medical Research*, 5(3): 183–6.

Thomas, K.J., Coleman, P. and Nicholl, J.P. (2003) 'Trends in access to complementary or alternative medicines via primary care in England: 1995–2001', *Family Practice*, 20: 5.

Turner, B.S. (2003) 'The history of the changing concepts of health and illness: outline of a general model of illness categories', in G.L. Albrecht, R. Fitzpatrick and S.C. Scrimshaw (eds), *The Handbook of Social Studies in Health and Medicine*. London: Sage.

Vickers, A.J. (1996) 'Research paradigms in mainstream and complementary medicine', in E. Ernst (ed.), *Complementary Medicine: An Objective Appraisal*. Oxford: Butterworth-Heinemann.

Vincent, C. and Furnham, A. (1996) 'Why do patients turn to complementary medicine? An empirical study', *British Journal of Clinical Psychology*, 35: 37–48.

Walker, M. (1994) *Dirty Medicine: Science, Big Business and the Assault on Natural Health Care*. London: Slingshot Publications.

Wiegant, F.A.C., Kramers, C.W. and van Wijik, R. (1991) 'Clinical research in complementary medicine: the importance of patient selection', *Complementary Medical Research*, 5(2): 110–15.

17

Researching the Health of Ethnic Minority Groups

MARK R.D. JOHNSON

Introduction

It is now widely recognized that the UK is a multicultural society. In consequence, there is interest in, and a need for, research into the health of ethnic minority groups. Minority populations are growing in both size and complexity and new groups of migrant origin continue to be added to the national community. In the 2001 decennial census of the population in England, nearly 1 in 10 of the population gave their ethnic origin as being from one of the 'black and minority ethnic groups' (see www.statistics.gov.uk/census2001/profiles/commentaries/ethnicity.asp). However, these figures may not include members of some white ethnic minorities, who may have found the new census categories inappropriate to their circumstances. The Office of National Statistics (ONS) Census form only offered 'British, Irish and Other White' as sub-categories of the White group. It is widely expected that the results of the 2011 census (due later in 2012) will show a much larger proportion of minorities, and also a growth in the numbers of those of faiths other than Christianity. The ONS estimates for 2009 suggest that at least 17.2 per cent of the population of England were not 'White British' (see www.ons.gov.uk/ons/publications/re-reference-tables.html?edition=tcm%3A77-50029).

(Continued)

(Continued)

- Particularly since the report of an official Commission of Inquiry in 1999, following the death of a young black man, Stephen Lawrence, both politicians and policy makers have given increasing attention to the needs of minorities. The Macpherson Report (1999) led to official recognition that many procedures and organizations were 'institutionally racist', as they did not take differences in ethnicity or culture into account. Subsequent legislation, including the Race Relations (Amendment) Act 2000, the European Human Rights Act and the Equality Act (2010), has placed the rights of minorities on a stronger base. Consequently, increasing attention has been focused on the health and social care needs of minority groups. Both Labour governments and senior health officials have stated that identifying and meeting the needs of these communities is a priority for the NHS (Crisp 2004) and under the Coalition government, similar expressions of intent have been included in the NHS Plan and the quality standards of the new Care Quality Commission (2010: 32), which state explicitly that:

> Equality, diversity and human rights ... Providers must consider equality, diversity and human rights in every aspect of their work. You should consider the needs of each person using a service against six key strands of diversity: Race, Age, Gender, Disability, Sexual orientation, Religion or belief. We sometimes refer to this as identifying a person's 'diversity' or 'diverse need'.

- This chapter argues that ethnicity is a key variable in explaining inequalities in health and therefore an important area of study. However, there are major challenges in identifying ethnic origin. Both narrow and broad definitions are considered, together with some of the approaches commonly used by social researchers. Some useful national sources of baseline data on ethnic minorities are given and the chapter concludes with a case study of an action research project where members of the community helped to develop research questions and carry forward the research process. Some general principles for conducting action research are suggested.

Key Variables in Patterns of Health and Disease

In recent decades, a consistent finding of research into health inequalities among ethnic minority groups has identified inequalities in access to care and in the outcomes of many health care interventions, with ethnic minority groups having less good access and poorer health outcomes (Johnson 2003; Williams and Johnson 2010). It has also been established that for certain conditions and diseases there are distinctive patterns of prevalence. The prognosis for the course of the disease may differ; and so may treatment needs between ethnic minority communities and those from other groups (Gill et al. 2002; Samanta et al. 2009).

In consequence, ethnic differences have attracted the attention of scientists seeking to understand disease, as ethnic variation provides the basis for a form of natural experiment: that is, cultural and genetic differences may explain variations in patterns of health and disease between groups within a population. There is a considerable literature that describes the patterns of health and disease associated with 'race' and 'ethnicity'.

'Race', culture and ethnicity are not the only factors that influence patterns of health and disease across groups. Social status or class factors have long been shown to affect health. However, there are difficulties in making a link between the class group to which people belong by virtue of their occupation and the ill health of particular individuals within that class. Social class is a crude label as class may be changed simply if occupation is changed. It does not reflect the lifetime experiences that contribute to health and ill health. Gender also affects health in many complex ways and some social analysts will describe women as effectively a minority, at least in terms of their relationship to the main dimensions of power in society. These are explored further in Chapter 18. Gendered inequalities in health – and also differences between gender groups in different ethnic or social communities – are very important, but cannot be fully explored here. However, no research into ethnic minority groups should assume that the health needs of men and women are identical. Both gender and class factors within ethnic minority groups will have an effect on health status.

Researching Ethnic Minority Health: Some Challenges

A number of problems occur when starting to research 'ethnicity' in health. A first and critical problem is one of definition: what is meant by ethnicity and what is an ethnic group? Second, particularly if a quantitative method is being followed, there is the problem of sampling. In order to sample, the size of the population to be sampled and the population characteristics must be known, yet such information may not be readily available. These two issues complicate the questions of choosing the most appropriate research design, whether quantitative or qualitative, and developing the most appropriate instruments in a situation where language, access and accessibility will require careful and informed thought. The challenges are explored in the following sections of this chapter.

Problems of definition

Since the late 1970s following a world conference of social and physical scientists, the term 'ethnic' has almost entirely replaced the word 'race' in most scientific discussions of population migration and mixing. Here, it was agreed that 'race' as a concept had no essential scientific validity (Banton 1977). In common parlance, the term 'ethnic' is also used as a form of shorthand to describe people and groups of people who are 'different'. However, we must recognize that the terms 'race and racism' continue to be used in both popular and political discussion. The existence of racism, defined as a belief, or action taken, based on the view that one's own group of origin is inherently superior to others, is a social reality. Indeed, many current tensions may be traced to the existence of racist ways of thinking and their consequences. The use of language, or terms used as categories, is therefore a matter for ethical reflection.

There is considerable uncertainty about the definition of ethnicity and how the term should be used in scientific, medical or health and social care research (LaVeist 1994). It is perhaps best to recognize, first, that 'ethnicity' is a complex, many-layered concept, and, second, that it is not fixed but dynamic. Culley (2000) observes that 'ethnicity' refers to a socially defined group of people who may be characterized by such factors as culture and language. However, ethnicity is also the ever-changing product of traditions and cultural practices. It is situational and contextual. Other key elements that mirror definitions in the legislation of the UK Race Relations Act include not only culture, language and religion, but also shared origins or at least a shared 'myth of origin'. These myths may be passed from generation to generation. For example, Jews may trace their ancestry to Abraham and Isaac. However, myths of origin can also be relatively modern creations (Cashmore 1982).

In health-related research, the key elements of ethnic identity have been shown to have direct relevance to health care needs and outcomes (Johnson 2003, 2008). When used to describe groups of a particular migrant origin, ethnicity may be associated with cultural factors that may affect health status, with exposure to specific risk factors. Migration itself may also affect health, as well as the ability of migrants to access health services in their new country. Culture itself is a multilayered concept that includes many aspects of belief and behaviour, some learned and some linked to cherished aspects of identity. It might include language, religion and exposure to, or preferences for, certain types of music and art. History, including a sense of the history of a family, group or nation, may be part of a culture, as well as shared experiences of discrimination or exclusion.

Language is usually learned from the parent (hence the term 'mother tongue') and language may help to unite or divide. On the Indian subcontinent, the use of different scripts is the main marker between those described as speaking 'Punjabi' (used by Sikhs and Hindus in certain parts of India) and 'Urdu' (a language essentially similar in vocabulary to Punjabi when spoken, but using a written language derived from Arabic or the Persian Farsi). In the UK, many families of South Asian people who settled in British cities came from the Mirpur District of Kashmir. This is a region divided between the nation states of India and Pakistan and there is a growing desire to describe the family language as 'Mirpuri'.

The politics of definition in researching ethnicity

The above discussion indicates that choices of terms are themselves political or ethical matters. Categories and labels change over time and differ across countries. Many studies now include a short description of their use of terms. For example, a common justification of using the word 'black' is that it is a collective term used to indicate groups that share a common history of social exclusion and discrimination. In North America, the terms used to describe 'Native Americans' or 'Indians' have undergone a long process of evolution. Some authors use terms such as 'First Nation' or 'Aboriginal'. The latter is also used in Australia rather than the more pejorative term 'Aborigine'. The 'tribal' name of the group may also be used for the same reason. In North America, the label 'Asian' tends to refer to people whose origins are in 'South-East Asia', in countries such as Vietnam, Cambodia/Khmer, Thailand or Korea. On the other hand, people from these countries may be grouped with those from the Pacific islands (Sadler et al. 2003).

In the absence of a scientific consensus, the most authoritative listing can be found in the National Institutes for Health (NIH) National Library of Medicine 'MeSH' (Medical Speciality Heading) catalogue used in PubMed and other databases. A recent revision states that the term 'Racial Stocks', pointing to categories of 'Australoid', 'Caucasoid', 'Mongoloid' and 'Negroid', has been abandoned because of the lack of scientific biological validity and its potentially offensive nature. Since 2004, 'Ethnic Groups' has been adopted as a term within the overall group heading of 'Continental Population Group origin'. This group includes an Oceanic Ancestry Group that refers to the Pacific islands and rim; European, African and Asian Ancestry Groups. The group formerly known as 'Black' in USA parlance is now recorded as African American, while Eskimos are generally known as Inuit (see www.ncbi. nlm.nih.gov/Entrez). In the UK, attempts have been made to break down the term Asian or South Asian (Bhopal et al. 1991). The exercise has been of some value in differentiating between the health experiences of some major groupings (Modood et al. 1997), although it could be criticized for being essentialist and/or creating adverse stereotypes. The majority of South Asian people living in the UK have fairly recent family connections to the larger states within the Indian subcontinent – notably India, Pakistan and Bangladesh. But many, including significant numbers of refugees and professionals, originally came from Sri Lanka, or were of 'Indian' origin when that was a single state under the English Raj. Some indeed had been settlers in various states in East Africa. Furthermore, India itself is one of the most populous and most diverse nations in the world, encompassing many distinctive languages and cultures, with significant numbers of followers for virtually every world religion.

The question of ethnic origin is important as UK data on health outcomes show that people of Muslim, particularly Bangladeshi and Pakistani, background have worse health and less satisfactory encounters with health services than those of other religions or national backgrounds (Acheson 1998). For this reason, it is necessary to consider precisely which system of ethnic categorization should be used in a particular health research project (Johnson 2008).

Self-identification and its limitations

One generally accepted approach among social scientists to the issue of 'ethnicity' is to insist that ethnic identity is a personal issue. The ascription of ethnic identity should therefore be made by the person being researched and not by the observer. For instance, an observer might easily ascribe a wrong label to a dark-skinned Devonian born in England or a light-skinned Pathan from Pakistan, if visual identification was used as a criterion, quite apart from any prejudices held by the observer. Guidance issued to the NHS and other bodies on 'ethnic monitoring', strongly supports the idea of self-identification (Johnson 2008). Public bodies are now required to collect data on ethnicity to overcome the disadvantages associated with racialized discrimination. However, a question such as 'To which ethnic group do you belong?' could create an almost infinite number of categories. It might also be impossible to compare any data collected with baseline data. This is a requirement for most scientific and health care related research.

There are also clinical reasons for wishing to identify members of certain ethnic groups who are at most risk of developing, or giving birth to children with, certain genetic conditions. A number of studies set out to test what category labels are most effective in identifying members of at-risk groups (Aspinall et al. 2003). These have found that it is possible to offer a selection of group labels which are meaningful to respondents and also have some predictive value for clinical purposes. Similarly, in epidemiological research it has been found possible to identify certain categorical labels that are recognized and accepted, and which also relate to clinical differences in health outcomes (Comstock et al. 2004). It is generally accepted that it is desirable when carrying out research to offer respondents a list of possible categories from which to choose, even if this restricts their choice. As in any social science research, the category 'other: please specify' provides a residual option.

The problem in data collection of shifting identities and social categories

National surveys and the decennial census are important sources of data on ethnic minority groups for researchers and, over the years, the Office of National Statistics (ONS) has devoted considerable effort to developing questions for these. The ONS notes that an individual's description of their ethnic group may change over time as, for quite legitimate reasons, a person may record themselves as belonging to one ethnic group at one time, and another when asked the same question on another occasion. Social and political attitudes change over time, as noted above in relation to North American studies. In Britain, 'black' was at one time an unacceptable term, but it is now widely used. For the groups concerned, it stands as a statement of political awareness and solidarity. In other words, any ethnic group label is only valid for the period and the context in which it is used. To overcome this problem, the ONS maintains a 'data-bridge' of categories to be used in surveys, including the census (National Statistics 2003; Afkhami and Acik-Toprak 2012). This provides a way of linking the terms used over time so that longitudinal work can be carried out.

In the UK, the decennial census is the major national set of data available to social science researchers. It incorporates data on 'ethnicity', and it has become the accepted wisdom to use the so-called 'Census Ethnic Question' drawn from the 2001 Census for England and Wales, and their subsequent update in 2011, as shown in Box 17.1. The question asked people to indicate 'which ethnic group' they felt best described their origins. The majority (over 85%) opted for 'White British' and thus, by definition, all other categories can be regarded as 'minority ethnic' groups. White British includes 'White Irish' and other white groups. The form makes it explicit that ethnicity is seen in terms of 'cultural background', rather than seeking to identify place of birth, nationality or even descent. The higher-level group headings, shown in italics below as 'Asian or Asian British', 'Black or Black British', make this point clearly. In Scotland and Northern Ireland, slightly different options were offered to take account of the much smaller numbers of people in the population from these minority groups.

Box 17.1 'Minority Ethnic Group' categories in the UK Census

What is your ethnic group? Tick the appropriate box to indicate your cultural background.

White:

White – British White – Irish (2011 adds Welsh/Scottish/Northern Irish/Gypsy-Traveller)

Any other White background (please write in)

Mixed:

Mixed – White/Black Caribbean Mixed – White/Black African Mixed – White/Asian

Any other mixed background (please write in)

Asian or Asian British:

Asian or Asian British: Indian – Asian or Asian British: Pakistani – Asian or Asian British: Bangladeshi

(2011 includes Chinese as an option under Asian or Asian British)

Any other Asian or Asian British background (please write in)

Black or Black British:

Black or Black British: Caribbean – Black or Black British: African

Any other Black or Black British background (please write in)

Chinese or other ethnic group: (in 2011 Chinese included under 'Asian')

Chinese or other ethnic group: Chinese (2011 offers Arab as tick-box option)

Any other ethnic group (please write in)

Source: Adapted from Office of National Statistics Census form for 2001 and 2011; Afkhami and Acik-Toprak (2012)

While this categorization has proved adequate for most national research and many local studies, it omits other identifiable groups such as Arab, Somali, Yemeni and Vietnamese. These population groups may be significant in particular localities or of interest for certain kinds of health care research. In 2011, Polish was added to Scottish census forms. It has been recognized that such groups should be included in local listings, and guidance is available from the ONS on the best ways to incorporate these categories into data to make projections compatible with the census data (National Statistics 2003, 2011). This still does not take account of many groups, especially those who may be defined as 'new migrants', including refugees and asylum seekers. There is at present no solution to this. As there are no nationally available data on the ethnic or national background or demographic composition of refugees and asylum seekers in Britain, the requirement to collect data which can be used to compare with a baseline estimate does not apply.

In many health research studies designed to identify health needs and behaviours, religion was the label used to identify certain groups: for example, Jews or Sikhs (Bonney 2004; Johnson 2004). Consequently, it is advisable for the researcher to include a separate question on religious adherence or membership. The ONS has collected some national data using a well-tested question to cover this matter, as have the Fourth National Study of Minority Groups (Modood et al. 1997) and the Health Survey for England (Erens et al. 2001). In yet other studies, the ability to communicate in a particular oral or written form has been a marker for cultural and ethnic identity. A question on language could be couched in terms of the 'preferred' language for communication, the 'mother tongue' or the language 'used at home', in order to explore the ways in which ethnic identity is constructed and expressed.

Researching Ethnic Minority Health in Practice

From a methodological perspective, it is clear that there is no single 'right answer' to the issue of researching the role and nature of ethnicity in health. The solution adopted by many researchers is therefore to use a 'mix of methods' (Creswell and Plano Clark 2010) and then triangulate the findings. The assumption is that using a variety of approaches will obtain a more rounded picture (see Chapter 22 for a discussion of triangulation). One particularly effective approach is the 'social action' research model. This combines elements of the survey with ethnographic or qualitative methods such as focus groups or unstructured interviews through 'action research' (see Chapter 8 for a discussion of action research). Research in this case is combined with capacity building and community or service development and incorporated into the research design (Fleming and Ward 1999, 2004). The advantages are that by working closely with members of the communities concerned, many of the problems of being an outsider can be avoided (Lloyd et al. 2007, 2008; Johnson and Borde 2009). Working with a community can increase a researcher's understanding of the significance of what is observed in terms of health behaviour and attitudes to health and illness. Questions may also be asked in a way that is relevant to the culture, as opposed to asking questions which have no relevance or cannot be answered within the terms of reference of the culture. Stages of the action research model developed by Morjaria-Keval and Johnson (2005) are shown in Box 17.2, which is followed by the inclusion of a case study.

Box 17.2 Using a social action model in researching ethnic minority health

Stage 1: Get started

A health research study working with minority communities should be based on a sound review of needs. Data from national and local sources should be obtained and consultations undertaken with the 'expert' community. A literature review of scholarly sources and the 'grey' literature is essential (see Chapter 3). Local reports often contain valuable information.

Stage 2: Recruit key worker(s)

Experience of working within minority cultural communities is necessary, as well as a commitment to change and to the community. Once appointed, key workers need extensive training and briefing in all aspects of the project, including their duty to observe ethical guidelines on confidentiality and being able to offer advice on health matters related to the project and the statutory and voluntary services provided locally.

Stage 3: Recruit and train community facilitators

The key element of the social action research model is the use of locally recruited community fieldworkers, who are given basic training in research and substantive issues including ethics and health promotion. If possible, this should be provided to a certificated level of competence. Our experience is that most local minority communities possess extraordinary reserves of well-qualified, highly committed and resourceful people. Some basic level of education and dual-language ability is essential, as well as personal qualities, such as respect for community members and other groups.

Stage 4: Develop survey questions/topic guide for interviews

Expert advice should be sought from community facilitators to test findings from the literature and identify the initial priorities of the project. During training sessions, community facilitators should be encouraged to comment on the research instruments and topic guides (see also the experiences of Johnson and Borde 2009).

(Continued)

(Continued)

Stage 5: Conduct interviews

The agenda or topic guide may be used to establish the views and perceptions of communities, service users and providers against a common template. It is likely that facilitators will use their community's own language and should provide a translated report on the discussions or interviews.

Stage 6: Review, analyse and feed back

It is essential to confirm or validate the analysis of transcripts from interviews with community facilitators and other informants. An opportunity to comment on the researchers' data analysis should be given prior to circulating reports to sponsors and service providers.

Stage 7: Take appropriate action – further intervention

It may be necessary to revise plans during the course of the project. The importance of assertive outreach and information giving is well established. Resources should be used flexibly to achieve this. It is essential to honour the pledge that the research will contribute positively to community development.

Stage 8: Evaluate and disseminate

The evaluation of outcomes and a dissemination strategy should be planned at the outset and modified as the project progresses. Key audiences include the communities that have taken part, as well as practitioners and academic peers. Findings should become part of an official record in order for others to learn from the research.

Source: Morjaria-Keval and Johnson (2005)

CASE STUDY

Case study: Ethnic minority health research using a social action approach

Background

In the 1990s, the NHS Executive Ethnic Health Unit was responsible for setting up a number of developmental projects, to bring about change in the way health care was provided and to promote improvements in the health status of minority groups across Britain (Chan 1997). One of the projects was the 'Sahara' project in Birmingham, designed to bring about change in the health behaviour of men in the Asian communities (Johnson and Verma 1998). In this case, 'Asian' was not defined. The project coordinators, including the author, interpreted their brief broadly. A central aim in the project was to explore existing perceptions of health and ill health and to find out the priorities of males as previous studies had focused on women. The project also aimed to enable local community organizations to conduct the research through providing training and support. From a very early stage, project researchers worked closely with community organizations such as neighbourhood centres and religious groups who were responsible for finding community facilitators and recruiting members for focus groups. Seven organizations were identified, which recruited 24 volunteers who were given training and paid as discussion group facilitators. Drawn from local groups, the interviewers were matched to the groups they were interviewing to ensure a better understanding of culturally specific concerns.

Refining the research questions

During the training, it became apparent that the men recruited represented, in their own terms, more than a dozen self-identified ethnic groups, so that the 'Pakistani' group contained representatives of people from the Kamalpuri/Campbellpur district, Pathans, Mirpuri or Kashmiri speakers, and people who described themselves as 'Pakistani Punjabi'. From the Indian side of the international border, there were also Hindu and Sikh Punjabis as well as Hindu Gujeratis.

Participants in the training were very vocal in discussing the appropriateness of certain questions and suggested ways in which questions could be phrased to ensure a worthwhile response. For instance, the normal practice in questionnaire design is to place the rather general question 'Are you happy with your health?' before a specific one: 'Are you happy with your level of energy?' We were advised by a representative that this would lead to a response for the second question, along the lines of: 'I have already said.' Placing the specific question first would allow the culturally appropriate response of 'no', while still expressing overall satisfaction with health. In other cases, we were advised to ask about 'some people' or 'others' in the community, on the grounds that there were certain cultural taboos that community members would not breach. For example, it would be difficult for Muslims to admit to drinking alcohol or Sikhs to say they used tobacco.

The social action research process

Following training, the community facilitators organized events and meetings in their community organizations, and obtained the agreement of groups of men to take part in focus group discussions that followed a predetermined topic guide. Discussions took place in a comfortable, familiar setting such as the community centre or someone's home. Discussions were tape-recorded, usually using the community language rather than English. The facilitators then wrote a report, transcribing relevant parts of the conversations, and added their comments on how these responses reflected community perceptions.

During and after the discussion, facilitators also gave information about health, or offered help with specific queries. In this way, particular issues were raised and debated. In consequence, information began to reach those who had previously been outside existing systems of health promotion. Furthermore, we obtained

(Continued)

(Continued)

extensive information on service use and, incidentally, the ease of access to, and use of, sport and exercise facilities that had not been included in the original survey design.

It became clear that the different 'ethnic groups' had distinctive perspectives on their health needs and priorities. A major complaint was that 'Asian' services did not meet their needs, and, frequently, that one sub-group or another had managed to hijack the local agenda and facilities. This feedback was later used to improve facilities and health promotion locally.

This study demonstrated the potential for using locally recruited, community-based informants as research workers, as have similar projects (Fleming and Ward 1999, 2004; Morjaria-Keval and Johnson 2005). Working with community members builds capacity, confidence and a sense of ownership within communities that can be sustained after a project has finished. It also combats the accusation that needs are being ignored. Joint or collaborative studies can combine the rigour expected from scientific research with virtues of insight from within the community.

Box 17.2 above illustrates the different stages of a social action research model, drawing on recent research in which the author was involved, supported by the Thomas Pocklington Trust and the Housing Corporation. The reader is also invited to reflect on the ethics of conducting research 'on' a community without their involvement (Lloyd et al. 2008), and to consider the advantages of conducting research 'with' a community and the ways in which this might be viewed by an ethics review committee, noting that the UK NHS National Institute for Health Research now no longer funds research which does not demonstrate 'user' involvement.

Conclusion

Research on health and access to health services is an important and relatively well-funded area of research, but full of pitfalls for the unwary. This chapter has looked at the problems of researching ethnicity, of which identifying the ethnic identity of research participants is a major issue. Various ways of thinking about, and determining, ethnicity have been discussed and key sources of baseline data identified.

Following up a theme addressed in Chapter 8 on action research, it is suggested that researchers in this area should aim to involve ethnic minority communities themselves in carrying out the various stages of research. Although this approach will require effective management of the research process, it has the advantage of working with, rather than on, communities, as well as helping to improve the research from a technical perspective. Great care should be taken to honour any promises made to provide feedback to communities or to seek service improvements as a consequence of the research.

Exercise: The take-up of services for the visually impaired from ethnic minority groups

The take-up of services for the visually impaired from ethnic minority groups is less than might be expected. Drawing on this chapter, consider from a health research perspective how you would address the following questions:

1 Why does it appear that people from ethnic minority groups are not taking up services for the visually impaired?

2 How would you raise awareness of and uptake of services currently being provided?

3 How far do we need to understand if 'needs' are the same or different from those of the majority community and whether different services or 'more of the same' are required?

4 Is the solution to work with communities to understand specific needs and generate materials to bring about change among service providers, as well as potential service users?

For more background information, see: www.pocklington-trust.org.uk or Joule and Levenson (2008)

Recommended Further Reading

Ingleby, D., Krasnik, A., Lorant, V. and Razum, O. (eds) (2012) *Health Inequalities and Risk Factors among Migrants and Ethnic Minorities.* Antwerp: Garant. (See especially the chapter by Johnson, M.R.D. 'Problems and barriers in the collection of ethnicity and migration related data')

Ingleby, D., Chiarenza, A., Devillé, W. and Kotsioni, I. (eds) (2012) *Inequalities in Health Care for Migrants and Ethnic Minorities.* Antwerp: Garant. (See especially the chapter by Johnson, M.R.D. 'User and community involvement in health and social care research: the case of migrants and ethnic minorities')

These two volumes represent the product of a five-year series of international European workshops looking at issues of health and care for migrant and minority ethnic groups across Europe, supported by the European Community 'Collaboration on Science and Technology' and 'Health of Migrants in Europe' projects.

Johnson, M.R.D. (2003) 'Research governance and diversity: quality standards for a multi-ethnic NHS', *Nursing Times Research*, 8(1): 2–10.

This article discusses the ethical issues lying behind the design of health care research to meet the needs of the wider population and especially the inclusion of minority ethnic groups in that objective.

Johnson, M.R.D. (2006) 'Engaging communities and users: health and social care research with ethnic minority communities', in J. Nazroo (ed.), *Health and Social Research in Multiethnic Societies*. London: Routledge.

This chapter considers the merits and problems of engaging with communities in participatory action for empowerment through the social action research model, in a Department of Health commissioned handbook covering the major issues involved in research with ethnic minority groups.

Johnson, M.R.D. (2006) 'Ethnicity', in A. Killoran, C. Swann and M. Kelly (eds), *Public Health Evidence: Changing the Health of the Public*. Oxford: Oxford University Press.

This chapter discusses the nature of ethnicity and the problems in defining, measuring and using it as a research category, in a volume addressing a wide range of issues by leading experts in public health research.

Online Readings

Mills, K. (2012) 'Under the radar: Impact of policies of localism on substance misuse services for refugee and asylum seeking communities', *International Social Work*, 55: 662–74.

How is ethnicity defined in this context? What are the different research methods used to identify health needs? What are the implications of using this type of method?

Coleman, L. and Testa, A. (2007) 'Sexual health knowledge, attitudes and behaviours among an ethnically diverse sample of young people in the UK', *Health Education Journal*, 66: 68–81.

How is ethnicity defined in this context? What are the different research methods used to identify health needs? What are the implications of using this type of method?

References

Acheson, D. (1998) *Independent Inquiry into Inequalities in Health*. London: The Stationery Office.

Afkhami, R. and Acik-Toprak, N. (2012) *Ethnicity: Introductory User Guide*. Colchester: ESDS Government. Available at: www.esds.ac.uk/government/docs/ethnicityintro.pdf (accessed 30 January 2012).

Aspinall, P.J., Dyson, S.M. and Anionwu, E.N. (2003) 'The feasibility of using ethnicity as a primary tool for antenatal selective screening for sickle cell disorders: pointers from the research evidence', *Social Science and Medicine*, 56: 285–97.

Banton, M. (1977) *The Idea of Race*. London: Tavistock.

Bhopal, R.S., Phillimore, P. and Kohli, H.S. (1991) 'Inappropriate use of the term "Asian": an obstacle to ethnicity and health research', *Journal of Public Health Medicine*, 13(4): 244–6.

Bonney, R. (2004) 'Reflections on the differences between religion and culture', *Clinical Cornerstone*, 6(1): 25–33.

Care Quality Commission (CQC) (2010) *Guidance about Compliance: Essential Standards of Quality and Safety* London: CQC.

Cashmore, E.E. (1982) *Rastaman: The Rastafarian Movement in England.* London: George Allen & Unwin.

Chan, M. (1997) *Achievements of the NHS Ethnic Health Unit.* Leeds: NHS Ethnic Health Unit.

Comstock, R.D., Castillo, E.M. and Lindsay, S.P. (2004) 'Four year review of the use of race and ethnicity in epidemiologic and public health research', *American Journal of Epidemiology*, 159(6): 611–19.

Creswell, J.W. and Plano Clark,V.L. (2010) *Designing and Conducting Mixed Methods Research.* London: Sage.

Crisp, N. (2004) Race Equality Action Plan. Available at Department of Health website: www.dh.gov.uk/PublicationsAndStatistics/Bulletins/BulletinArticle/fs/en?CONTENT_ID=4072494&chk=1e/oI7

Culley, L. (2000) 'Working with diversity: beyond the factfile', in C. Davies, L. Finlay and A. Bullman (eds), *Changing Practice in Health and Social Care.* London: Sage.

Erens, B., Primatesta, P. and Prior, G. (eds) (2001) *Health Survey for England 1999 Volume 1: Findings. Volume 2: Methodology and Documentation.* London: The Stationery Office.

Fleming, J. and Ward, D. (1999) 'Researcher as empowerment: the social action approach', in W. Shera and L. Wells (eds), *Empowerment Practice in Social Work.* Toronto: Canadian Scholars' Press.

Fleming, J. and Ward, D. (2004) 'Methodology and practical application of the social action research model', in F. Maggs-Rapport (ed.), *New Qualitative Research Methodologies in Health and Social Care: Putting Ideas into Practice.* London: Routledge.

Gill, P., Kai, J., Bhopal, R.S. and Wild, S. (2002) *Black and Minority Ethnic Groups in Healthcare Needs Assessment: Epidemiologically-based Needs Assessment Reviews, Third Series.* Oxford: Radcliffe Medical. Available at: http://hcna.radcliffe-oxford.com/bemgframe.htm

Johnson, M.R.D. (2003) 'Ethnic diversity in social context', in J. Kai (ed.), *Ethnicity, Health and Primary Care.* Oxford: Oxford University Press.

Johnson, M.R.D. (2004) *Towards an Epidemiology of Ethnic Diversity.* Module in ENB/DH/Nursing & Midwifery Council Online Course for Cultural Competence. Available at: www.rcn.org.uk/Resources/Transcultural/Index.php

Johnson, M.R.D. (2008) 'Making difference count: ethnic monitoring in health (and social care)', *Radical Statistics*, 96: 38–45.

Johnson, M.R.D. and Borde, T. (2009) 'Representation of ethnic minorities in research: necessity, opportunity and adverse effects', in L. Culley, N. Hudson and F. van Rooij (eds), *Marginalized Reproduction: Ethnicity, Infertility and Reproductive Technologies*. London: Earthscan.

Johnson, M.R.D. and Verma, C. (1998) *It's Our Health Too: Asian Men's Health Perspectives*, CRER Research Paper 26, Southern Birmingham Community Health NHS Trust and NHS Executive Ethnic Health Unit, Coventry: University of Warwick.

Joule, N. and Levenson, R. (2008) *People from Black and Minority Ethnic (BME) Communities and Vision Services: A Good Practice Guide*. London: Thomas Pocklington Trust.

LaVeist, T.A. (1994) 'Beyond dummy variables and sample selection: what health services researchers ought to know about race as a variable', *Health Services Research*, 29: 1–16.

Lloyd, C.E., Johnson, M.R.D., Mughal, S., Sturt, J.A., Collins, G.S., Roy, T., Bibi, R. and Barnett, A.H. (2008) 'Securing recruitment and obtaining informed consent in minority ethnic groups in the UK', *BMC Health Services Research*, 8: 68. Available at: www.biomedcentral.com/1472-6963/8/68

Lloyd, C.E., Johnson, M.R.D., Sturt, J., Collins, G.S. and Barnett, A.H. (2007) 'Hearing the voices of service users: reflections on researching the views of people from South Asian backgrounds', in A. Williamson and R. DeSouza (eds), *Researching with Communities: Grounded Perspectives on Engaging Communities in Research*. Auckland, NZ: Muddy Creek Press.

Macpherson, W. (1999) *The Stephen Lawrence Inquiry: Report of an Inquiry*. London: Home Office.

Modood, T., Berthoud, R., Lakey, J., Nazroo, J., Smith, P., Virdee, S. and Beishon, S. (1997) *Ethnic Minorities in Britain: Diversity and Disadvantage*, PSI Report 843. London: Policy Studies Institute.

Morjaria-Keval, A. and Johnson, M.R.D. (2005) *Our Vision Too: Improving the Access of Ethnic Minority Visually Impaired People to Appropriate Services*. Seacole Research Paper 4. Leicester: MSRC with Housing Corporation and Thomas Pocklington Trust.

National Statistics (2003) *Ethnic Group Statistics: A Guide for the Collection and Classification of Ethnicity Data*. London: Stationery Office/Office of National Statistics.

National Statistics (2011) *Measuring Equality: A Guide for the Collection and Classification of Ethnic Group, National Identity and Religion Data in the UK*. London: Office of National Statistics. Available at: www.ons.gov.uk/ons/guide-method/measuring-equality/equality/ethnic-nat-identity-religion/index.html (accessed 30 January 2012).

Sadler, G.R., Ryujin, L., Nguyen, T., Oh, G., Paik, G. and Kustin, B. (2003) 'Heterogeneity within the Asian American community', *International Journal for Equity in Health*, 2: 12. Available at: www.equityhealthj.com/content/2/1/12

Samanta, A., Johnson, M.R.D., Guo, F. and Adebajo, A. (2009) 'Snails in bottles and language cuckoos: an evaluation of patient information resources for South Asians with osteomalacia', *Rheumatology*, 48(3): 299–303.

Williams, C. and Johnson, M.R.D. (2010) *Race and Ethnicity in a Welfare Society*. Maidenhead: Open University Press/McGraw.

18

Gender and Health Research

ELLEN KUHLMANN AND ELLEN ANNANDALE

Introduction

- In this chapter, we bring a gender lens to health research and highlight three main areas: gender and health status; gender and health care; and gender and health policy. We seek to explore why gender matters and how a gender lens can be applied. This includes drawing attention to the challenges of gender-sensitive research, such as the distinction between 'sex' and 'gender', and the intersections between biological and social dimensions of health.

- Flanked by international organizations, such as the World Health Organization (WHO) and legal requirements in many (Western) countries, gender-sensitive perspectives have now entered into the mainstream of health research. It is increasingly recognized that a gender lens is important for men's health as well as women's health (and for boys and girls). This is not only a matter of social justice and equality, but also a strategy for increasing the quality and efficiency of health systems and services. At the same time, gender bias and unfair and unequal treatment of men and women persist. In our chapter, we provide some general guidance on how to enhance gender-sensitive health research. We then use health policy assessment of new models of care for coronary heart disease as an illustrative case, taking into account the benefits of mixed methods approaches and multiple data sources.

Why Is a Gender Lens Important in Health Research?

Gender-sensitive health research has moved from the margins into the mainstream of health research. Thus, 'gender' is no longer merely a matter of feminist concern and a synonym for women, but includes the rapidly expanding field of men's health research (Broom and Tovey 2009). In this chapter, we argue that a gender-sensitive lens is important in the entire field of health research in order to improve the equality and quality/efficiency of health systems and services, to elucidate how health and illness are experienced and to explore the social patterning of health and illness. Box 18.1 below shows how a gender lens can assist in our analyses.

Box 18.1   The value of a gender lens in health research

- *Associations between gender and health status*: this includes research on patterns of morbidity and mortality; individual health-related behaviours, like smoking, drinking, exercise and eating disorders; and public health measures (for examples, see Annandale and Hunt 2000; Bird et al. 2012).
- *Lay concepts of health and the experience of illness:* this encompasses the study of lay epidemiology, such as people's beliefs about how the causes and distribution of illness vary by gender, how representations of illness can be gendered, as well as how gender expectations can influence how people care for themselves and others when ill or incapacitated (for examples, see Macintyre et al. 2005; Kempner 2006; Riska and Heikell 2007).
- *Gender and health care*: this refers to wide-ranging issues of the governance, organization and management of care, including access to, and accessibility of, services, as well as the attitudes and performance of health professionals and lay carers. It also includes the governance of health human resources, including the workforce skill-mix and planning measures (for examples, see Kuhlmann and Annandale 2012a).
- *Gender and health policy:* this refers to equal opportunity and gender-specific policies and increasingly to the assessment of the development, implementation, monitoring and evaluation of all health policies regardless of their focus of concern. This may also include policies beyond health that are assumed to have a strong impact on health status and/or health care, such as education, labour market, or environmental policies (for examples, see WHO 2011; Abdool et al. 2012; Lin and L'Orange 2012).

There is no one-size-fits-all recipe for 'getting health research right' from the viewpoint of gender sensitivity. Instead, context-sensitive approaches and critical reflection on the methodological paradigms of social science and the ways in which sex and gender are connected in health-related research can help to avoid the negative impact of gender-blind health research.

Methodological paradigms

Bringing gender into health research inevitably means that we must engage with epistemology and methodological 'paradigm wars' (see Chapter 2 of this volume). Initially tacked on to feminist approaches, gender perspectives have challenged the epistemological basis of science, something which is especially true for health and biomedical research. Women writers and women's health activists were among the first researchers to highlight the critical relevance of social dimensions of health and illness as far back as the early decades of the nineteenth century. Gender is not a given, rather, as West and Zimmerman (1987: 126) put it in their oft-cited article, it 'is a routine, methodical, and recurring accomplishment'.

This way of thinking shifted research towards interpretivist and social constructivist theoretical approaches and to qualitative methods. These were deemed better able to capture the lived experience of health, illness and health care. During the 1970s and 1980s in particular, feminist theories and women's health research criticized the limitations of positivism and related claims for the neutrality and objectivity of science (for an overview, see Lagro-Janssen 2012). At the same time, feminist research does not fundamentally oppose the search for 'objectivity' in science but calls for power-sensitive approaches (Harding 1986; Haraway 1988).

Here, it is also important to appreciate that gender is not simply a 'variable' or a 'role' that can be adopted flexibly by men and women. It is argued here that gender is:

- Fundamentally an organizing principle of societies and science.
- A part of situated experience.

Traditionally, medical science and practice have played a key role in the exclusion of women in the name of 'neutrality' and 'objectivity' of science and bolstered the hegemonic claims of the predominantly white male actors who claim authority within science (Haraway 1988). More recently, it has been recognized that men's own health can suffer from conventional expectations of normative masculinity (Riska 2010). Gender also does not simply add to other dimensions of social inequality, like, for instance, ethnicity (see Chapter 17). How then can health be researched in such a way that takes the health needs and interests of men and women into account?

First and foremost, it is important to be aware that gender-sensitive research is not linked to any specific method or research design. The assumption made by some authors during the formative phase of feminist health research in the 1970s and 1980s, that qualitative methods such as open-ended interviews and varieties of participant observation have a natural affinity with 'researching women' and are liberatory by design, cannot be supported. Neither can the corollary that quantitative research, such as large-scale survey trials, is inherently exploitative.

Here, it is important to appreciate that a long tradition of feminist-oriented quantitative research on health inequalities stems back to the 1960s (Annandale 2009). As Oakley

(2005a: 249) has argued, looking back, many feminists had 'mistakenly thrown at least part of the baby out with the bathwater', because without large-scale comparative data it is hard to 'distinguish between personal experience and large scale oppression'. As she also argues through a study of pregnancy, randomized controlled trials (RCTs) may be the only way to fully assess whether or not the availability of a social support intervention improved things for women and their babies (Oakley 2005b). Research on men's health and gender, which often acknowledges the feminist methodological heritage, has been more receptive to a range of research methods. This perhaps reflects a loosening of the 'paradigm wars' during its period of formative development in the 1990s.

Today, gender research employs the entire spectrum of types of research and of data collection techniques. Moreover, researchers are increasingly comfortable with a perspective that different research questions call for different methodological approaches and with the merits of 'mixed methods' (see Chapter 22). In the case of gender and health, this involves not only the now conventional data collection techniques such as interviews, focus groups, participant observation and surveys, but also the newer methods of the analysis of texts and images and participant-generated data such as photographs and written materials (for examples, see Bourgeault et al. 2010).

In a similar vein, like all health research, gender-sensitive research is a matter of social justice and fairness and hence an ethical issue. However, there is no demand for specific ethical guidelines for gender research, except ethical matters in relation to the reproductive rights of women and the protection of the foetus. These are especially relevant in the area of drug testing and research.

In summary, gender-sensitive research calls for a critical reflection of traditional methodological paradigms, such as the purported neutrality and objectivity of science. This is relevant for qualitative, quantitative and mixed methods, as well as for all types of research design at all stages, from the development of research questions and aims through to data collection, analysis and interpretation. Unsurprisingly, a gender lens is not easily applied in health research, not least because the study of gender itself embodies a number of challenges such as how to study the relationship between biological and social dimensions of health that are encompassed within the sex/gender distinction.

How sex and gender matter

The concepts of biological sex and social gender originated in psychiatry some half a century ago. They were subsequently taken up by feminist scholars as an attempt to counteract biologism and the devaluation of women. Within this binary framework, 'sex' marks the biological and 'gender' the social category. For many years, this distinction has served well to challenge biological explanations for social conditions of health and illness and to bring the social constructions and configurations of health-related inequality into sight. At the same time, the 'gender binary' has always been a matter of controversy in feminist theory (Kuhlmann and Annandale 2012a).

As explained in more detail elsewhere (Annandale and Kuhlmann 2012), until recently the most problematic area was the marked tendency to use the concepts of sex and gender to divide men and women (and boys and girls) into two distinct groups, and then to read social and biological differences off these distinctions. This binary division of all human beings not only provokes essentialist approaches to men and women, boys and girls as homogeneous, opposed groups, but also excludes transgender individuals. Ironically, binary thinking has been necessary in order to collect sex-disaggregated data to make any inequities in health and health care transparent. This has been exacerbated by the rapidly emergent field of 'gender medicine' (also labelled 'gender-specific' or 'sex-specific' medicine), which typically involves the search for differences between men and women that are seen as biologically fixed. In consequence, it has encouraged men and women to think about their health in inappropriately fixed, gender-specific ways (Annandale and Hammarström 2011).

Sex or biological differences may sometimes matter, such as in the context of reproductive health or illnesses related to anatomical differences like prostate or ovarian cancers. Yet in most, if not all, areas of health and illness, the reduction of gender to biological difference can actually be quite dangerous. As Epstein (2007: 248) has argued, it risks 'improper medical treatment of a patient who doesn't conform to the stereotype of his or her group'.

Gender often intersects with other factors, such as ethnicity, social class, sexuality and age, which can also be associated with vulnerability or resistance to ill health, with access to care and with the quality of care that is provided. For example, oppressions connected with gender, class, age, sexuality and race are not simply additive, nor do they necessarily act together, rather they often interact in complex ways (for an overview, see Bates et al. 2012). At the same time, some of the recent approaches to the intersecting dimensions of inequality at best risk losing sight of gendered inequalities and at worse question the viability of gender as an overarching 'master status' in the construction of health and health care inequalities.

A further challenge is to better understand how the social and biological dimensions of health intersect with sex and gender. Here, it is important to appreciate that both are sensitive to changes in the societies within which men and women live out their lives.

Although we tend to think of social gender as being the most amenable to change, the biological body is not fixed either. As Fausto-Sterling puts it, 'we *acquire* a body rather than a passive unfolding of some preformed blueprint' (2003: 131, emphasis in original). The circumstances of our social lives get written on our bodies and, consequently, the social and the biological dimensions of health and gender also intersect (Krieger and Davey Smith 2004). Research into gender and health has neglected the biological dimensions of health. Thus, the achievements of gender research 'have been secured at the cost of limiting the analysis of interactions between health and social context to what happens beyond the skin, outside of the body' (Kuhlmann and Babitsch 2002: 438). Ironically, the wheels may now turn to the other extreme, as the sexing of cells and tissues in the emergent field of 'gender medicine' may lose sight of the wider 'social constraints' on health.

These points are of more than theoretical interest. How we approach sex and gender matters because they have become an indispensable part of policy formulation in relation to gender, health and health care.

Gender Policy and Politics

The concept of gender mainstreaming has been a significant driver towards the establishment of gender-sensitive research, providing both a legal framework and a methodological toolset. Taking a definition adopted by WHO (2002: 6):

> ... [gender mainstreaming] is a strategy for making women's as well as men's concerns and experiences an integral dimension in the design, implementation, monitoring and evaluation of policies and programmes in all political, economic and social spheres, such that inequality between men and women is not perpetuated. The ultimate goal is to achieve gender equality.

Based on the 1995 Beijing platform of the fourth International World Conference of Women, the concept of gender mainstreaming originated from feminist activism but is also closely linked with new management and governance within the public sector. Gender mainstreaming is important because it expands the scope of attention from women's health alone to encompass men's health care and male actors (Annandale and Riska 2009). It provides a flexible methodological 'toolset' for the institutions of national health care states and local communities, and may therefore be translated in different ways – in women's health care, for instance, in the areas of sexual violence or maternity care; in men's health care in areas that counteract traditional masculinities, such as in seeking help for mental health care problems; and in gender-sensitive health care in areas that may benefit either men or women, or both, as social groups (Kuhlmann and Annandale 2012b).

Gender indicators may be linked directly to financial incentives and gender budgeting, and also to performance management and existing models of organizational and professional self-governing controls (for an overview, see Abdool et al. 2012; Lin and L'Orange 2012). The development and implementation of indicators thus serves as the 'grease' in gender-sensitive research and as a connecting tie between health policy and health care research on the one hand, and health status and inequalities on the other.

In summary, while gender mainstreaming has helped to further gender-sensitive health research and has significantly improved its acceptance, it severs research on health from its original feminist linkages, thus reducing the focus on problems with the sex/gender distinction and the embedded social relations of power. Hence, gender mainstreaming and the tools provided do not necessarily solve the challenges of applying a gender lens in ways that reduce gendered health inequalities and poor service quality.

Studying sex, gender and health

There is growing agreement that sex and gender need to be taken into account in research, but it is often not clear how this can be done. Thus, many questions arise: When are men-only and when are women-only studies of health and health care useful? When must research include comparisons of men and women? Are sex and gender binary attributes? How do we capture gender as an experience that is complex and variable? How do we study diverse and intersecting social dimensions of health without losing sight of any overarching influence of gender as a 'master' category? As Saltonstall (1993) has demonstrated, doing health is a form of doing gender. But there is no one-to-one association between being a man or woman, boy or girl, and certain health problems, attitudes, behaviours or expressions of symptoms. So how do we identify when sex and gender do and when they do not matter? This is a key question to be considered when designing and carrying out research.

As a general rule, research should be designed to be as gender-inclusive as possible (Annandale and Hunt 2000). Single-sex studies are, without doubt, relevant in some areas, but justifications for them need to be critically evaluated and reflected upon in order to avoid the unthinking reproduction of gender differences in research. This can result in gender stereotyping. Research into help-seeking is a useful illustration.

Gender Inclusive and Comparative Research: The Case of Help-seeking

Gender differences in help-seeking have repeatedly been reported in qualitative and in quantitative studies, revealing a general pattern of more positive attitudes and higher levels of consultation in the group of women when compared to men. These findings may be a result of an 'overemphasis of differences' and gender stereotypes of women as the 'weaker' sex (and subsequently in need of help) and men as the 'lonely heroes' ('men/boys do not cry'). As Hunt et al. (2012) argue, there is an urgent need to reconsider such findings, especially because men's supposed 'under-use', or delayed use, of health care is often taken to be a key part of the explanation for men's shorter life expectancy. The difference with women's life expectancy has moved high up on the policy agenda in many countries.

Using a gender comparative approach enabled Hunt et al. (2012) to draw a more nuanced picture. Their research reveals that although, on average, women consult in primary care more than men, particularly during the peak reproductive years, there is little robust evidence comparing rates of consultation for men and women experiencing the same illnesses. Their gender-comparative perspective counteracts widespread assumptions on differences and instead highlights that men do not delay longer in seeking help for conditions that are not gender-specific, such as colorectal cancer, a major contributor to premature mortality.

Cross-country comparison with a focus on older people reveals 'Western' bias in research into help-seeking. For example, findings reported by Roy and Chaudhuri (2012) show that, in developed countries, older women generally either report better self-assessed health than men or levels of health that are comparable to men, but with higher utilization of health care services. By comparison, in developing countries, it is women who tend to report worse health than men, as well as having lower utilization of services.

Contextualized and intersectional approaches: the case of health inequalities

When looking at inequalities in health status, gender is clearly relevant but it is difficult to assess in what ways sex or gender or both may play a role (Annandale 2009). Across the globe, with very few exceptions, women live longer than men, even if by only a few years. This finding is robust and enduring, despite the wide-ranging geographical, cultural and socio-economic differences in life expectancy in different parts of the world. But women's 'choices' for health are at the same time often more constrained than those of men, as women in most societies achieve lower average incomes than men and work more hours (in paid and domestic work). They are clustered in lower status segments of the labour market or even excluded from paid work, but assigned higher responsibility for reproductive tasks (Bird et al. 2012). And to add even more puzzles, women also often report more ill health and receive poorer health treatment, even in countries committed to equal opportunity policies (Sen et al. 2007).

There is as yet no convincing explanation for gender gaps in life expectancy and in health status during life, but there are good reasons to give up the search for any one-to-one association with either biology (sex) or societal factors (gender). In Western societies in particular, traditional binaries of sex and gender – for example, distinct male and female bodies, and distinct male and female social experiences in work and family life – persist. They have even become hyper-accentuated, but also exist alongside fluidity and diversity, especially among younger people. For example, consumption patterns, which were traditionally very highly gendered such as smoking (male) and dieting (female), have increasingly become 'opened up' to both men and women. This is not to say that men and women are now equal (though that may be the case for some, in some domains of life), but rather that far more complex patterns of equality and inequality are apparent (Annandale 2009). This highlights the need for both large-scale survey research and qualitative studies that approach women and men as creative agents in time and place, who act on and shape the world around them (Popay and Groves 2000).

What to learn from this research?

The examples we have given stress the need to unpack the sex/gender distinction and relocate the gender category more systematically in its social context, including structural, cultural and action dimensions and to examine how they intersect. They draw attention to the importance of capturing the different analytical dimensions of gender and how their connectedness plays out differently in the various fields of health research. In summary, we can conclude that:

- Gender inequality may result from essentialist assumptions about existing differences not based on empirical evidence or may overemphasize difference. They may similarly overemphasize either biological/sex or social/gender dimensions of health. Classic examples of this are studies that fail to include both men and women when this is necessary and/ or oversimplify what are in effect complex intersections of sex and gender in relation to health and health care.
- Gender inequality may be produced by 'gender neutral' research designs that ignore the different biological and socially constructed needs of men and women and specific vulnerable groups. One example of this is that clinical trials, until very recently, have focused on men. RCTs have shown that some standard diagnostic processes and treatments such as medication for coronary heart disease (CHD) have been found to be less effective in women when compared to men.

It is therefore important that researchers automatically assume neither gender differences nor gender neutrality. Instead, they need to design research and devise data collection methods that avoid potentially biased assumptions about both men and women. In this chapter we have stressed the need for gender-inclusive and comparative approaches in order to make any problematic bias visible (for more on general comparative research, see Chapter 21 in this book).

Assessing the impact of new health policies in the area of coronary heart disease care through the lens of gender

Health policy assessment through the lens of gender is closely linked to the politics of mainstreaming and the toolset provided by the new management and governance of performance. At the same time, gender sensitivity has been very poor when it comes to health reform and policy making. Hence, there is an urgent need for more careful assessment, monitoring and evaluation of health policies that may inform future policy making so that it does not obscure gender difference (Kuhlmann and Annandale 2012b).

This case study uses empirical material from an expert report by one of the authors on mainstreaming a gender perspective into programmes for chronic illness in Germany, focusing on so-called Disease Management Programmes (DMPs) for

CASE STUDY

(Continued)

(Continued)

CHD (funded by the Federal Ministry for Family, Elderly, Women and Youth; Kuhlmann 2004). DMPs were first introduced in 2002, but fully came into force in 2006; they marked a radical change in health policy with the state taking a more interventionist role. DMPs seek to improve the standardization of care for certain chronic illnesses, the coordination of services and collaboration between general practitioners (Hausärzte) and specialist doctors. It is furthermore important to know that gender mainstreaming policies were introduced in 2000 as a legal obligation in the public sector, complementing existing equal opportunity policies (for further details, see Kuhlmann and Annandale 2012b).

The research design comprised three main steps and combined secondary and primary sources and qualitative and quantitative methods, vis-à-vis:

- A scoping review of the international literature and available German data.

- Document analysis and additional expert interviews and written statements from key stakeholders.

- Secondary analysis of material from qualitative and quantitative research comprising data on attitudes towards gender-sensitive CHD care in groups of doctors and information drawn from an expert workshop with key stakeholders and policy entrepreneurs.

Step 1 assessed whether gender differences in CHD and CHD care exist and whether these need to be considered when developing new programmes and policies. The analysis was primarily descriptive and based on secondary sources focusing on gender differences. International evidence was complemented with analysis of German data disaggregated for sex, including epidemiological data, and published reports and statistical data on diagnoses and drug treatments. The findings showed that significant gender differences exist in Germany similar to those in other countries that cannot be explained by biological differences such as age differences between women and men. The German data broadly mirrored international trends, revealing wide variations in the treatment of women and men with CHD. Women were less seldom treated in accordance with evidence-based medicine and were less likely than men to receive the entire range of diagnostic and surgical procedures. Thus, existing data clearly highlighted the need for policy interventions to improve the quality of CHD care for women to ensure equity in health care.

Step 2 assessed whether and, if so, how a gender-sensitive approach was included in new programmes for CHD care. Here, a more analytical and exploratory approach was adapted combining secondary and primary sources. Document analysis of new health policies and legal statements made it clear that the DMP for CHD used a gender-neutral approach and fundamentally failed to take into account existing evidence on how gender can matter. Additional qualitative data were gathered in order to expand the analysis beyond policy documents and to include a broader range of stakeholders from top-level management. These included representatives of sickness funds and medical associations of generalists and specialists involved in CHD care; patient representatives and scientists; and feminist activists

(24 written statements and additional expert information and interviews). Here, the research objective moved towards an exploratory approach and beyond assumptions of gender differences. The analysis brought possible alliances with more gender-sensitive stakeholders and opportunities for the inclusion of gender in the DMPs into perspective. This was further explored in Step 3.

Finally, Step 3 explored more subtle barriers that cannot be captured by looking at policy documents and legal requirements for gender equality and how such barriers could be reduced. Here, the approach was exploratory using mixed methods and a more experimental design. A survey with doctors (n = 3,200) provided data on their attitudes. The analysis revealed positive attitudes and knowledge of gender differences on CHD and CHD care in approximately half of those surveyed. A workshop (comprising the same stakeholders referred to in Step 2) made it possible to explore further the reasons for either positive or negative attitudes towards gender issues. Interestingly, there was a wide call among respondents for better data and information on what 'gender' actually means when applied to CHD care. Obviously, there were supportive actors in nearly all institutions, even if gender issues did not play any significant role in the institutions or associations.

In summary, this illustrative case study highlights how various different types of research types, research methods and data sources can be combined creatively in order to assess new models of care, even under conditions that are common for consultancy or expert reports, namely a low budget and an expectation of fast delivery of results in order to have a chance of impacting on the policy process. Linking the analysis of gender differences with an exploration of how gender matters helped to bring opportunities for mainstreaming gender issues into policy and practice into view and also revealed barriers. Alongside ignorance of gender issues, respondents often also demonstrated a lack of knowledge of what gender actually means and how it can be researched and 'measured'. This establishes the crucial relevance of effective systems of knowledge transfer from research into practice and policy.

Conclusion

This chapter has highlighted the need for gender-sensitive approaches in health research. We have discussed the methodological challenges of gender research and raised the concern that simplistic binary notions of sex and gender difference are difficult to get away from. They are easily fixed in the research and practice imagination and lend themselves to naive and potentially risky associations between certain health conditions, attitudes, beliefs and behaviours, and being either a man or a woman.

Although there is no easy answer and specific method or 'standard approach' as to how to get gender-sensitive health research right, there are a number of helpful tools and guidelines. We have suggested, first, that the meanings of sex and gender (biological and social conditions) and the connections between them – as well as intersections with other dimensions of potential social inequality – need to be subject to ongoing reflection so that sterile and ineffective conceptions do not get fixed in research design. Second, it is important that research designs and methods, where appropriate, should be gender-inclusive and comparative in order to dismantle gender stereotypes and bias in research. Third, we have illustrated how new health policies may be assessed through the lens of gender, combining secondary and primary data effectively.

Exercise: Evaluate health care services for coronary heart disease through the lens of gender

Carry out a literature review or scoping review (see Chapter 3 of this book) and explore whether the data point towards relevant social inequalities in relation to health outcomes, and, if so, (how) does gender matter?

What are the key intersecting dimensions of social inequalities, for example between age and gender, ethnicity/culture and gender?

What are the explanations for your findings? Discuss theoretical approaches and empirical data for potential explanations, including macro and micro level influences (institutional and actor-centred approaches) and quantitative and qualitative studies.

Reflect especially on sex and gender dimensions and how they might intersect:

- Is your research descriptive and focused on 'sex' differences, or explorative and concerned with revealing 'gendered' dimensions of health care?
- Do the data focus on women, on men or on both?
- Does the research take an integrated and gender-comparative approach?

Are there any data that point towards gender bias in relation to health service provision, the organization of care and health policies?

Are there any data that point towards relevant gender differences in the attitudes of both providers and users, such as, for example, gendered preferences and behaviour in relation to help-seeking?

Are there any systematic health policy interventions targeted at improving gender-sensitive health research and health outcomes?

On the basis of your findings, what are the policy recommendations for improving gender-sensitive health care for citizens, including recommendations for further research and methodological investigation?

Recommended Further Reading

Kuhlmann, E. and Annandale, E. (eds) (2012) *The Palgrave Handbook of Gender and Healthcare*, 2nd edition. Basingstoke: Palgrave.

This authoritative book addresses the main issues and core debates related to gender and healthcare in one accessible volume, including in research in this area.

WHO (2011) *Human Rights and Gender Equality in Health Sector Strategies: How to Assess Policy Coherence.* Geneva: World Health Organization.
This publication aims to provide a tool to increase policy coherence in relation to human rights and gender equality.

The following are useful websites on gender and health:
Gendered Innovations in Science, Health and Medicine, and Engineering. Available at: www.genderedinnovations.eu (accessed 20 February 2012).
Gender Summit (2011) *Manifesto for Integrated Action on the Gender Dimension in Research and Innovation.* Available at: www.gender-summit.eu (accessed 20 February 2012).

Online Readings

Annandale, E. and Hammarström, A. (2011) 'Constructing the "gender-specific body": A critical discourse analysis of publications in the field of gender-specific medicine', *Health*, 15 (6): 571–587.
According to the authors, what problems arise when taking a 'gender-specific' approach to the study of the health of men and women?

Kuhlmann, E. and Annandale, E. (2012) 'Mainstreaming gender into healthcare: A scoping exercise into policy transfer in England and Germany', *Current Sociology*, 60 (4): 551–568.
According to the authors, how are gender equality and gender mainstreaming policy translated into health policy and, in turn, implemented in European healthcare systems? How does this impact in the provision of healthcare for women and men?

References

Abdool, S.N., García-Moreno, C. and Amin, A. (2012) 'Gender equality and international health policy planning', in E. Kuhlmann and E. Annandale (eds), *The Palgrave Handbook of Gender and Healthcare*, 2nd edition. Basingstoke: Palgrave.

Annandale, E. (2009) *Women's Health and Social Change.* London: Routledge.

Annandale, E. and Hammarström, A. (2011) 'Constructing the "gender-specific body": a critical discourse analysis of publications in the field of gender-specific medicine', *Health: An Interdisciplinary Journal for the Study of Health, Illness and Medicine*, 15(6): 577–93.

Annandale, E. and Hunt, K. (2000) 'Gender inequalities in health: research at the cross-roads', in E. Annandale and K. Hunt (eds), *Gender Inequalities in Health*. Buckingham: Open University Press.

Annandale, E. and Kuhlmann, E. (2012) 'Gender and healthcare: the future', in E. Kuhlmann and E. Annandale (eds), *The Palgrave Handbook of Gender and Healthcare*, 2nd edition. Basingstoke: Palgrave.

Annandale, E. and Riska, E. (2009) 'New connections: towards a gender-inclusive approach to women's and men's health', *Current Sociology*, Special Issue, 7(2): 123–33.

Bird, C.E., Lang, M.E. and Rieker, P.P. (2012) 'Changing gendered patterns of morbidity and mortality', in E. Kuhlmann and E. Annandale (eds), *The Palgrave Handbook of Gender and Healthcare*. Basingstoke: Palgrave.

Bourgeault, I., Dingwall, R. and De Vries, R. (eds) (2010) *The Sage Handbook of Qualitative Methods in Health Research*. London: Sage.

Broom, A. and Tovey, P. (2009) 'Introduction: men's health in context', in A. Broom and P. Tovey (eds), *Men's Health: Body, Identity and Social Context*. Chichester: Wiley-Blackwell.

Epstein, S. (2007) *Inclusion: The Politics of Difference in Medical Research*. London: Chicago University Press.

Fausto-Sterling, A. (2003) 'The problem with sex/gender and nature/nurture', in S. Williams, L. Birke and G. Bendelow (eds), *Debating Biology*. London: Routledge.

Haraway, D.J. (1988) 'Situated knowledge: the science question in feminism and the privilege of a partial perspective', *Feminist Studies*, 14(2): 583–90.

Harding, S. (1986) *The Science Question in Feminism*. New York: Cornell University Press.

Hunt, K., Adams, J. and Galdas, P. (2012) 'Gender and help-seeking: towards gender-comparative studies', in E. Kuhlmann and E. Annandale (eds), *The Palgrave Handbook of Gender and Healthcare*, 2nd edition. Basingstoke: Palgrave.

Kempner, J. (2006) 'Gendering the migraine market: do representations of illness matter?', *Social Science and Medicine*, 63: 1986–97.

Krieger, N. and Davey Smith, G. (2004) '"Bodies count" and body counts: social epidemiology and embodying inequality', *Epidemiological Reviews*, 26(1): 92–103.

Kuhlmann, E. (2004) *Gender Mainstreaming in den Disease Management-Programmen – das Beispiel Koronare Herzkrankheiten*. Expert Report for the Federal Coordination Women's Health (BKF/AKF). Bremen.

Kuhlmann, E. and Annandale, E. (2012a) 'Bringing gender to the heart of health policy, practice and research', in E. Kuhlmann and E. Annandale (eds), *The Palgrave Handbook of Gender and Healthcare*, 2nd edition. Basingstoke: Palgrave.

Kuhlmann, E. and Annandale, E. (2012b) 'Mainstreaming gender into healthcare: a scoping exercise into policy transfer in England and Germany', *Current Sociology*, 60(4), Special Issue, 551–68.

Kuhlmann, E. and Babitsch, B. (2002) 'Bodies, health, gender: bridging feminist theories and women's health', *Women's Studies International Forum*, 25(4): 433–42.

Lagro-Janssen, T. (2012) 'Sex, gender and health: developments in medical research', in E. Kuhlmann and E. Annandale (eds), *The Palgrave Handbook of Gender and Healthcare*, 2nd edition. Basingstoke: Palgrave.

Lin, V. and L'Orange, H. (2012) 'Gender-sensitive indicators for healthcare', in E. Kuhlmann and E. Annandale (eds), *The Palgrave Handbook of Gender and Healthcare*, 2nd edition. Basingstoke: Palgrave.

Macintyre, S., McKay, L. and Ellaway, A. (2005) 'Who is more likely to experience common disorders: men, women, or both equally? Lay perceptions in the west of Scotland', *International Journal of Epidemiology*, 43: 461–6.

Oakley, A. (2005a) 'Paradigm wars: some thoughts on a personal and public trajectory', in A. Oakley (ed.), *The Ann Oakley Reader*. Bristol: Policy Press.

Oakley, A. (2005b) 'Who's afraid of the randomized controlled trial? Some dilemmas of the scientific method and "good" research practice', in A. Oakley (ed.), *The Ann Oakley Reader*. Bristol: Policy Press.

Popay, J. and Groves, K. (2000) '"Narrative" in research on gender and inequalities in health', in E. Annandale and K. Hunt (eds), *Gender Inequalities in Health*. Buckingham: Open University Press.

Riska, E. (2010) 'Gender and medicalization theories', in A. Clarke, L. Mamo, R.J. Fosket, J.R. Fishman and J.K. Shim (eds), *Biomedicalization: Technoscience, Health and Illness in the US*. London: Duke University Press.

Riska, E. and Heikell, T. (2007) 'Gender and images of heart disease in Scandinavian drug advertising', *Scandinavian Journal of Public Health*, 35: 585–90.

Roy, K. and Chaudhuri, A. (2012) 'Gender differences in healthcare utilization in later life', in E. Kuhlmann and E. Annandale (eds), *The Palgrave Handbook of Gender and Healthcare*, 2nd edition. Basingstoke: Palgrave.

Saltonstall, R. (1993) 'Healthy bodies, social bodies: men's and women's concepts and practices of health in everyday life', *Social Science and Medicine*, 36(1): 7–14.

Sen, G., Östlin, P. and George, A. (2007) *Unequal, Unfair, Ineffective and Inefficient. Gender Inequality and Health Care: Why It Exists and How We Can Change It*. Final report to the WHO Commission on Social Determinants of Health, Karolinska Institute. Available at: www.eurohealth.ie/pdf/WGEKN_FINAL_REPORT.pdf

Springer, K.W., Hankivsky, O. and Bates, L.M. (2012) 'Gender and health: relational, inter-sectoral and biosocial approaches', *Social Science and Medicine*, 74(11): 1661–6.

West, C. and Zimmerman, D. (1987) 'Doing gender', *Gender and Society*, 1(2): 125–51.

World Health Organization (WHO) (2002) *Integrating Gender Perspectives in the Work of WHO*. Geneva: WHO.

World Health Organization (WHO) (2011) *Human Rights and Gender Equality in Health Sector Strategies: How to Assess Policy Coherence*. Geneva: WHO.

19

Public Health Research

STEPHEN GILLAM, PENNY CAVENAGH AND PETER BRADLEY

Introduction

- This chapter focuses on research design and methodology in the field of public health. Public health is classically defined by Winslow (1920) in terms of 'preventing disease, prolonging life and promoting health' through organized efforts and informed choices made by society, public and private bodies and communities which in large part mirrors more contemporary definitions (for example, Acheson 1988). It is a field which includes a wide range of research questions from the investigation of the impact on health of food-borne outbreaks of disease to the analysis of the effect of specific programmes on lifestyle choices.
- Overall, there is an emphasis in public health research on populations or groups, rather than individuals. Public health research is used to develop clear recommendations to enhance and protect population health by assessing data on population health and the causes of disease (epidemiology); collecting evidence of effective interventions; and improving knowledge of current services and gaps in service. The latter is known as health needs assessment and requires a wide variety of data sources (for the range of issues covered by public health, see Griffiths and Hunter 1999).
- Primary public health research employs generic qualitative and quantitative techniques. Consideration of health needs assessment and public health research methodology is the starting point for the chapter, which is followed by a case study of a Health Improvement Scheme and its subsequent evaluation. The case study sets the scene for exploring concepts such as social marketing and the use of focus groups, as well as how these have influenced public health research methodologies.

Central to Public Health: Epidemiology

Rational public health policy requires a sound basis in epidemiology: the study of the distribution and determinants of disease in human populations. Early studies of the geographical distribution of infectious diseases led to preventive measures being implemented through the proposing and testing of hypotheses about how epidemics start. Exactly the same principles apply today to important non-infectious diseases such as cancer and coronary heart disease (Gillam et al. 2007).

The epidemiological analysis of a disease from a population perspective is vital in order to organize and monitor effective preventive, curative and rehabilitative services. An awareness of epidemiology takes the researcher beyond questions relating to individuals such as 'What should be done for this patient now?' to challenging fundamentals such as 'Why did this person get this disease at this time?', 'Is the prevalence of the disease increasing and, if so, why?' and 'What are the causes or risk factors for this disease?' There are many accounts of how epidemiology has responded to these questions, on which the contents of this section on epidemiology as part of public health research are drawn (see, for instance, Rothman et al. 2008; Carneiro and Howard 2011).

Time, place and person

Epidemiologists seek answers to a range of questions, as outlined in Box 19.1.

Box 19.1   Key questions for epidemiology

- How does the pattern of this disease and well-being vary over time in this population?
- How do lifestyle choices or exposure to environmental hazards influence patterns of disease and well-being?
- How does the place in which the population lives affect patterns of disease and well-being?
- How do the personal characteristics of people such as gender, ethnicity, income or family networks affect patterns of disease and well-being in the population?
- What is the relative importance of genetic and environmental influences in bringing about population differences in disease or creating well-being?

In large populations, genetic make-up as a factor in causing disease is relatively stable. Changes in disease frequency in large populations over short periods of time are almost wholly due to environmental factors. Conversely, in individuals as opposed to populations, genetic make-up is profoundly important in shaping risk of disease, as genetic variation between individuals is great. Disease is, of course, caused by the interaction of the genome and the environment. From a public health perspective, a decline in a disease is as worthy of investigation as a rise. International differences in disease patterns mainly, though not wholly, reflect the fact that populations are at different stages in their demographic and epidemiological transitions. International variations are reducing as these transitions take place, just as migrant populations' disease patterns converge towards those of the populations they join (Mathers and Loncar 2005).

Epidemiological variables: some definitions

Disease patterns are influenced by the interaction of factors (or variables) at social, environmental and individual levels. Consideration of these factors aids the depiction, analysis and interpretation of differences in disease patterns within and between populations. Age, sex, economic status, social class, occupation, country of residence or birth, and racial or ethnic classifications may be used to show variations in health status. Most variables used in epidemiology are likely to be markers for complex, underlying phenomena that cannot be measured so easily.

What qualities should an exposure variable have to make it worth pursuing in epidemiology? These are outlined in Box 19.2 below.

Box 19.2   Qualities of a good epidemiological variable

A good epidemiological variable should:

- Have an impact on health in individuals and populations.
- Differentiate populations in their experience of disease and health.
- Differentiate populations in terms of underlying characteristics relevant to health, for example income or behaviour.
- Be measurable and generate testable aetiological hypotheses.
- Help to develop health policy, plan and deliver health care, and prevent and control disease.

Measures of frequency

One essential component of epidemiological measures is measuring frequency. It is a count of the number of cases of a disease occurring in a population. This can be a measure of disease frequency, the frequency of a lifestyle choice, or the frequency of exposure to a given risk factor to health, such as pollution. For the sake of brevity, in this chapter we will limit the following description to those of disease frequency and/or lifestyle choice. However, the number of cases or the proportion of people adopting a lifestyle choice alone is not particularly informative. Account must also be taken of the size of the population and usually the length of time over which it, or its members, are observed. This gives rise to a comparison between the number of cases in the population and the size of the population, often expressed as a 'rate'. The numerator of a rate is the number of 'cases'. Specifically defining a case can be difficult and requires a great deal of care. For example, some disease descriptions, such as for rabies, are clear-cut; others, such as hypertension or safe alcohol consumption, show a spectrum of severity. Arbitrary criteria must be imposed to distinguish people with a disease from the non-diseased. The limits of 'normality' may be defined in different ways, such as by statistical criteria or clinical importance. The denominator of a rate is the 'population at risk' and this too must be carefully defined. However, the following definitions are then derived:

Prevalence is a measure of the burden of disease or lifestyle choice in a population. It is the number of cases of disease in a population at a given time.

$$\text{Prevalence} = \frac{\text{Number of diseased persons or number of persons adopting a lifestyle habit in a defined population at one point in time}}{\text{Number of persons in the defined population at the same moment in time}}$$

Prevalence is a proportion and, unlike the measures of incidence discussed below, does not involve time. Prevalence is a measure that is frequently used in planning the allocation of resources to improve public health. In research into the aetiology of disease, measures of disease incidence are of primary interest.

Incidence refers to the new cases of a disease, lifestyle behaviour or exposure to a risk factor that occur in a defined period of time, or that occurred first during that time.

Risk is defined as the number of cases of a disease or lifestyle choice or exposure to a risk factor that occur in a defined period of time, as a proportion of the number of people in the population at the beginning of the period. Deaths in the population may be measured in this formula rather than the number of cases.

$$\text{Risk in defined period of time} = \frac{\text{Number of persons who become diseased (or die) or adopt a lifestyle choice or are exposed to a risk factor during the period}}{\text{Number of persons in the population at the beginning of the period}}$$

For epidemiologists, the association between risk of disease and both individual and social characteristics (risk factors) is the usual starting point for causal analysis.

Incidence rate is defined as the number of cases (or deaths) occurring in a defined period of time in a defined population. In this equation, the person-time at risk is the sum of the periods of time for each individual when they are disease-free, but may develop the disease.

$$\text{Incidence rate} = \frac{\text{Number of persons who have become diseased}}{\text{Person-time at risk}}$$

In the example in Figure 19.1 below, the person-time at risk in population A is clearly smaller than that for population B – resulting in the incidence rate for A being greater than for B. Note, however, that the risk at time t (the end of the period) is the same in A and B.

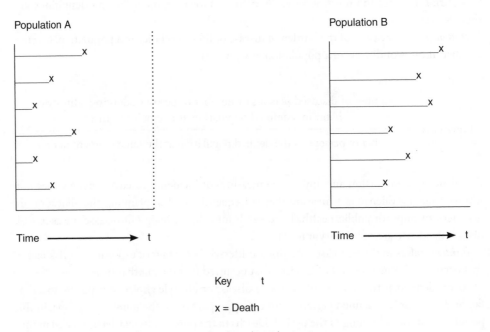

FIGURE 19.1   Depiction of person-time at risk and incident rate

Causation

Much epidemiology seeks to relate causes to the effects they produce. Epidemiological evidence by itself is rarely sufficient to establish causality, but it can provide powerful circumstantial evidence. A statistical association between two or more events or other variables may be produced in various circumstances. The presence of an association does not necessarily imply a causal relationship.

To learn more about aetiology – that is, associations between the disease and the hypothesized cause – natural experiments must be observed. Causality is more likely if the association fits the template in Box 19.3.

Box 19.3 Strengthening the case for causality

Causality is more likely, if the association can be shown to be:

- Strong.
- Dose-related.
- In the right time sequence.
- Independent of recognized confounding factors.
- Consistent between different studies.
- Plausible.
- Reversible.

The association between cigarette smoking and lung cancer provides a classic illustration of the relevance of understanding causality in the service of human health (see, for example, Doll et al. 2005).

This consideration of key concepts in epidemiology takes us neatly on to a discussion of the related area of health needs assessment, which follows.

Health Needs Assessment

Health needs are often measured in terms of demand, particularly when we are thinking of health care. However, demand is to a great extent 'supply-induced' – that is, if a service is provided, people tend to use it. For example, geographical variations in surgical intervention rates may have less to do with the health status of the populations served than with the availability of specialist services (Abel-Smith 1994).

There is no generally accepted definition of 'need'. Bradshaw (1972), however, has highlighted four types of need as set out in Box 19.4.

Box 19.4 Types of need

Types of need include:

- Expressed needs (needs expressed by action, for instance visiting a doctor).
- Normative needs (defined by experts).
- Comparative needs (comparing one group of people with another).
- Felt needs (those needs people say they have).

Source: Bradshaw (1972)

Drawing on this definition of needs and discussions of health needs assessment in the literature (see, for example, Wright 1998; East et al. 2000), this section of the chapter explores the area in more detail.

Formerly, a thorough investigation of the benefits of health interventions in clinical trials was not routinely undertaken. This situation has rapidly changed and the benefits of new health interventions are now routinely considered in randomized controlled trials (RCTs). Even now, many services on offer in health care do not have a research base to show that they actually work or are effective. This is a major concern as many treatments have known side-effects (as highlighted by Le Fanu 2011).

Public health tries to ensure that a balanced view of benefits and harms is given to decision makers, and information on the impact and cost of interventions quantified. Cost-effectiveness is an important concept and is discussed in Chapter 14. The aim of this activity is to inform decision makers so that they can prioritize within their finite budgets. The ethical conflicts raised are not easily resolved. The tension between what is best for the individual and what may be best for society will always present a dilemma for clinicians. In reality, a complex range of considerations, of which cost-effectiveness is but one, will determine both clinical and strategic decision making.

Planning

The planning cycle should originate in an assessment of needs: that is, address where we are now and where we want to get to. The rest of the cycle is mostly concerned with how to get there and is shown in Figure 19.2. Comprehensive needs assessment will generate a bewildering array of possible needs. There are many ways of identifying priorities more objectively. These often involve a form of ranking. Various criteria may be used to rank priorities, which include size of the health problem (prevalence and incidence); its severity in terms of morbidity or mortality; the availability of effective interventions; the feasibility of the work entailed; the level of group interest; and the costs and resources required. Audit and evaluation (seeing whether we have got to where we want to go) is the final stage in the cycle and therefore integrally related to needs assessment.

The aim of a health needs assessment is therefore to describe health problems in a population and detect differences within, and between, different groups in order to determine unmet need. The first step is to identify health priorities by defining the population under scrutiny and collecting and analysing routine data: that is, carrying out a comparative needs assessment. Routine data of the sort described below indicate what it is that people are dying from and why they consult general practices, hospitals and social services. This will help to prioritize topics for local discussion with a range of other local agencies and professionals. These data allow comparisons to be drawn between local services and those available in other geographical areas. It is also possible to compare these data with previously set standards.

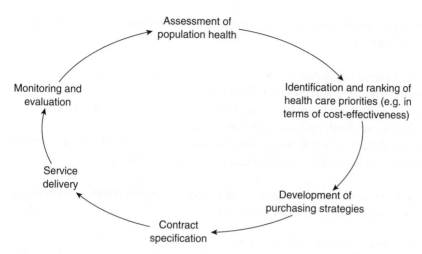

FIGURE 19.2   The planning cycle

Corporate needs assessment is a term used to describe how local priorities are agreed by involving other agencies, users and the public. Many of the techniques used, such as focus groups, are described elsewhere in this book. Finally, a more detailed epidemiological approach to assessing health needs involves three kinds of measurement, outlined in Box 19.5.

Box 19.5   Measures made on an epidemiological approach to health needs

- *The size of the problem*: how much illness or ill health there is in the community by assessing incidence and prevalence.
- *The current services that exist to meet this burden:* how local provision compares with other areas; whether services meet needs and whether they are over- or under-provided.
- *Whether services are effective*: whether new services are required to meet unmet need, what is known about what works, whether it will make a difference and how is 'effectiveness' measured?

The Health Status of the Population

This takes us on to consider the health status of the population from a public health research perspective. Imagine you are asked to describe the health status of your local population to a new minister of health with no previous background in the health field. What kinds of measures would you choose to portray the health of your community? Consider not only specific types of data, but also the qualities of the data you would seek out. The health status data required need to:

- Describe both health and disease.
- Include qualitative and quantitative measures.
- Be both self-reported (subjective) and measured (objectively verified).
- Include actual death rates and anticipated disease trends.
- Include details of health service structure (such as number of doctors), processes (for example, admission rates) and outcomes (for instance, death).

Various representations of health status can be used to compare one population with another. Some of these are given below in Table 19.1.

TABLE 19.1   Representations of health status

Indices	Definitions
Life expectancy	Year of life in a population expected on basis of current mortality rates ÷ population
Maternal mortality rate	Deaths from puerperal causes during pregnancy or within 42 days ÷ live births
Stillbirth rate	Stillbirths per 1,000 total births
Perinatal mortality rate	Stillbirths + 1st week deaths ÷ total births
Infant mortality rate	Deaths at <1 year ÷ live births
Birth rate	Live births ÷ population
Fertility rate	Live births ÷ women 15–44 years
Abortion rate	Number of abortions ÷ women 15–44 years
Consultation rate	Number of consultations ÷ registered population
Hospitalization rate	Discharges and deaths ÷ population

Specialists in public health must identify those areas where work will produce results beneficial to the health of the population. The concept of need is important here and has been described above. The 'perceived' need of the population by a lay person may be very different from need as identified by a planner. Numerous measures of mortality and morbidity are used to assess the health needs of a community and the priorities that must be addressed.

Measuring mortality

One of the most commonly used epidemiological measurements, because of the widespread availability of data, is the incidence of death. For comparative purposes, it is usual to express the number of deaths as a rate:

The *crude death rate* is the average number of deaths in a given population, usually expressed per thousand population (for example, 10.6/1,000 for all causes in England and Wales in 2009). Differences in the age structure of populations affect crude rates and for most epidemiological purposes it is usual for them to be refined. One way is to compare *age and sex-specific death rates*. In order to have a single summary figure which allows for different age or sex distributions, *standardized death rates* are used. These make use of a standard (or *reference*) population (for instance, the population of England and Wales in 2001).

The *standardized mortality ratio* (SMR) is the ratio of deaths observed in the study population to the number of deaths that would have occurred if it had the age- and sex-specific death rates of the reference population, multiplied by 100. This is used to compare populations differentiated by such factors as geographical region, time and social class.

Measures of morbidity

Morbidity is defined as any departure, subjective or objective, from a state of physiological or psychological well-being. Morbidity statistics cover, for example:

- Infectious diseases.
- Hospital data.
- General practitioner data.
- Cancer registries.
- Congenital malformations.
- Abortions.
- Population surveys.

Sources of data in the UK will include those from the main constituent countries of England, Wales and Scotland (forming Great Britain) with Northern Ireland. The Office for National Statistics (ONS) covers England and Wales, with separate organizations for Scotland and Northern Ireland. Data sets are available at the health and social care section of the ONS website (www.ons.gov.uk/ons/taxonomy/index.html?nscl=Health+and+Social+Care).

Research Questions and Research Design in Public Health Research

Research questions should determine the choice of research methodology and study design, not least in relation to health status. For example, a public health specialist may want to find out whether current services are meeting local health needs for people with epilepsy.

As highlighted in this book, there are a range of common research methods – ranging from experiments using the RCT to economic analysis – each of which is best suited to answer a particular type of research question. This is particularly true for public health research where, depending on the research question and accessibility to populations, some problems are best addressed by quantitative techniques such as closed questionnaires and the collection of numeric data. Two methods used recently in health promotion are experimental methods to test for the efficacy of a programme and social marketing which places greater emphasis on qualitative methods and consultation with users.

Experimental methods, including RCTs, have been used to test the efficacy of different techniques to encourage behaviour that promotes the common good by 'nudging' people or by consulting with them. 'Nudge' techniques are about framing choices. They include giving cues and signals, introducing small incentives, exerting peer pressure, providing information and/or consulting in different ways. RCTs have been used to test which interventions are most effective. An account of these experiments including the public can be found in John et al. (2011). The approach is an interesting one as it provides an example of a way of comparing and testing small scale, local level interventions in public policy using a rigorous method.

The public health researcher may also draw on qualitative methods (Ulin et al. 2005), as well as more quantitative methods classically used in medicine and the biological sciences (see Laake et al. 2007 and Chapter 1 of this book). Qualitative methods explore more subjective areas of the patient experience, such as perceptions and motivation. These involve the collation of non-numeric material such as certain types of interview data (for example, Henwood and Pidgeon 1995) and data generated through focus groups (for instance, Bloor et al. 2001) which allow for more personal reflection and opinion to emerge. Both quantitative and qualitative methods may be used in social marketing.

Social marketing is a concept taken from commercial market research where a company work with consumers to identify their needs and preferences. It has been introduced into the public services to support behaviour changes for the social good and, in doing so, provides an alternative to top down directives and regulation. Social marketing draws on theories, concepts and models from psychology, sociology, ethnography and behavioural economics. It is also based on communication and behavioural theory, theories of motivational change and social cognitive theories. While the concept of social marketing has been in existence for some decades, the techniques have only been employed in public health for the last twenty years (Grier and Bryant 2005). It has moved health promotion from simply providing information to using other methods such as focus groups and group interviews to engage with groups and communities, identify incentives and tailor interventions in ways that lead to behaviour changes that are sustainable (Department of Health 2004).

Social marketing has been described as 'the art and science of promoting planned, targeted, social change' (Lowry et al. 2004: 240). It is seen as a powerful tool that can promote innovation in services and better use of resources by focusing on mechanisms to achieve behavioural change. Successful social marketing initiatives have tackled a variety of issues including smoking cessation in pregnant women, increasing physical activity and encouraging children to make healthy food choices at school. This demonstrates how research that enables a thorough understanding of people and their circumstances can be one of the most significant and powerful components in effective health promotion. The implementation of social marketing through rigorous techniques places the health care user or consumer at the heart of decision making. It allows health professionals to work with health care users to encourage changes in behaviour that will improve health. According to Hastings and Haywood (1991:140):

> It is the consumer who ultimately guides the health promoter through problem definition and setting objectives, to segmenting the market and achieving objectives by means of the marketing mix.

Both social marketing, particularly if it offers financial incentives, and trials of techniques that 'nudge' people into good behaviour, have been criticized for being manipulative or only leading to changes in the short term. However, if we are to find out what interventions work in health promotion policy and those which do not, the experiment that seeks to separate cause from effect through the RCT should not be ruled out, provided that the ethical principles outlined in Chapter 15 are followed. Social marketing techniques too can be evaluated through research. The case study below reports on the evaluation of a social marketing project.

CASE STUDY

The Evaluation of a Health Enhancement Reward Scheme

This case study describes the public health evaluation of a Health Enhancement Reward Scheme (HERS) that was run in a county in the East of England for one year during 2009, in which two of the authors of this chapter were involved. It will focus on the selection of methods used to evaluate the extent to which the scheme was successful from the point of view of participants, health care professionals and other stakeholders.

The origins of the scheme

The scheme aimed to engage pregnant women who were current smokers in a smoking cessation programme. Smoking during pregnancy can have negative consequences. It is associated with an increased risk of complications during pregnancy and labour (Castles et al. 1999), and may result in perinatal mortality, low-birthweight babies and enduring health problems for the child (Windham et al. 2000). The scheme was initiated by the county Stop Smoking Service and ran in two small market towns. It was developed in response to an advisor's observation that midwives were too busy to offer stop smoking advice to their patients and that specialized stop smoking support was needed.

(Continued)

(Continued)

The programme aimed to identify and engage pregnant women who smoked as early as possible in their pregnancy. The objective was for women to be smoke-free when the child was delivered and to remain smoke-free post-partum. Two stop smoking advisors produced clinical guidelines for HERS following the National Institute for Health and Clinical Excellence (NICE 2010) guidelines for pregnancy. These highlighted the need to explain the risks and benefits of using nicotine replacement therapies (NRT) for both pregnant and breast-feeding women. In addition, the scheme offered education sessions in order to maximize the benefits of NRT.

The scheme was developed using principles informed by social marketing. With the support of an NHS Primary Care Trust Health Improvement Facilitator, focus groups were run that enabled the views and perspectives of potential service users to be sought and then used to further develop the scheme. Financial incentives were offered to pregnant women who were asked to provide evidence that they had stopped smoking. They were also requested to take carbon monoxide tests and were encouraged to attend education sessions on, for example, healthy eating and breast feeding. Midwives in the two market towns were asked to promote the scheme to the target group – pregnant women who smoked – in their areas. There were no formal criteria for inclusion or exclusion. Participants were told about the programme and could participate if they wished. Some women chose not to do so.

The evaluation of the scheme

Researchers at a local university were asked to carry out an evaluation of the programme and began work in the last few months of the scheme. They had not previously been involved in its design or implementation. The researchers decided to use various methods to evaluate the scheme that drew on social marketing.

The first step in the evaluation was to undertake a systematic review of other smoking cessation schemes. The researchers undertaking the review concluded that general smoking cessation interventions in pregnancy can reduce the proportion of women who continue to smoke in late pregnancy, and reduce low-birthweight and pre-term births (Lumley et al. 2009).

There was also some evidence to support the use of incentives for pregnant women who are smokers to stop smoking. Providing incentives appeared from the review to be most effective in the short term. Studies indicated that approximately 24 per cent of women gave up smoking during their pregnancy if incentives were offered. However, there was little evidence that incentives encouraged people to stop smoking in the longer term. Trials to date suggest that early success in stopping smoking can dissipate when rewards are no longer offered (Cahill and Perera 2011). The systematic review also showed that social marketing campaigns can be effective in encouraging young people not to smoke, but again there is little research on the impact of such campaigns for pregnant women (Stead et al. 2007).

The second step was to decide on a design for the evaluation. This was informed by a social constructivist methodology in which action is taken by an individual in response to their understanding of an experience. Qualitative methods were used for the evaluation, including focus groups and semi-structured interviews, to assess how women in the project understood the risks of smoking in pregnancy and what they thought were the most appropriate methods for changing behaviour. In the event, only one of the market towns recruited enough women to run a focus group, so a combination of semi-structured face-to-face and telephone interviews were primarily used.

Face-to-face interviews were also held with representatives of the five partner organizations (including local authorities, housing associations and children's centres) and stop smoking advisors. Other contributors to the scheme (for example, those who ran education sessions) were asked to complete an electronic survey that made use of open-ended questions which could then be analysed according to themes.

Seventeen women participated in the evaluation of the HERS project. This included eight pregnant women currently on an initial pilot scheme, eight graduates of the scheme and one woman who had left the scheme early. The schedule of topics used in both the focus groups and semi-structured interviews covered areas including how participants thought women could be motivated to give up smoking; how they viewed the role of midwives as stop smoking advisors in stop smoking schemes; the part played by the partner/family/children in encouraging women to stop smoking; the role of group meetings in providing support; and the effect of financial incentives.

The semi-structured format of the interviews and focus groups helped to ensure consistency and flexibility across the methods used. In order to encourage participation, the focus group took place during a scheduled stop smoking session and transport, child care and refreshments were provided. An additional incentive was the offer of a £10 voucher for attendance. The focus group meanwhile was audio-recorded and the recordings transcribed in full. Notes were also taken in interviews and typed up immediately afterwards. Additionally, two researchers ran the focus group; one led the discussion, ensuring the schedule questions were asked, while the second took notes of the proceedings.

Thematic analysis involving coding and categorizing data was undertaken, in which the codes and themes used were informed by the systematic review carried out at the start of the evaluation (for more details of this process, see Chapter 7). Following data collection, a report was written aimed at commissioners, including evidence of return on investment and recommendations should the scheme be implemented on a wider scale The evaluation suggested that the scheme had some success in terms of smoking cessation for 16 of the 17 women consulted (quitting completely; quitting during pregnancy; and cutting down during pregnancy). The social support delivered through the monthly group sessions was particularly successful and the most appreciated aspect of the scheme for the majority of women. The education component of HERS was also well received and may have a longer-term impact for the women and their families. Although the financial incentives were a key factor in terms of recruitment to the scheme, they were not a guarantee of reduction in smoking. Discussion on further development and expansion of the scheme suggested the need for a dedicated project lead in the east of the county. The evaluation report was delivered in early 2010.

Commentary

The following reflections were made on the research:

- One of the limitations of the project was that the evaluation team was not involved in the initial stages of the project and therefore was unable to influence the design. This was a contributing factor to the decision to use qualitative

(Continued)

(Continued)

methods, including focus group and semi-structured interviews. The small size of the scheme was also among the reasons that a quantitative approach was not used as part of a comprehensive evaluation strategy.

- As noted in Chapter 7, focus groups have limitations. They can be difficult to organize; they are time-consuming; and may require incentives to encourage attendance. As Reed and Payton (1997) note, the role of the facilitator is critical in managing the group so that it is not dominated by a single person. Yet the facilitators may themselves lead the discussion in such a way as to bias a group's conclusions. External validity may also be enhanced by integrating data from focus groups with data using other methods (Sale et al. 2002). For this reason, in this evaluation, the focus group findings were checked against the findings using data provided, among other things, from the semi-structured interviews.
- A further limitation of the focus groups and interviews was that the participants were asked to self-report their smoking behaviour. This presents significant problems for the evaluation of the project. It is known that people tend to both under- or over-report smoking behaviour. Self-reporting therefore may be unreliable. A preferable approach may have also been to use objective data, such as blood carbon monoxide levels.

More broadly, an experimental design could have been considered for this project with one group receiving the intervention – the participants of the HERS programme – and another group of pregnant women smokers receiving normal care from a midwife.

Conclusion

Researching public health questions is complex and requires methodological dexterity on the part of the researcher. Techniques such as health needs assessment are used to apply this research in practice. This requires a combination of quantitative and qualitative research methods, epidemiological data and knowledge of existing services to inform future policy. Even the best research methods give results which are open to interpretation. At best, each individual research project constantly increases and modernizes knowledge of how to achieve complex change. The evaluation of HERS gives one example of the complexities of such research in the public health arena. This said, public health research importantly complements other forms of research into health and health care. An exercise which further underwrites its significance follows.

Exercise: Public health and inequalities

It is well known to the public health department of a county council that there are significant health inequalities between two adjacent districts within the county. This is evidenced by indicators such as life expectancy rates and the prevalence of long-term conditions – for example, asthma, diabetes, chronic obstructive airways disease and levels of obesity.

You are asked to design a research study to investigate why these inequalities might exist, and suggest what could be done to address the disparity in health outcomes, and to improve these in both districts.

It is suggested that you start with a hypothesis about why these health inequalities exist and develop your design around testing this.

Questions to consider include:

1 What has informed the development of your hypothesis and where will you search for secondary data to inform your hypothesis?
2 Why is this research necessary and what contribution may it make?
3 What are your research aims and objectives?
4 Which research methodology and methods will you use and why?
5 How would you disseminate your findings – to whom and why?

Acknowledgement

Thanks are due to the following: Dr Will Thomas, University Campus Suffolk, and Dr Mirjam Southwell for The Health Enhancement Reward Scheme research funded by Suffolk NHS Primary Care Trust. Thanks are also given to Judy Rainer from Suffolk County Council for her advice on social marketing and Dr Amanda Burls for her work on the Critical Appraisal Skills Programme, on whose activity the quantitative research methods section is based.

Recommended Further Reading

Gillam, S., Yates, J., and Badrinath, P. (eds) (2007) *Essential Public Health: Theory and Practice*. Cambridge: Cambridge University Press.
This book gives a lucid overview of critical perspectives and tools to aid both understanding and action in public health.

Laake, P., Benestad, H.B. and Olsen, B.R. (2007) *Research Methodology in the Medical and Biological Sciences*. Amsterdam: Elsevier-AP.
This text covers a range of scientific methodologies and methods that may be drawn upon in public health research.

Ulin, P.R., Robinson, E.T. and Toller, E.E. (2005) *Qualitative Methods in Public Health: A Field Guide for Applied Research*. San Fransisco, CA: Jossey-Bass.
This clearly presented and jargon-free book is a key guide for students in applying qualitative methods in public health research.

Online Readings

Figueira, H., Figueira, A., Cader, S., Guimarães, A., Oliveira, R., Figueira, J., Figueira, O., and Dantas, E. (2012) 'Effects of a physical activity governmental health programme on the quality of life of elderly people', *Scandinavian Journal of Public Health*, 40: 418–22.
How is public health defined in this context? What epidemiological factors is this research attempting to cover?

Fagan, D., Kiger, A. and Teijlingen, E. (2012) 'Faith communities and their assets for health promotion: The views from health professionals and faith leaders in Dundee, in Scotland', *Global Health Promotion*, 19: 27–36.
How is public health defined in this context? What epidemiological factors is this research striving to account for?

References

Abel-Smith, B. (1994) *An Introduction to Health, Policy, Planning and Financing*. Englewood Cliffs, NJ: Prentice Hall.

Acheson, D. (1988) *Public Health in England*. London: HMSO.

Bloor, M., Frankland, J., Thomas, M. and Robson, K. (2001) *Focus Groups in Social Research*. London: Sage.

Bradshaw, J. (1972) 'A taxonomy of social need', in G. McLachlan (ed.), *Problems and Progress in Medical Care: Essays on Current Research*. London: Oxford University Press.

Cahill, K. and Perera, R. (2011) 'Competitions and incentives for smoking cessation'. Editorial Group: Cochrane Tobacco Addiction Group. Chichester: Wiley & Sons.

Carneiro, I. and Howard, N. (2011) *Introduction to Epidemiology*, 2nd edition. Maidenhead: Open University Press.

Castles, A., Adams, E.K., Melvin, C.L., Kelsch, C. and Boulton, M.L. (1999) 'Effects of smoking during pregnancy: five meta-analyses', *American Journal of Preventive Medicine*, 16(3): 208–15.

Department of Health (2004) *Choosing Health: Making Healthy Choices Easier*. London: Department of Health.

Doll, R., Peto, R., Boreham, J. and Sutherland, I. (2005) 'Mortality from cancer in relation to smoking: 50 years' observations on British doctors', *British Journal of Cancer*, 92: 426–9.

East, L., Hammersley, V. and Hancock, B. (2000) 'Health needs assessment', in M. Saks, M. Williams and B. Hancock (eds), *Developing Research in Primary Care*. Oxford: Radcliffe Medical.

Gillam, S., Yates, J. and Badrinath, P. (eds) (2007) *Essential Public Health: Theory and Practice*. Cambridge: Cambridge University Press.

Grier, S. and Bryant, C.A. (2005) 'Social marketing in public health', *Annual Review of Public Health*, 26: 319–39.

Griffiths, S. and Hunter, D. (1999) *Perspectives in Public Health*. Oxford: Radcliffe Medical.

Hastings, G. and Haywood, A. (1991) 'Social marketing and communication in health promotion', *Health Promotion International*, 6(2): 135–45.

Henwood, K.L. and Pidgeon, N.F. (1995) 'Grounded theory and psychological research', *The Psychologist*, 8: 115–18.

John, P., Cotterill, S., Moseley, A., Richardson, L., Smith, G., Stoker, G. and Wales, C. (2011) *Nudge, Nudge, Think, Think. Experimenting with Ways to Change Civic Behaviour*. London: Bloomsbury Academic Publishing.

Laake, P., Benestad, H.B. and Olsen, B.R. (2007) *Research Methodology in the Medical and Biological Sciences*. Amsterdam: Elsevier-AP.

Le Fanu, J. (2011) *The Rise and Fall of Modern Medicine*, 2nd edition. London: Abacus.

Lowry, R.J., Hardy, S., Jordan, C. and Wayman, G. (2004) 'Using social marketing to increase recruitment of pregnant smokers to smoking cessation service: a success story', *Journal of the Royal Institute of Public Health*, 118: 239–43.

Lumley, J., Chamberlain, C., Dowswell, T., Oliver, S., Oakley, L. and Watson, L. (2009) 'Interventions for promoting smoking cessation during pregnancy'. Editorial Group: Cochrane Pregnancy and Childbirth Group. Chichester: Wiley & Sons.

Mathers, C.D. and Loncar, D. (2005) *Updated Projections of Global Mortality and Burden of Disease, 2002–2030: Data Sources, Methods and Results*. Geneva: World Health Organization.

NICE (2010) *Public Health Guidance PH26: Quitting Smoking in Pregnancy and Following Childbirth*, June 2010. Available at: http://guidance.nice.org.ukPH26/Guidance/pdf/English

Reed, J. and Payton, V. R. (1997) 'Focus groups: issues of analysis and interpretation', *Journal of Advanced Nursing*, 26: 765–71.

Rothman, K.J., Greenland, S. and Lash, T.L. (eds) (2008) *Modern Epidemiology*, 3rd edition. Philadelphia, PA: Lippincott, Williams and Wilkins.

Sale, J.E.M., Lohfeld, L.H. and Brazil, K. (2002) 'Revisiting the quantitative-qualitative debate: implications for mixed-methods research', *Quality and Quantity*, 36: 43–53.

Stead, M., McDermott, L., Hastings, G., Lawther, S. and Angus, K. (2007) 'Research to inform the development of a social marketing strategy for health improvement in Scotland'. Edinburgh: NHS Health Scotland. Available at: www.healthscotland.com/uploads/documents/3915-SMHI_FINAL_REPORT_19JAN07.pdf

Ulin, P.R., Robinson, E.T. and Toller, E.E. (2005) *Qualitative Methods in Public Health: A Field Guide for Applied Research*. San Fransisco, CA: Jossey-Bass.

Windham, G.C., Hopkins, B., Fenster, L. and Swan, S.H. (2000) 'Prenatal active or passive tobacco smoke exposure and the risk of preterm delivery or low birth weight', *Epidemiology*, 11: 427–33.

Winslow, C.A. (1920) 'The untilled fields of public health', *Science*, 51: 23–33.

Wright, J. (ed.) (1998) *Health Needs Assessment in Practice*. London: BMJ Books.

20

Involving the User
in Health Research

SOPHIE HILL

Introduction

- Users of health services not only produce their health but, increasingly, help to produce health knowledge through participation in health research. At face value, this represents a fundamental shift in social power. Is it a real phenomenon or is lip service being paid to participation by patients and the public in health research? It may not be possible to answer this question conclusively but I address it by exploring some key terms and the nature, features, advantages and disadvantages of user involvement in research. I draw on documents, mainly from the UK and Australia, concerned with promoting participation.

- The involvement of users in health research represents the intersection of two phenomena – on the one hand, the emergence of health social movements (Brown and Zavestoski 2004) and, on the other, the development of theories, methods and knowledge in the clinical sciences. In this chapter, I first outline how this intersection is played out in ways that often defy easy description, categorization or analysis. The task is made more difficult by the developmental, voluntary and political nature of community participation, which in many instances is not well documented or researched.

- Second, I assess the effect or impact of participation by outlining potential advantages and disadvantages from different perspectives. In the course of the chapter, I will present the views and experiences of members of the Consumer Network who have been involved in research in The Cochrane Collaboration, an international health research organization. This allows me to illustrate the ways in which participation in research is happening in practice and to document some of the major barriers to participation. Individuals may have an illness that affects their ability to attend meetings; they may lack the knowledge and skills to represent the lay view; and there are likely to be language differences between experts and lay people, as well as a lack of the financial resources to take part in activities. I will also explore how these barriers may be overcome.

Research Issues: Definitions and Categorizations

From patient to health consumer to health care user

In recent decades across a number of countries, many health advocacy or patients' groups have not only raised awareness of problems with the quality and delivery of health services and health policies, but also turned their attention to conduct and priorities in health and medical research. This shift in critical stance reflects a desire to influence health care, but also demonstrates an increasingly sophisticated understanding of science and its methods by groups representing health care users (see, for instance, Coulter 2011).

This shift is evident in language. In recent decades, many terms have been used to refer to the person at the receiving end of health care. This partly reflects the range of roles that a person can inhabit at any one time as patient, advocate, family carer, lay person, volunteer, citizen or member of the public (Hill 2011), but also ideological differences some commentators take as implicit in the terms health care consumer and health care user. The change in terms reflects the fertile political discourse and debate. The use of the term 'consumer' is contested, reflecting various political, economic and social assumptions that have changed over time (Herxheimer and Goodare 1999; Boote et al. 2002; Henderson and Petersen 2002). A further complication is that the scope of health services has broadened. There is greater attention paid to illness prevention and health promotion. This means that the recipient of services is commonly not a sick person: that is, not a patient in the traditional sense of the term. There are also differences between countries in the English-speaking world in terminology, even though similar policies for participation are being adopted.

For this chapter, I will use the terms 'health care user', which is more widely employed in the UK when considering participation in research, and 'health care consumer', a term that is commonly used in policy documents in Australia interchangeably. Both terms include patients and potential patients; people who use health, social and community services; carers, parents and guardians; people with disabilities; members of the public targeted by health promotion programmes; organizations that represent the interests of the public; communities that are affected by health, public health or social care issues; and groups asking for research because they believe they have been exposed to potentially harmful circumstances, products or services (National Health and Medical Research Council and Consumers' Health Forum of Australia 2001; INVOLVE 2007).

Participation or involvement, and by whom?

Australians use the term participation while the British literature favours involvement. The implied meaning is much the same. In the past, user involvement in research occurred through participation by patients and members of the public as subjects in research carried out by professional or clinical researchers. Typically, they gave their informed consent to being a subject in a research project, but had no part in setting up the research or contributing to the design process. Nor were they necessarily informed of the outcomes.

The emphasis has now shifted to a more 'active involvement' or 'partnership' in all stages of the research process from setting priorities to assessing outcomes (Consumers in NHS Research Support Unit 2000; Williamson 2001). The meaning of these terms reflects subtle shifts in power with health care users undertaking a range of new activities in health care settings. In the UK, INVOLVE is a national advisory group that supports greater public involvement in NHS, public health and social care research. It defines 'public involvement in research as research being carried out "with" or "by" members of the public rather than "to", "about" or "for" them' (INVOLVE 2011, their emphasis). According to an Australian joint consumer-researcher publication, this is 'where consumers and researchers work in partnership with one another to shape decisions about research priorities, policies and practices' (National Health and Medical Research Council and Consumers' Health Forum of Australia 2004a: 9). The policy implies that people have the right to be represented and have some power to shape the decisions made.

This level of involvement cannot occur without some reorganization and structuring within the health sector to harness the contribution of active and informed citizens and the expansion and diversification of health consumer groups and associated organizations in the health sector. Consumers of health care have been classified by Boote et al. (2002), as shown in Box 20.1.

Box 20.1   The classification of consumers

Classification of consumers in health research

Individuals may participate as:

- Service users and carers.
- Patient representatives.
- Patient advocates.
- Citizens.
- Members of the public who are potential users of health services.

Local groups may participate through:

- Population groups.
- Support groups.
- Groups convened to discuss health matters, such as citizens' juries.
- (Inter)national consumer organizations.
- Statutory bodies.
- Charities.
- (Inter)national support groups.

Source: Boote et al. (2002)

In what kinds of research are health care users involved?

INVOLVE in the UK uses a straightforward definition of research, describing it as 'finding out new knowledge that could lead to changes to treatments, policies or care' (INVOLVE 2012). In Australia, the National Health and Medical Research Council and Consumers' Health Forum of Australia (2004b) categorized health research into various health domains under the following headings in Box 20.2.

Box 20.2   Health research categories

- *Basic research:* research that happens in the laboratory, using test tubes and microscopes and operating at the level of cells, not people. Consumer involvement could occur at a policy level, such as reviewing the ethics of specific tests and procedures. At the level of the research body, consumers could donate specimens such as blood, sperm or ova for study.

(Continued)

(Continued)

- *Clinical research:* research that is seeking to understand the causes of, or treatments for, ill health and that may happen in the laboratory or in other health settings in contact with people. At the macro level, consumers could be involved in identifying priorities for research. Within clinical research, they could be involved in identifying important outcomes or advising on how results should be disseminated. This is the domain in which they are most commonly subjects.
- *Public health research:* research involving the study of communities or populations, which aims to identify factors that contribute to ill health and how those factors can be influenced to reduce ill health, which commonly happens outside health care settings. Consumers could be involved by helping to formulate research questions by raising questions about potential cause and effect relationships. At the other end of the spectrum, they could advise researchers and governments on how findings could be used to change practice and programmes – for instance, providing advice on the implications of social diversity.
- *Health services and health systems research:* research that aims to improve the delivery of health care, which may focus on issues of access, equity, cost and effectiveness. Consumers could review recruitment strategies, such as how to recruit people from 'hard to reach' groups, or they could participate in the development of training programmes to be used for consumer advocates for review of the quality of care.

The National Health and Medical Research Council and Consumers' Health Forum of Australia (2004b) define the stages of research as follows: deciding what to research; deciding how to do it; doing it; letting people know the results; and then deciding what to research next. Recent attention to the science of implementation adds a further phase: getting research into practice. The list emphasizes that users should be involved at all stages and that research is an ongoing, cyclical process. Furthermore, who is involved, their role and the methods used will depend on the stage and the activity.

What are the different models and methods of involvement?

Oliver et al. (2004, 2008) have developed a comprehensive framework for categorizing involvement in research. It has eight key features that explore a range of roles, functions and methods, and has wide applicability (see Paterson 2004; Nilsen et al. 2006). The framework can assist in analysing the dimensions of consumer involvement in a particular project by using a checklist that covers a number of characteristics. These are set out in Box 20.3 below.

Box 20.3   Categorizing involvement in research

- Who is involved: individuals or people representing a consumer organization?
- Who initiated the involvement: consumers or researchers?
- What was the degree of involvement: did this take the form of information giving and consultation or was there some form of power sharing through collaboration or consumer control?
- What are the forums for exchanging ideas: for example, citizens' juries, focus groups or consensus conferences?
- What are the methods used for collective decision making? As an example, this can be through developing a method for ranking research priorities.
- What are the practical arrangements for user involvement in terms of, for instance, transport, financial resources, opportunities for training and skill development?
- What is the context for agenda setting in terms of institutional type, geographical coverage or the background of participants in consumer activism?
- What particular theory underpins the strategy for consumer involvement? Is this researcher-led, consumer-led or even professionally led?

Source: Oliver et al. (2004, 2008)

The framework provides a structure for analysing consumer involvement that makes explicit reference to the power relationships and dynamic nature of participation in health research. Thus, for example, the third item above suggests a power continuum from 'consultation', a process for seeking or inviting views, through to 'collaboration', an active and ongoing relationship, to 'consumer-controlled research', where the process is led by consumers.

The National Health and Medical Research Council and Consumers' Health Forum of Australia (2004a) placed an emphasis on developing the conditions for effective consumer participation. These include developing organizational leadership and capacity; integrating participation into the structure of organizations; earmarking resources for participation; and recognizing that time is needed to change attitudes. However, while there has been some recognition by governments and research bodies of the need for consumer participation in research policy making (Department of Health 2007), grant-making bodies such as research councils, research institutes, professional bodies and universities are semi-autonomous research institutes and have not seen the need to involve a wider public in setting priorities (Dickersin and Schnaper 1996; National Health and Medical Research Council and Consumers' Health Forum of Australia 2004a).

The Challenge: What Do Advocates Hope To Achieve and Why?

There are several intertwined strands in what advocates hope to achieve through increasing user participation in health research. First, social movements that represent women, people with HIV/AIDS and indigenous people and particular health social movements have aimed to challenge medical authority and autonomy and laid the ground for extending that challenge to health and medical researchers (Dickersin and Schnaper 1996; Sepkowitz 2001; Brown and Zavestoski 2004). A more 'patient-centred health care' has been embraced by politicians for some decades.

A second and related point is that it cannot be taken for granted that health researchers understand or reflect the perspective of the people who ultimately 'consume' research knowledge, in terms of ultimate treatments and services (Entwistle et al. 1998). Indeed, users have different priorities from those who research (Tallon et al. 2000). For this reason, lay people and their representatives have asked for a 'seat at the table' where decisions on research priorities are made (Breast Cancer Network Australia; see www.bcna.org.au/speak-out). This claim to be involved has been most fully acknowledged by the James Lind Alliance based in Oxford, England. This organization has established a partnership between health professionals and patient and carer groups, to stimulate new research questions (see Elwyn et al. 2010 for research questions on asthma).

Third, it has been argued that better quality decisions will be made if users participate in research and are in a position to influence how findings are applied (O'Donnell and Entwistle 2004). Moreover, research where users take part in the formulation and conduct of the study is more likely to measure outcomes of importance to those who may be affected by the research results (Sakala et al. 2001).

Fourth, in developing an ethical framework for public involvement, supporters have argued that people have a right to influence the development of new knowledge and the procedures or processes that affect what happens to their own bodies or those of future patients (National Health and Medical Research Council and Consumers' Health Forum of Australia 2001; Williamson 2001). This argument is strengthened by the disclosure that some research has breached ethical codes and harmed those who have participated (Goodare and Smith 1995). In recent years, research malpractice, as well as large-scale system failures in health care systems, have led to closer scrutiny of research practice. The prevailing view is that researchers should be accountable for their research practice, both upwards to professional bodies and government departments and downwards to local communities and groups representing health care users (Cartwright Inquiry 1988; Bristol Inquiry 2001; National Health and Medical Research Council and Consumers' Health Forum of Australia 2001).

Finally, consumer and community groups and researchers have argued that society benefits from having a knowledgeable public, aware of research, how it is done and what findings imply. User participation is seen as a means to inform patients and consumer organizations so that findings can be disseminated to the wider community (National Health and Medical Research Council and Consumers' Health Forum of Australia 2001). This argument has been developed particularly in relation to what the public should know about research undertaken by pharmaceutical companies and the activities they undertake to promote a market for their products (Moynihan 2005).

Pharmaceutical companies themselves have a commercial interest in informing users about their products and involving them in deciding on research priorities (Oliver et al. 2004). Market opportunities are expanded if products are tailored to the needs of end-users, especially with the development of designer drugs, but the rules governing involvement should be developed to prevent special interests distorting priorities. The debate about user involvement is both dialectic and reflexive.

As well as having a 'self-interest', citizens and groups have been drawn into the policy arena to serve governmental interests in developing a more responsive health policy. In consequence, other interests – professional, commercial and institutional – have seen consumer involvement in research as a 'policy requirement' and also an advantage in achieving their own particular policy aim (O'Donnell and Entwistle 2004).

In summary, a great deal rides on user involvement in research. It may produce research that reflects the health problems of the community, conducted with the community and not on the community. This can improve health outcomes within the context of an accountable and ethical system.

The Advantages of User Involvement: What Effects and Impacts Have Been Demonstrated?

A Cochrane systematic review of trials of methods of consumer participation across a broad range of domains including research shows that little has been done to evaluate the effects of involving users in health care decisions at the population level. A review by Nilsen and colleagues summarized the available evidence up to 2009 in an update to their 2006 review (Nilsen et al. 2006). Results from randomized controlled trials illustrated the patchiness of the evidence. The review reported 'low quality evidence that using consumer interviewers instead of staff interviewers in satisfaction surveys can have a small influence on the survey results'. Furthermore, there was 'low quality evidence that an informed consent document developed with consumer input (potential trial participants) may have little if any impact on understanding compared to a consent document developed by trial investigators only'. Research techniques may change the data collected because there was 'very low quality evidence that telephone discussions and face-to-face group meetings engage consumers better than mailed surveys in order to set priorities for community health goals' and 'result in different priorities being set for these goals' (Nilsen et al. 2006).

The review of consumer involvement in the process of agenda setting for research by Oliver et al. (2004) provides some evidence on impact, although their conclusions are tentative. They suggest that the extent of influence in terms of identifying and prioritizing research topics is related to the degree of consumer participation and control. Collaborative approaches where interaction is active and ongoing appear more effective in influencing the agenda than consultation alone. To be effective, consumer involvement requires an investment of time; training for skill development for consumers and researchers; establishing effective working practices for committees; involving consumers who are well networked; and providing them with information, resources and support for consulting with their peers. Dialogue, to be constructive, must be ongoing with frequent reflection and review.

There are also certain organizational requirements (Oliver et al. 2004). The activity should be endorsed by senior staff; staff should be experienced in consultation and collaboration techniques; there should be a commitment to building ongoing and constructive relationships with communities; the knowledge and experience of consumers should be valued; and whatever representative mechanisms are put in place should recognize different groups within the communities.

Advocates working towards 'user-controlled' research have noted three reasons for this more 'radical' form of user involvement: 'to make change happen; to highlight the needs of marginalized groups; and because "No-one else will do it"' (INVOLVE 2010). This reaches directly into the issue of power to define the problems and to stimulate change.

What Are the Disadvantages of User Involvement?

The disadvantages of consumer involvement may be seen from the perspective of the various interests involved. For example, within medicine concerns have been expressed that users will be insufficiently knowledgeable; may be biased in their views; and would only 'represent' themselves and not others (Entwistle et al. 1998). Moreover, they might be simply troublesome and hinder decision making. From the perspective of research-funding bodies, given the lack of consensus and uncertainties about the benefits of the process, there have been concerns that users may dominate a project. This may occur, for example, in the context of public lobbying for new treatments in association with powerful pharmaceutical or manufacturing interests (O'Donnell and Entwistle 2004). In consequence, guides to user involvement have proliferated in recent years. INVOLVE surveyed people leading patient and public involvement initiatives, including health managers. Training and finding and involving people were the main priorities, but respondents also noted the need to avoid tokenism and the importance of researcher recognition of public involvement (INVOLVE 2011). This is not surprising, given that a team from Sheffield in England who conducted interviews with researchers have documented apprehension and uncertainty on the part of researchers about involving members of the public (Thompson et al. 2009).

From the point of view of users, a disadvantage may be token involvement. Users have identified the following problems: feeling outnumbered and isolated on committees full of professionals; not being listened to; being manipulated; and having no real opportunity to influence the research agenda, the research project itself and the research process (National Health and Medical Research Council and Consumers' Health Forum of Australia 2001). The review by Oliver et al. (2004) identified problems associated with poor-quality consumer representation, poor communication and dysfunctional relationships within committees and serious time constraints. In a review of consumer involvement in research to promote best practice in the use of medicines in Australia, Kirkpatrick et al. (2005) showed that most research projects were dominated by health professionals, despite a policy commitment to consumer involvement. The authors also highlight the importance of adequate resources and a robust infrastructure to support the development of initiatives from consumer groups.

It should also be stressed that most research has a long lead time. Oliver (1999) argues that a contribution to research is an evolutionary process. Knowledge of the user perspective is cumulative and must be created, shared and applied within a consultative framework that includes people's experiences (see www.healthtalkonline.org – a database of people's experiences of health-related conditions and illnesses). Moreover, researchers may have to understand differences in experience in terms of culture, class and age, and gender differences in terms of life experience, as well as the differing perspectives of the ill person and the carer. Undoubtedly, there is a tension between the individual experience and the way that research questions are structured and addressed (Ong and Hooper 2003; Beard 2004).

There are also inherent inequalities in access to resources between research professionals and consumers. Participation by users is commonly on a voluntary basis. Many consumer groups are resource poor. They juggle with many competing objectives and must choose their policy priorities carefully. In this context, it is not surprising that the study by Baggott et al. (2005) of health consumer groups in the UK showed an increase in active relationships between consumer groups and pharmaceutical companies.

For health consumer groups, collaboration with a pharmaceutical company may provide additional funds for projects and activities and provide access to information on recent developments, research or products. Some groups, such as those representing people with a disease where management or cure is dependent on the company's products, may have a shared agenda with pharmaceutical interests. However, the dilemma is the potential for loss of integrity and independence in a relationship where there is inequality in terms of power and wealth, and where profit is the overriding goal for companies. There have been concerns about the lack of transparency. In the UK, the Parliamentary Health Select Committee (2005) recommended that companies should disclose donations and funding to health consumer groups, and this is also endorsed in guidelines by the Association of the British Pharmaceutical Industry (2002).

For their part, peak or national organizations in the UK have developed codes of practice for their members in relation to funds received from companies (Herxheimer 2003; Baggott et al. 2005). Similarly in Australia, the Consumers' Health Forum, together with the peak body for research-based pharmaceutical companies, have produced a guide, *Working Together*, to inform consumer groups about relationships they may form with pharmaceutical companies (Consumers' Health Forum of Australia and Medicines Australia 2008). The two organizations recognize the increasing number and complexity of these relationships and provide guidance through posing a series of questions such as: Will any funding arrangement be perceived as appropriate? Have we considered the benefits and risks of the type of funding or sponsorship involved? A study of disclosure by health consumer groups and pharmaceutical companies concluded that consumer groups in the UK were not 'captured' by industry interests, but full disclosure was not apparent (Jones 2008). Greater transparency, it was argued, would improve the legitimacy of consumer groups.

CASE STUDY

The Cochrane Collaboration

Many of the advantages and disadvantages of consumer participation may be illustrated by reference to the international Cochrane Collaboration which is provided as a case study of consumers in research in practice.

The aim of The Cochrane Collaboration

Established in 1993, The Cochrane Collaboration (www.cochrane.org) is an international non-profit and independent organization set up to ensure that up-to-date, accurate information about the effects of health care interventions is readily available worldwide. This is achieved by coordinating and publishing systematic reviews of studies on the effects of interventions in an Internet-based library of specialized databases called *The Cochrane Library*. The Collaboration's 2005 Strategic Plan includes the principle 'Enabling wide participation in the work of The Cochrane Collaboration by reducing barriers to contributing and by encouraging diversity'. This principle is realized through various structures and processes. These include setting up a network so that consumers can participate (see the Cochrane Consumer Network at http://consumers.cochrane.org/); introducing consumer representation from the network at steering group level; the active encouragement of consumer involvement in organizations producing reviews; and support and funding for consumers to participate in annual scientific meetings and training programmes (Ghersi 2002). Table 20.1 lists the main functions carried out by consumers.

TABLE 20.1   The functions carried out by consumers in The Cochrane Collaboration

Different stages of research	The roles and tasks of consumers
Deciding what to research	Identifying review topics or priorities
Deciding how to do it	Identifying issues from a consumer's perspective and important outcomes Commenting on drafts of Cochrane reviews and protocols as referees
Doing it	Hand-searching journals for research missed by database searching Translating documents Researching and writing a review, as co-reviewers Working as editors and coordinators Running training courses
Letting people know the results	Writing lay versions of reviews for simultaneous publication with full reviews Disseminating the results, giving presentations, writing newsletters, linking to consumer groups
Deciding what to do next	Representing consumer members on the organization's management and working groups Encouraging others to participate

Source: Horey (2002)

A survey identified that many consumers wanted to be more involved in The Cochrane Collaboration, yet faced a range of personal and structural barriers. Personal barriers included the financial costs of participation such as wages forgone, the cost of attending meetings, health costs for those with chronic illness, language barriers and the feeling of being isolated from other consumers (Horey 2002: 18–19).

Structural barriers included the lack of clarity within The Cochrane Collaboration of the roles of consumers and communication about changes; the lack of access to computers and other technology to enable some people to participate; the complexity of the scientific language and concepts; poor communication between the institutions contributing to The Cochrane Collaboration and consumers; the short timescale in which to complete complex tasks; and the patronising or insensitive attitudes of professionals and researchers (Horey 2002).

Overcoming barriers to participation

A small number of Cochrane groups have written up their experiences, documenting their strategies to establish consumer involvement in the research and the measures taken to overcome barriers to participation. The Cochrane Musculo-skeletal Group, which coordinates the production of reviews of treatments for musculoskeletal conditions and is based in Ottawa, Canada, provides dedicated resources to consumers in all stages of its work, with roles, functions and tasks similar to those listed above. Access to people who might be interested in volunteering was made easier by the Group's close relationship with the Arthritis Society of Canada, which itself had built a broad network of interested people with arthritis. Despite these advantages, the Group reported difficulties in maintaining its consumer membership as people faced health problems, competing priorities in their lives or both. People also complained about the costs for individuals of participation (Shea et al. 2005).

The Haematological Malignancies Group based in Cologne, Germany, faced similar difficulties that in its case were compounded by language barriers and serious illness. It was found that the appointment of a dedicated consumer coordinator, one-to-one support for consumer representatives, time spent on consulting and listening, and training programmes for participants assisted the process (Skoetz et al. 2005). Most of the consumer representatives came from a self-help group relevant for people with haematological malignancies. Individuals had an interest in research, but also wanted to take back what they had learned to the consumer group.

Both of these groups had the benefit of significant support at a senior level for consumer participation and dedicated resources. They established or improved relationships to existing organizations which already had consumers involved. Both also emphasized the importance of intensive and ongoing interaction to sustain commitment. Once established, the relationship enables both consumers and researchers to report back to consumers more generally on the influence or impact of consumer participation in terms of ideas or actions taken, a process for

(Continued)

(Continued)

improving transparency of research and accountability of researchers. The findings suggest, though, that while The Cochrane Collaboration is global in coverage, local or regional support is necessary to sustain activity.

Supporting user involvement in health research

The Cochrane Collaboration has expected health researchers to support consumer participation and to respond to the issues raised by consumers. The intellectual dominance within The Cochrane Collaboration of questions on the effectiveness of clinical and pharmaceutical interventions raises the question: Is the impact of consumer participation important enough to warrant the investment in time and resources?

This attractive, but facile, question obscures other and broader challenges within health research. Brown and Zavestoski (2004: 680–1) write: 'Science and technocratic decision-making have become an increasingly dominant force in shaping social policy and regulation.' They suggest that one cost to society for the dominance of science is that: 'Scientists are asked to answer questions that are virtually impossible to answer scientifically due to data uncertainties or the infeasibility of carrying out a study.' A second cost is that: 'The scientization of decision-making delegitimizes the importance of those questions that may not be conducive to scientific analysis.' These processes, they argue, diminish the capacity of the public to participate as citizens in framing and contributing to policy debates.

I would argue that these processes in fact provide a compelling rationale and justification for seeking effective ways of enabling users to participate in the production of knowledge. After all, it is their bodies and their lives that are affected by the uncertainties. Their participation may enable impossible questions to be reframed and to be addressed in meaningful ways.

Conclusion

This chapter has summarized some of the ways in which user involvement in research is taking place. In conclusion, there are two important questions that will require further exploration. First, for researchers, the question is how to establish and sustain a meaningful relationship that accommodates epistemologically and practically the intersection of the experience of illness with producing new knowledge about illness and health (Hess 2004). Second, for health care users, the challenge is how to move from critique to constructive participation. Effective participation must balance a critical viewpoint and independence with understanding and involvement in the concerns of researchers. These are exciting questions to explore, but to be answered they require more than token commitment to user participation, and a greater awareness that the process is more complex than has been assumed. Readers can test the latter point further by attempting the exercise below on developing a policy for user participation for a health research organization.

Exercise: Develop a policy for user participation in research for a health research institute

Imagine you are working in a health research institute and the board has decided that it needs a user participation policy. Further, all new projects are expected to involve lay people. The board asks you to develop a user participation policy, to identify where users could be 'found', their roles and some indication of achievements for the first 1–2 years.

1 The evidence base and the social setting: identify sources of evidence that will assist you to develop a policy position paper. Consider searching using all the relevant terms for user. In addition to the sources in the references, you may wish to check the following:

   • The Cochrane Library, including the databases of the Cochrane Database of Systematic Reviews and the Database of Reviews of Effectiveness, to identify recent reviews of evidence.
   • Medical and health research databases, in addition to databases of activities and projects for user involvement in research.
   • The websites of local or national consumer groups who would have an interest in the research in your institute.

2 The development of a plan: consider using the framework for consumer involvement developed by Oliver et al. (2004), to form a plan for user participation in your institute. Against the eight main features, document your proposed strategies. Remember to identify what type of research is undertaken in your Institute and for whom. Consider whether you would consult consumer groups and researchers to identify their interest in user participation, the prospect for ongoing relationships and the skills that people may require. Build this into your plan. Identify realistic achievements for the first 1–2 years, using the available literature to substantiate your proposals where possible. Formulate a strategy for obtaining support for your plan and the outcomes from the board and chief executive officer.

3 Evaluation: the policy should have an evaluative component that establishes a process of reflexive practice involving users and researchers. Identify indicators of success or impact and how these will be measured.

Acknowledgement

My thanks go to Dr Dell Horey for her thoughtful comments on the practicalities of consumer participation in research, and in particular for her insights into pharmaceutical funding for consumer groups, and to Professor Sandy Oliver for showing me a connection between research and change.

Recommended Further Reading

Brown, P. and Zavestoski, S. (2004) 'Social movements in health: an introduction', *Sociology of Health and Illness*, 26(6): 679–94.
This is good reading for those interested in acquiring a sociological understanding of health social movements.

Nilsen, E.S., Myrhaug, H.T., Johansen, M., Oliver, S. and Oxman, A.D. (2006) 'Methods of consumer involvement in developing healthcare policy and research, clinical practice guidelines and patient information material', *Cochrane Database of Systematic Reviews*, Issue 3. Art. No.: CD004563.
This key reference is a Cochrane systematic review of evaluation studies relevant to consumer participation in research, which is regularly updated.

Oliver, S., Clarke-Jones, L., Rees, R., Milne, R., Buchanan, P., Gabbay, J., Gyte, G., Oakley, A. and Stein, K. (2004) 'Involving consumers in research and development agenda setting for the NHS: an evidence-based approach', *Health Technology Assessment*, 8(15). Available at: www.ncchta.org/fullmono/mon815.pdf
This provides a detailed background on the development of the framework for analysing consumer participation in research.

Williamson, C. (2010) *Patients' Experiences and the Patient Movement*. Bristol: Policy Press.
This book provides an up-to-date account of the achievements and shortcomings of the patient movement in the UK.

 ## Online Readings

Rose, D., Fleischmann, P. and Schofield, P. (2010) 'Perceptions of user involvement: A user-led study', *International Journal of Social Psychiatry*, 56: 389–401.
How is user involvement defined in this context? To what extent did users control the research process? What are the advantages/disadvantages of such an approach?

Perkins, P., Booth, S., Vowler, S. and Barclay, S. (2008) 'What are patients' priorities for palliative care research? A questionnaire study', *Palliative Medicine*, 22: 7–12.
How is user involvement defined in this context? To what extent did users control the research process? What are the advantages/disadvantages of such an approach?

References

Association of the British Pharmaceutical Industry (ABPI) (2002) *The Code of Practice for the Industry*. London: ABPI.

Baggott, R., Allsop, J. and Jones, K. (2005) *Speaking for Patients and Carers: Health Consumer Groups and the Policy Process*. Basingstoke: Palgrave Macmillan.

Beard, R.L. (2004) 'Advocating voice: organisational, historical and social milieux of the Alzheimer's disease movement', *Sociology of Health and Illness*, 26(6): 797–819.

Boote, J., Telford, R. and Cooper, C. (2002) 'Consumer involvement in health research: a review and research agenda', *Health Policy*, 61: 213–36.

Bristol Inquiry (2001) *Learning from Bristol: The Report of the Public Inquiry into Children's Heart Surgery at the Bristol Royal Infirmary 1984–1995*. Available at: www.bristol-inquiry. org.uk/final_report/the_report.pdf

Brown, P. and Zavestoski, S. (2004) 'Social movements in health: an introduction', *Sociology of Health and Illness*, 26(6): 679–94.

Cartwright Inquiry (1988) *The Report of the Committee of Inquiry into Allegations Concerning the Treatment of Cervical Cancer at the National Women's Hospital*. Auckland: WHA.

Consumers' Health Forum of Australia and Medicines Australia (2008) *Working Together: A Guide to Relationships between Health Consumer Organisations and Pharmaceutical Companies*. Revised edition. Available at: www.chf.org.au/497-working-together-guide-manual-2008.chf (accessed 12 March 2012).

Consumers in NHS Research Support Unit (2000) *Involving Consumers in Research and Development in the NHS: Briefing Notes for Researchers*. Eastleigh: Consumers in NHS Research Support Unit.

Coulter, A. (2011) *Engaging Patients in Health Care*. Buckingham: Open University Press.

Department of Health (2007) *Best Research for Best Health*. London: Department of Health. Available at: www.dh.gov.uk/en/Publicationsandstatistics/Publications/Publications PolicyAndGuidance/Browsable/DH_4127225 (accessed 12 March 2012).

Dickersin, K. and Schnaper, L. (1996) 'Reinventing medical research', in K.L. Moss (ed.), *Man-made Medicine: Women's Health, Public Policy and Reform*. Durham, NC, and London: Duke University Press.

Elwyn, G., Crowe, S., Fenton, M., Firkins, L., Versnel, J., Walker, S. et al. on behalf of the JLA Asthma Working Partnership (2010) 'Identifying and prioritizing uncertainties: patient and clinician engagement in the identification of research questions', *Journal of Evaluation in Clinical Practice*, 16: 627–31.

Entwistle, V.A., Renfrew, M.J., Yearley, S., Forrester, J. and Lamont, T. (1998) 'Lay perspectives: advantages for health research', *British Medical Journal*, 316: 463–6.

Ghersi, D. (2002) 'Making it happen: approaches to involving consumers in Cochrane reviews', *Evaluation and the Health Professions*, 25(3): 270–83.

Goodare, H. and Smith, R. (1995) 'The rights of patients in research', *British Medical Journal*, 310: 1277–8.

Henderson, S. and Petersen, A. (2002) 'Introduction: consumerism in health care', in S. Henderson and A. Petersen (eds), *Consuming Health: The Commodification of Health Care*. London: Routledge.

Herxheimer, A. (2003) 'Relationships between the pharmaceutical industry and patients' organizations', *British Medical Journal*, 326: 1208–10.

Herxheimer, A. and Goodare, H. (1999) 'Who are you and who are we? Looking through the eyes of some key words', *Health Expectations*, 2: 3–6.

Hess, D.J. (2004) 'Medical modernisation, scientific research fields and the epistemic politics of heath social movements', *Sociology of Health and Illness*, 26(6): 695–709.

Hill, S. (2011) 'Preface', in S. Hill (ed.), *The Knowledgeable Patient: Communication and Participation in Health*. Chichester: Wiley-Blackwell.

Horey, D. (2002) *'It Takes Time to Find Your Role': A Survey of Consumers in the Cochrane Collaboration in 2002*. Email survey available at: http://consumers.cochrane.org/reports (accessed 12 March 2012).

INVOLVE (2007) *Promoting Public Involvement in NHS, Public Health and Social Care Research: Strategic Plan 2007–2011*. National Institute for Health Research, UK.

INVOLVE (2010) *Changing our Worlds: Examples of User-controlled Research in Action: Summary*. By A. Faukner. Available at: www.invo.org.uk/resource-centre/publications-by-involve/ (accessed 12 March 2012).

INVOLVE (2011) *INVOLVE Survey of Priorities for Public Involvement across the NIHR: September 2011*. Available at: www.invo.org.uk/resource-centre/publications-by-involve/ (accessed 12 March 2012).

INVOLVE (2012) *Research*. Available at: www.invo.org.uk/posttypejargon/research/ (accessed 12 March 2012).

Jones, K. (2008) 'In whose interest? Relationships between health consumer groups and the pharmaceutical industry in the UK', *Sociology of Health and Illness*, 30(6): 929–43.

Kirkpatrick, C.M.J., Roughead, E.R., Monteith, G.R. and Tett, S.E. (2005) 'Consumer involvement in Quality Use of Medicines (QUM) projects: lessons from Australia', *BMC Health Services Research*, 5: 75. Available at: www.biomedcentral.com/1472-6963/5/75

Moynihan, R. (2005) 'The marketing of a disease: female sexual dysfunction', *British Medical Journal*, 330: 192–4.

National Health and Medical Research Council and Consumers' Health Forum of Australia (2001) *Statement on Consumer and Community Participation in Health and Medical Research*. Commonwealth of Australia, Canberra. Available at: www.nhmrc.gov.au/publications/synopses/r22syn.htm

National Health and Medical Research Council and Consumers' Health Forum of Australia (2004a) *A Model Framework for Consumer and Community Participation in Health and Medical Research*. National Health and Medical Research Council, Commonwealth of Australia, Canberra. Available at: http://gov.au/publications/synopses/r22syn.htm

National Health and Medical Research Council and Consumers' Health Forum of Australia (2004b) *Resource Pack for Consumer and Community Participation in Health and Medical Research*. National Health and Medical Research Council, Commonwealth of Australia, Canberra. Available at: www.nhmrc.gov.au/publications/synopses/r22syn.htm

Nilsen, E.S., Myrhaug, H.T., Johansen, M., Oliver, S. and Oxman, A.D. (2006) 'Methods of consumer involvement in developing healthcare policy and research, clinical practice guidelines and patient information material', *Cochrane Database of Systematic Reviews*, Issue 3. Art. No. CD004563.

O'Donnell, M. and Entwistle, V. (2004) 'Consumer involvement in research projects: the activities of research funders', *Health Policy*, 69: 229–38.

Oliver, S. (1999) 'Users of health services: following their agenda', in S. Hood, B. Mayall and S. Oliver (eds), *Critical Issues in Social Research*. Buckingham and Philadelphia, PA: Open University Press.

Oliver, S., Clarke-Jones, L., Rees, R., Milne, R., Buchanan, P., Gabbay, J., Gyte, G., Oakley, A. and Stein, K. (2004) 'Involving consumers in research and development agenda setting for the NHS: an evidence-based approach', *Health Technology Assessment*, 8(15): 1–148. Available at: www.ncchta.org/fullmono/mon815.pdf

Oliver, S.R., Rees, R.W., Clarke-Jones, L., Milne, R., Oakley, A.R., Gabbay, J., Stein, K., Buchanan, P. and Gyte, G. (2008) 'A multidimensional conceptual framework for analysing public involvement in health services research', *Health Expectations*, 11: 72–84.

Ong, B.N. and Hooper, H. (2003) 'Involving users in low back pain research', *Health Expectations*, 6(4): 332–41.

Parliamentary Health Select Committee (2005) *(HC 42-1) 4th Report 2004/5: The Influence of the Pharmaceutical Industry*. London: The Stationery Office.

Paterson, C. (2004) '"Take small steps to go a long way": consumer involvement in research into complementary and alternative therapies', *Complementary Therapies in Nursing and Midwifery*, 10: 150–61.

Sakala, C., Gyte, G., Henderson, S., Neilson, J.P. and Horey, D. (2001) 'Consumer – professional partnership to improve research: the experience of the Cochrane Collaboration's Pregnancy and Childbirth Group', *Birth*, 28(2): 133–7.

Sepkowitz, K.A. (2001) 'AIDS: the first 20 years', *New England Journal of Medicine*, 344(23): 1764–72.

Shea, B., Santesso, N., Qualman, A., Heiberg, T., Leong, A., Judd, M. et al. (Cochrane Musculoskeletal Consumer Group) (2005) 'Consumer-driven health care: building partnerships in research', *Health Expectations*, 8(4): 352–9.

Skoetz, N., Weigart, O. and Engert, A. (2005) 'A consumer network for haematological malignancies', *Health Expectations*, 8(1): 86–90.

Tallon, D., Chard, J. and Dieppe, P. (2000) 'Relation between agendas of the research community and the research consumer', *Lancet*, 355: 2037–40.

Thompson, J., Barber, R., Ward, P.R., Cooper, C.L., Armitage, C.J. and Jones, G. (2009) 'Health researchers' attitudes towards public involvement in health research', *Health Expectations*, 12: 209–20.

Williamson, C. (2001) 'What does involving consumers in research mean?', Editorial, *Quarterly Journal of Medicine*, 94(12): 661–4. Available at: http://qjmed.oxfordjournals.org/cgi/reprint/94/12/661

21

Comparative Health Research

VIOLA BURAU

Introduction

- Health, health care and policies have become more international over recent decades, reflecting a number of factors. The development of mass media and communication technologies means that information about health problems and health services in individual countries has become more readily and widely available. This trend is also supported by the work of international organizations such as the World Health Organization (WHO) and the Organization for Economic Cooperation and Development (OECD), which not only gather but also disseminate information about health care across a wide range of countries. Health policies are also increasingly made at the international level. For example, the European Union is now involved in a wide range of areas from public health to pharmaceutical policies. Finally, many health problems are shared across countries, such as HIV/AIDS. Industrialized Western countries also share a concern about how to respond to ageing populations and how to control infectious diseases, such as the respiratory disease SARS, that cross country borders.
- With the internationalization of health care, the cross-country, comparative perspective has become increasingly significant in understanding contemporary issues in health. Although there are methodological challenges, comparative health research allows the evidence from more than one country to be used in a systematic way. The notion of comparison may be incorporated into a flexible research design and draw on a range of different methods.

Approaches to Comparative Health Research

Comparative health research can deal with a wide range of substantive areas in health and take a range of perspectives. Researchers should be aware of different approaches prior to embarking on a study and Øvretveit (1998) and Clasen (2004) provide useful overviews. One area of study is to focus on the health needs of particular patients. For example, the needs of asthma patients could be approached in two ways: either through an analysis of how the organization of health services across different countries addresses the needs of asthma patients or, alternatively, through focusing on health professionals. How do doctors and nurses across different countries respond to asthma patients and what services do they provide?

Studies can also be undertaken at three different organizational levels:

- Macro-level studies may test a hypothesis and use statistical analysis.
- Meso-level studies tend to focus on the organization of health services.
- Micro-level studies are concerned with specific aspects of health care behaviour and practice.

This is illustrated by Box 21.1 below.

Box 21.1   Examples of comparative health research

- *Macro-level studies*: Huber (1999) compared OECD health figures from 29 countries over nearly three decades to examine whether there are any distinct trends in the development of health care expenditure. The analysis suggests that health care expenditure levelled off in the 1990s, although countries continue to fall into three groups in terms of the overall level of health care expenditure.
- *Meso-level studies*: there is a large literature on health policy and reform. Freeman (2000) and Moran (1999), for example, use the categories of funding, provision and regulation of health care to understand why policy responses to health problems vary across countries. They, as well as other authors, suggest that public control over provision and funding offers states better leverage in relation to containing costs and pursuing organizational reform.
- *Micro-level studies*: in their analysis of care arrangements of older people in Britain and Germany, Chamberlayne and King (2000) use qualitative methods to study the biographies of individual carers and identify different 'cultures of care' within particular countries.

The Purpose of Comparison

Beyond the choice of substantive area and level of analysis, another important consideration is the purpose of comparison. Comparison may be about:

- Exploration.
- Explanation.
- Evaluation.

Exploratory studies

Exploratory comparative health research aims to investigate the same 'phenomenon' in different countries. This can be anything from the organization of palliative care and public health policies to cancer survival rates and public expenditure on hospital care. Here, the aim is to broaden the 'basis of evidence' by considering cases from very different contexts to get a better idea of the potential variation in service delivery.

Exploratory studies help to avoid both false particularism ('everywhere is unique') and false universalism ('everywhere is the same') as they aim to identify what is different and what is similar. In this respect, studies may adopt a static perspective and focus on the differences and similarities as such. For example, Raffel (1997) analyses the differences and similarities in the organization of health services across 10 industrialized countries. A study may adopt a more dynamic perspective and analyse how countries are becoming more different, or similar. This approach is particularly dominant in studies that analyse processes of convergence, whereby health problems, services or policies tend to become more similar over time. Schmid et al. (2010) analyse health reforms across OECD countries and suggest that there are increasing similarities across different types of health system, with individual health systems becoming more hybrid in form.

Explanatory studies

Explanatory studies investigate deeper questions, notably about why it is we find certain differences and similarities (Klein 2009). For example, a study by Haug (1995) of the division of labour between doctors and nurses in Britain and Germany starts with the observation (based on OECD health statistics) that the ratio between doctors and nurses in the two countries differs significantly. She uses the remainder of her study to examine various explanations for this difference. Although exploratory studies give an indication of findings, explanatory studies make better use of the analytical potential of the comparative research design. The particular explanations considered depend on the specific theories underlying the research questions. For example, theories of policy making are the basis for the central assumption of Haug (1995) that the influence nurses enjoy at both the macro and micro levels of organization explains the different ratio of doctors to nurses within different systems.

Evaluation studies

Finally, there are health studies using comparison as a method of evaluation. Here, the main aim is to assess the impact of health care and policies in different countries against specific criteria of relative success or failure. An important example is the World Health Report by the WHO (2000). The report compares the performance of different health systems and makes recommendations about how the performance of health systems can be improved within available resources. Evaluative studies build on two more or less explicit assumptions. First, the evaluation of health involves making judgements, often by identifying exemplary cases or so-called 'best practice'. This suggests implicitly that there is a best way of doing things, and the promotion of market-based mechanisms in health care is a prominent example. Second, evaluative studies assume that best practice can be transferred across countries and that in this way countries can learn from each other in very practical ways. However, both assumptions are problematic as the next section shows.

The Politics of Comparative Health Research

The interest of both governments and international organizations in comparative health research has led to an increasing politicization of comparative studies. This is reflected particularly in more applied studies where the aim is explicitly to evaluate evidence from different countries in order to identify what works best in relation to, for example, the use of medical technologies or in particular care pathways. A clinical or care pathway refers to an evidence-based protocol for treating a group of patients with a specific condition. It is used as a management tool and aims to reduce variations in care to improve outcomes. In relation to the former, there is a well-established methodology of 'health technology assessment', which Stargardt (2008), for instance, uses to assess the costs of hip replacement in nine European Union countries. An example of the latter is the survey by Vanhaecht et al. (2006) of 23 countries to identify the specific uses of clinical pathways. This leads the authors to call for more international benchmarking of clinical pathways. Governments identify existing problems and seek 'solutions' by looking at other health systems (Rose 2000). For instance, in the UK, the NHS has been seen as 'underfunded' when compared with other countries which spend higher levels of GDP on health care (Dunne 2002). For policy makers, the attraction of cross-country comparison lies in the fact that it resembles a kind of 'natural experiment', which allows for 'testing' individual reform instruments and assessing their relative suitability and success.

This is especially attractive in two respects. First, policy making informed by comparative research potentially allows learning from the mistakes of others, and thereby holds the implicit promise of avoiding policy failure altogether. This is an attractive promise in any policy area, not least health, which is high on the political agenda of many countries, reflecting the importance of health services to the general public. Second, policy making informed by comparative research enjoys greater credibility because it is informed by more than the personal judgement of policy makers. As such, comparison can be part and parcel of a more 'evidence-based' style of policy making. In the case of the increase in NHS funding referred to above, it was precisely the comparison with other countries that devoted a higher proportion of GDP to health care, which offered additional credibility to an otherwise controversial policy decision. This is also in line with the distinctively anti-ideological and pragmatic approach of the previous New Labour government in the UK (Rose 2000).

The process of 'comparing for policy making' is not a neutral, but a highly politicized, activity and the literature on policy learning and transfer identifies different dimensions of this complexity (Dolowitz and Marsh 1996; Klein 2009) as follows:

- The process of policy learning itself is selective and more often than not reflects the specific, domestic agendas of policy makers. For example, the internal market reforms of the British NHS in the early 1990s were influenced by health care practice and thinking in the USA, precisely because of the common neo-liberal market orientation of the two governments at the time. Policy learning from other countries therefore is often concerned with finding additional arguments for a political decision already made.
- Best practices are deeply embedded in highly specific national, social, economic and political contexts and therefore cannot be transferred easily. Indeed, the literature suggests that health policies follow country-specific paths and reflect existing institutional frameworks in health care and the broader political system (Wilsford 1994) and past policy choices may constrain the scope for policy learning (Peterson 1997). This also means that the relative success of individual best practices is highly conditional and depends on specific organizational settings. Any transfer is likely to be partial and require some adaptation. For example, although market mechanisms were the central focus of health reforms in the 1990s across Europe, countries implemented market mechanisms in very different ways. This reflects differences in specific policy goals, in political institutions and in the structure of health systems (Harrison 2004).

What are the implications of these political factors for the researcher undertaking comparative health research? The literature suggests that researchers must be aware of the limitations of research for policy. They should recognize that the most desirable comparative research design for policy makers may not necessarily be the most fruitful analytically. Researchers also need to be sensitive to the specific contexts and conditions under which best practices may be considered as 'best'.

The Methodological Challenges of Comparative Health Research

Sampling: choosing cases

The first challenge is related to sampling. Sampling requires clarifying the rationale for comparison. What is it that comparison is supposed to explain? Individual studies should focus on either differences or similarities, depending on what it is they aim to analyse and/ or explain. For example, a study looking at the effect of the introduction of market forces in health care cannot, in the same study, both analyse convergence towards market mechanisms in health care reforms and analyse differences in the implementation of health care markets.

Sampling is about choosing suitable countries or more generally 'cases' for comparison – that is, cases from which one can learn most in terms of what the study aims to analyse and explain. The choice of cases is closely tied to the underlying theoretical framework of a study (Ebbinghaus 2005). For example, the widespread reference to 'market forces' in health reforms may reflect processes of policy learning and transfer. Relevant theories suggest that such cross-country learning is more likely where there are similarities in the mode of health care delivery between countries. Thus, Britain and Sweden, with their tax-funded national health systems, can be used as comparators (Glennerster and Matsaganis 1994).

In contrast, if the focus of attention is on analysing why markets in health care have been implemented in very different ways across European countries, it would be more appropriate to include countries with contrasting or dissimilar health systems (Verspohl 2012). In terms of theory, neo-institutionalist theories suggest that differences in policy outcome reflect differences in the institutional setting. However, both research designs require that the cases chosen are comparable in the first place and the literature identifies with different strategies to achieve this. From a variable-oriented perspective, Lijphart (1975) defines comparability as a strategy, whereby the theoretically insignificant 'background variables' are held constant. This means choosing countries with comparable levels of economic wealth, with stable democratic political systems and with developed welfare states. From a context-oriented perspective, comparability is established by thoroughly analysing the specific contexts the individual cases are embedded in, in order to identify the multiple similarities (and differences) among them (Mangen 2004).

Equivalence: ensuring comparability

A second challenge relates to 'equivalence', which can be understood as identifying comparable units for cross-country comparison (see Øyen 2004). This question arises at the research design phase – however, comparing 'apples with apples' rather than 'pears' is less straightforward than it appears. The units of comparative health research can be anything from specific health workers to professional practices, disease patterns, health services, health policies or health outcomes.

Identifying such units of comparison across countries is complicated as it involves being aware not only of differences in the use of language, but also differences in the specific cultural meaning and the related function of such units. In the literature, this is referred to as the difference between 'formal' and 'functional' equivalence. For instance, units that have similar cultural meanings (and functions) may have different names; conversely, units with the same name may have very different cultural meanings (and functions). Health care is culturally embedded within society (Freeman 1999) – as highlighted by Box 21.2 below.

Box 21.2   Formal vs. functional equivalence – the case of the hospital

Although the English term 'hospital' can be translated directly into other European languages (as *hôpital* in French, *Krankenhaus* in German or *sygehus* in Danish), this disguises differences in cultural meaning and function. For example, English hospital trusts are providers of specialist health care and cover both inpatient and outpatient services, whereas their German counterparts focus on inpatient specialist care only. This reflects the fact that the majority of outpatient specialist care is delivered by office-based specialists.

To secure the validity of a piece of comparative research, it is essential to identify similar units for comparison. It is, however, a complex process requiring translation of both words and meanings and an acknowledgement of the social construction of concepts (Barbour 2010). One way of taking account of linguistic and cultural differences while ensuring comparability is to work with 'functional equivalents'. This means the researcher makes a choice of the unit of analysis on the basis that its substantive functions are comparable. For example, a British–German comparison of hospital care could use the unit 'inpatient specialist care' as a focus of study.

Managing complexity: processing and interpreting data

A third challenge of comparative health research is to manage the quantity, diversity and complexity of the data collected in a systematic and theoretically meaningful way. This must be achieved through all the phases of the research from data collection to data processing and interpretation where more than two countries are included. It is especially important to process the material emerging from comparative health research in a systematic way by specifying clearly what material is relevant and in what way. This is about labelling and categorizing, but is more than a technical exercise. Instead, processing comparative research material is at the centre of the interpretation itself. To be done systematically, analysis must be theory-led. Processing has to reflect the specific hypotheses that are expected to explain differences or similarities across countries.

The use of ideal types

One method used for data processing and interpretation is to cluster explanatory factors into 'ideal types'. These are constructs that can be understood as the basic variants of a particular phenomenon and have been a particularly important tool in meso-level comparative health research (Burau and Blank 2006). For example, a commonly used typology of health systems defines them as representing specific sets of macro-institutional characteristics, and such a typology can be used to explain specific variations of health policies across different countries. In this case, the typology is based on variations in the funding of health care and corresponds to differences in the organization of health care provision (OECD 1987). It distinguishes three basic models of health systems:

- The national health service model with funding out of general taxation.
- The social insurance model with compulsory social insurance funded out of employer and employee contributions.
- The private insurance model funded by individual and/or employer contributions.

The underlying assumption of this typology of health systems is that the public funding of health care, or lack of it, is the defining characteristic of the extent of state involvement in health care. Thus, Freeman (2000) uses the typology to explain specific variations in the politics and policies of health care across a number of European countries. The ideal type model of health systems helps not only to describe and categorize the organization of health care, but also to explain why countries respond to health problems in certain ways. In consequence, the analysis moves beyond the specificity of individual countries, towards more insight into the health system in general.

The limitations of typologies

Using typologies is not without its problems, many of which arise from the ambiguous relationship between ideal types and real systems. Ideal types of the health system are abstractions drawn from real health systems and are meant to help in understanding the organization of health care. Typologies aim to simplify reality but, in doing so, they may limit understanding of actual systems. In Singapore, for example, health care funding comes from private sources in the form of personal savings accounts, although payment into such accounts is mandatory. The health system of Singapore therefore fits poorly into the typology of health systems referred to above. In this case, the typology raises more questions than it answers (see Blank and Burau 2010).

Another danger is that analyses become divided by individual ideal types and do not effectively compare across different countries. An example is the international literature on health professions, which is often based, more or less explicitly, on a typology centred on the Anglo-American professions (Collins 1990). Its limited explanatory power has resulted in single-country case studies dominating the literature. Cross-country comparative studies have been few (see, for example, Hellberg et al. 1999).

In comparative health research, there is an underlying tension between uniqueness and generalization. As Mabbett and Bolderson (1999) point out, broad-brush characterizations often do not hold up when confronted with the complex detail of actual arrangements. Yet the dilemma is that once one departs from such characterizations, research can become merely descriptive, which militates against identifying clear and all-encompassing contrasts. Thus, classification is at the heart of comparative health studies (Freeman and Frisina 2010), illustrated further in the case study below.

CASE STUDY

Comparative health research in practice

The following discussion is based on a comparative study of nursing in Britain and Germany (Burau 1999a, 1999b, 2005). The initial interest in the study arose from the following puzzle. Although nursing is the single largest occupation in most health systems in Europe, relatively little is known about nursing across countries. The comparative literature on health care and policy is notable for its silence on nursing. The study addressed the following research questions: What are the different strategies used for governing nursing as an occupation? How can the differences between nursing in Britain and Germany be explained? The study used two sets of theories. Theories of the professions were used to identify the main strategy for occupational governance and the substantive focus for occupational governance. Typically, the literature associates occupational governance with strategies for 'professional closure' through state-licensed self-regulation in relation to overseeing education and maintaining a register of the qualified. In addition, strategies for occupational governance are used to explain intra-professional dynamics. However, as feminist writers have noted, the state often plays an influential role in the governance of women-dominated occupations such as nursing. The study therefore also used institutionalist theories to explain the specific strategies of occupational governance of nursing. These theories suggest that institutional rules backed by coercion as well as norms and values shape the interests and resources of actors involved in the governance of nursing. In this instance, actors included nurses themselves, both individually and collectively, health care providers as employers of nurses and the state. The interplay of these various interests shaped the strategies for the occupational governance of nursing.

The research questions and the choice of theoretical framework had implications for the design of this cross-country comparative study. The effect of institutions is relatively easy to identify where institutions are different, and the study focuses on Britain and Germany, where the institutional arrangements for the occupational governance of nursing differ, as does the organization of health care and the role of the state. Britain has a tax-funded, publicly provided health service with the highly centralized political system providing important levers in relation to the occupational governance of nursing. In contrast, the health system in Germany is funded by social insurance contributions and health service provision is a public/private mix. This provides the basis for extensive joint self-governance by providers and insurers. Moreover, the federal structure devolves governance to the more local level. In consequence, the role of the state in health care organization, and the occupational governance of nursing, is limited.

To examine how strategies for occupational governance had been shaped by different institutional arrangements required a two-part analysis:

- An analysis of the structures of occupational governance in the two countries.
- A case study of the strategies for occupational governance of nursing.

For the case study, comparable units of analysis had to be chosen to deal with issues of equivalence. This proved to be challenging. Although in both countries there is a policy emphasis on providing nursing care outside hospital, there was no equivalent to 'primary' or 'community care' in Germany. Nor was there a category of 'practice nurse'. Primary care remains highly medically oriented. However, in both countries home-based nursing services exist, albeit organized in different ways. In Britain, specialist 'district nurses', general nurses and health care assistants deliver care to patients in their homes. In Germany, general nurses, geriatric carers (*Altenpfleger*) and care assistants provide home-based care and there is no specific term for nurses delivering this type of care.

In this study to ensure functional equivalence, the research focused on the occupational field of home-based (nursing) care rather than on individual occupational groups. To allow for the different meanings of home-based (nursing) care, the study used the term 'district nurses' only in the British context. When referring to Germany or both countries, the more neutral term 'community nurses' or 'community nursing staff' was used.

As with most comparative research, complex data had to be gathered, managed and analysed. The study used existing meso-level typologies of health systems and health care states to order the material on the structure of nursing occupational governance. The distinction between 'Anglo-American' and 'Continental' types of professions was less useful as this was developed on the basis of influential, male-dominated professions.

Conclusion

In attempting to carry out a piece of comparative research, a number of choices have to be made in terms of strategy and this chapter has aimed to provide a structured approach to making those choices and to negotiate the pitfalls of a complex field. First, a choice must be made about the unit for comparison across countries. It has been suggested that there should be functional equivalence in what is being compared. Second, in choosing the countries in a study, the best strategy is to compare countries that have some broad similarities. Here, typologies or ideal types are a useful device, although one that should be used cautiously as real systems rarely conform fully to a concept that is based on an abstraction. Third, the researcher should then decide whether in making comparisons their strategy is to look for lines of difference or lines of similarity. They should also decide whether the study they are undertaking is exploratory, explanatory or evaluative. Finally, any analysis of similarity or difference should be theory-led; that is, the researcher should identify a general proposition or hypothesis about the way in which policies, organizations, groups or individuals function that they are seeking to explain. To conclude the chapter, a practical exercise for the reader follows.

Exercise: Comparing health care expenditure and cost containment policies

In principle, health policy in most developed capitalist democracies has been based on achieving three goals: the provision of high-quality services; equal access for all citizens to health care; and cost-efficient provision (Blank and Burau 2010). In the first two decades following the Second World War, health policy initiatives were particularly concerned with the first two goals. Since the 1970s, cost efficiency and containment have become dominant across countries. With this in mind, examine the OECD's data on the total expenditure on health as a percentage of GDP (see Table 21.1) and answer the three questions below:

TABLE 21.1   Total expenditure on health as a percentage of GDP

	1980	2009
Austria	7.4	11.0
France	7.1	11.8
Germany	8.7	11.6
Italy	7.7*	9.5
Netherlands	7.5	9.9**
New Zealand	5.9	10.3
Spain	5.4	9.5
Sweden	9.1	10.0
UK	5.6	9.8
USA	8.7	17.4

*Figure for 1985; **Figure for 2008

Source: OECD (2011)

(Continued)

(Continued)

1   Looking at the figures for 2009, rank countries in order of the percentage of GDP spent on health care.

- What is the difference in percentage points between the country at the top and the bottom of the list?
- Are countries spread evenly or do they cluster into separate groups? Are there any clear outliers?

TABLE 21.2   The health care systems in Britain, Germany and Sweden

	Germany	Britain	Sweden
Funding	• Access to health services mainly on basis of social insurance membership • Funding primarily through social insurance contributions raised by statutory, non-profit insurance funds, complemented by taxes and co-payments • Allocation of funding based on contracts between insurance funds and providers through various mechanisms; federal legislation as framework	• Access to health services on basis of social citizenship • Funding through general taxation raised by central government • Allocation of funding based on national global budget and through local budget allocations embedded in a central framework	• Access to health services on basis of social citizenship • Funding through income tax raised by regional governments • Allocation of funding based on regional global budget but through a variety of mechanisms
Provision	• Hospitals in public, non-profit or private ownership; service delivery based on contracts; control jointly by insurance funds and providers • Hospital doctors are salaried employees, office-based doctors work as independent contractors • Decisions about medical technology are part of budget negotiations between insurance funds and providers	• Hospitals are independent non-profit trusts; service delivery on basis of contracts, embedded in centralized structures with performance management and planning • Hospital doctors are public employees, GPs work as independent entrepreneurs in public primary care trusts • Decisions about medical technology by regional government agencies based on local applications within central framework	• Most hospitals are run by regional governments; service delivery subject to national framework and monitoring • Most hospital doctors and GPs (working in health centres) are public employees • Decisions on medical technology on a case-by-case basis by regional governments

(Continued)

(Continued)

2 Looking at the development of health care expenditure between 1980 and 2009, rank countries in order of the relative increase in percentage of GDP spent on health care.

- What is the difference in percentage points between the country at the top and the bottom of the list?
- Are countries spread evenly or do they cluster into separate groups? Are there any clear outliers?

3 Using your analysis of OECD health expenditure data, list those observations you find particularly interesting, striking and/or surprising. Use this as a basis for formulating two or three research questions, which you feel require further comparative analysis.

With your questions for comparative research in mind, read the summaries in Table 21.2 of the health systems in Britain, Germany and Sweden. Based on the summaries, make a list of the factors relating to the organization of health care and the state, which facilitate and mitigate against successful cost containment respectively.

Designing a comparative study of cost containment policies: With your insight into the factors making for more/less successful health care cost containment in mind, re-read the research questions you have formulated and address the following issues:

1 Which one research question do you think is the most important and why?

2 Which two countries would it be most useful to compare to answer your research question and why?

3 What additional aspects of the institutional context for health care provision would you look at in each of the countries you have chosen, and why do you think these are important in answering your research question?

Recommended Further Reading

Blank, R.H. and Burau, V. (2010) *Comparative Health Policy*, 3rd edition. Basingstoke: Palgrave Macmillan.
This introductory comparative text analyses key issues in health policy from a research viewpoint and assesses how far policy problems and responses in different countries have common or diverse origins.

Freeman, R. and Frisina, L. (2010) 'Health care systems and the problem of classification', *Journal of Comparative Policy Analysis*, 12: 163–78.
This recent article discusses the strengths and weaknesses of different approaches to understanding the country-specific contexts of health care and health policies.

Mabbett, D. and Bolderson, H. (1999) 'Theories and methods in comparative social policy', in J. Clasen (ed.), *Comparative Social Policy: Concepts, Theories and Methods*. Oxford: Blackwell.
This chapter discusses different approaches to comparative international research and the implications of the comparative approach for the research process.

 ## Online Readings

Sussman, J., Barbera, L., Bainbridge, D., Howell, D., Yang, J., Husain, A., Librach, S., Viola, R. and Walker, H. (2012) 'Health system characteristics of quality care delivery: A comparative case study examination of palliative care for cancer patients in four regions in Ontario, Canada', *Palliative Medicine*, 26: 322–35.
What type of comparative research is this (see PPS2/3)? What are key features of this methodological approach? How useful was comparative research in this context?

Astin, F., Atkin, K. and Darr, A. (2008) Family support and cardiac rehabilitation: A comparative study of the experiences of South Asian and White-European patients and their carer's living in the United Kingdom', *European Journal of Cardiovascular Nursing*, 7: 43–51.
What type of comparative research is this (see PPS21.2/21.3)? How useful was comparative research in this context?

References

Barbour, R.S. (2010) 'Using qualitative methods in comparative research', *Salute e Società*, 9: 65–79.

Blank, R.H. and Burau, V. (2010) *Comparative Health Policy*, 3rd edition. Basingstoke: Palgrave Macmillan.

Burau, V. (1999a) 'Occupational governance and the dynamics of change: a comparative analysis of nursing in Britain and Germany', PhD thesis, University of Edinburgh.

Burau, V. (1999b) 'The politics of internal boundaries: a comparative analysis of community nursing in Britain and Germany. Some preliminary observations', in I. Hellberg, M. Saks and C. Benoit (eds), *Professional Identities in Transition: Cross-cultural Dimensions*. Södertälje: Almqvist & Wiksell.

Burau, V. (2005) 'Comparing professions through actor-centred governance: community nursing in Britain and Germany', *Sociology of Health and Illness*, 27(1): 114–37.

Burau, V. and Blank, R.H. (2006) 'Comparing health policy: an assessment of typologies of health systems', *Journal of Comparative Policy Analysis*, 8(1): 63–76.

Chamberlayne, P. and King, A. (2000) *Cultures of Care: Biographies of Carers in Britain and the Two Germanies.* Bristol: Policy Press.

Clasen, J. (2004) 'Defining comparative social policy', in Patricia Kennett (ed.), *A Handbook of Comparative Social Policy.* Cheltenham: Edward Elgar.

Collins, R. (1990) 'Changing conceptions in the sociology of professions', in R. Torstendahl and M. Burrage (eds), *The Formation of Professions: Knowledge, State and Strategy.* London: Sage.

Dolowitz, D. and Marsh, D. (1996) 'Who learns what from whom: a review of the policy transfer literature', *Political Studies*, 44: 343–57.

Dunne, R. (2002) 'Will extra billions cure NHS ills?', *BBC News.* Available at: http://news.bbc.co.uk/1/hi/health/1935417.stm

Ebbinghaus, B. (2005) 'When less is more: selection problems in large-N and small-N cross-national comparisons', *International Sociology*, 20: 133–52.

Freeman, R. (1999) 'Institutions, states and cultures: health policy and politics in Europe', in J. Clasen (ed.), *Comparative Social Policy: Concepts, Theories and Methods.* Oxford: Blackwell.

Freeman, R. (2000) *The Politics of Health in Europe.* Manchester: Manchester University Press.

Freeman, R. and Frisina, L. (2010) 'Health care systems and the problem of classification', *Journal of Comparative Policy Analysis*, 12: 163–78.

Glennerster, H. and Matsaganis, M. (1994) 'The English and Swedish health reforms', *International Journal of Health Services*, 24(2): 231–51.

Harrison, M. (2004) *Implementing Change in Health Systems: Market Reforms in the UK, Sweden and the Netherlands.* London. Sage.

Haug, K. (1995) *Arbeitsteilung zwischen Ärzten und Pflegekräften in deutschen und englischen Krankenhäusern oder warum arbeiten doppelt so viel Krankenschwestern pro Arzt in englischen wie in deutschen Krankenhäusern?* Konstanz: Hartung-Gorre.

Hellberg, I., Saks, M. and Benoit, C. (eds) (1999) *Professional Identities in Transition: Cross-cultural Dimensions.* Södertälje: Almqvist & Wiksell.

Huber, M. (1999) 'Health care expenditure trends in OECD countries, 1970–1997', *Health Care Financing Review*, 21(2): 99–117.

Klein, R. (2009) 'Learning from others and learning from mistakes: reflections on health policy making', in T.R. Marmor, R. Freeman and K.G. Okma (eds), *Comparative Studies and the Politics of Modern Medical Care.* New Haven, CT: Yale University Press.

Lijphart, A. (1975) 'The comparable-bases strategy in comparative research', *Comparative Political Studies*, 8(2): 158–77.

Mabbett, D. and Bolderson, H. (1999) 'Theories and methods in comparative social policy', in J. Clasen (ed.), *Comparative Social Policy: Concepts, Theories and Methods.* Oxford: Blackwell.

Mangen, S. (2004) '"Fit for purpose?" Qualitative methods in comparative social policy', in P. Kennett (ed.), *A Handbook of Comparative Social Policy.* Cheltenham: Edward Elgar.

Moran, M. (1999) *Governing the Health Care State: A Comparative Study of the UK, the USA and Germany.* Manchester: Manchester University Press.

OECD (1987) *Financing and Delivering Health Care: A Comparative Analysis of OECD Countries.* Paris: OECD.

OECD (2011) *OECD Health Data 2011: Health Expenditure and Financing.* OECD Health Statistics. Available at: http://dx.doi.org/10.1787/hlthxp-total-table-2011-1-en

Øvretveit, J. (1998) *Comparative and Cross-cultural Health Research: A Practical Guide.* Abingdon: Radcliffe Medical Press.

Øyen, E. (2004) 'Living with imperfect comparisons', in P. Kennett (ed.), *A Handbook of Comparative Social Policy.* Cheltenham: Edward Elgar.

Peterson, M.A. (1997) 'The limits of social learning: translating analysis into action', *Journal of Health Politics, Policy and Law*, 22(4): 1077–114.

Raffel, M.W. (ed.) (1997) *Health Care and Reform in Industrialized Countries.* University Park, PA: Pennsylvania State University Press.

Rose, R. (2000) 'What can we learn from abroad?', *Parliamentary Affairs*, 53: 628–43.

Schmid, A., Cacace, M., Götze, R. and Rothgang, H. (2010) 'Explaining health care system change: problem pressure and the emergence of "hybrid" health care systems', *Journal of Health Politics, Policy and Law*, 35: 455–86.

Stargardt, T. (2008) 'Health service costs in Europe: cost and reimbursement of primary hip replacement in nine countries', *Health Economics*, 17(1): S9–20.

Vanhaecht, K., Bollmann, M., Bower, K., Gallagher, C., Gardini, A., Guzeo, J., et al. (2006) 'Prevalence and use of clinical pathways in 23 countries: an international survey by the European Pathway Association', *Journal of Integrated Care Pathways*, 10: 28–34.

Verspohl, I. (2012) *Health Care Reforms in Europe: Convergence Towards a Market Model?* Baden-Baden: Nomos.

Wilsford, D. (1994) 'Path dependency, or why history makes it difficult but not impossible to reform health care systems in a big way', *Journal of Public Policy*, 14: 251–83.

World Health Organization (WHO) (2000) *The World Health Report 2000. Health Systems: Improving Performance.* Geneva: WHO.

PART V
Applying Health Research

22

Mixed Methods and Multidisciplinary Research in Health Care

JONATHAN TRITTER

Introduction

- The key aim of this chapter is to examine the benefits and limitation of mixed methods and multidisciplinary research in health care and the implications these have for project management. This will include describing mixed methods and multidisciplinary research; outlining the strengths and weakness of mixed methods and multidisciplinary research; considering the implications for research design and project management; and providing an illustrative example and a problem-solving exercise.
- Increasingly, those who fund research and publishers of professional journals require health research that is based on data collected through different methods and draws on expertise from both the biomedical and social sciences. A project may draw on physiological measurement and epidemiological data, as well as data that explore people's understanding of their illness – collected, for example, from illness diaries or narratives. As researchers, one of the initial questions we face in designing a study is the nature and type of data we wish to collect and the methods we use to do so – and frequently projects use a range of different methods and types of data. These data often require analysis using various disciplinary frames of reference and knowledge. This chapter explores some of the reasons for adopting mixed methods in research and illustrates a number of typical research designs. It identifies some of the difficulties that can arise in multidisciplinary research and suggests ways of meeting the challenge. Fundamental to this is careful forethought and a strategic approach to research.

Mixing Methods: Some Typical Approaches

Beginning with qualitative enquiries

As earlier chapters have discussed, different research methods are associated with different kinds of research question. However, the same method may serve different purposes depending on the order in which it is applied within a research project. Often research in an area about which little is known begins with an open approach that seeks to identify relevant issues or topics. Exploratory research rarely has explicit questions or a hypothesis to be tested. Instead, these are developed in the initial phase using a qualitative method such as observation, in-depth interviews or focus group discussions. This should yield the key dimensions that can then be used to frame a later stage of the project that will adopt other methods.

For example, we know from epidemiological studies that asthma has become more prevalent, and the incidence is increasing among children. In order to understand the experience of children with asthma of different ages, say in secondary schools, initially research might begin with observing playground activities or physical education lessons. Another approach might be to convene a number of focus groups to include children of the same age for a discussion of how they think asthma affects their life in school. Each strategy would yield different information, but both provide a way of identifying key issues for research participants. Other methods could be used to measure these more precisely.

Interviews or focus group discussions can also help to develop and refine research instruments. For example, the focus group discussion could be used to identify five key areas where children felt their school experience was affected by asthma. These could provide a basis for an unstructured interview topic guide or be used to design a questionnaire.

This type of approach can ensure that research is grounded in the experience of those who are the object of study. Research that builds on the health needs expressed by a population group being studied is especially relevant when the objective is to evaluate or develop a health service. It has been argued that the increased policy emphasis on user involvement in research (Lowes and Hulatt 2005) and on patient and public participation in health policy (Tritter and McCallum 2006) may privilege studies that adopt such approaches.

Laying the groundwork with quantitative methods

A different approach is to undertake a survey of a sample population to establish the frequency of a certain phenomenon. Using the example of asthma from above, a survey could be used initially to identify the number of children with asthma in secondary schools in a given area. The data could then be used to provide a sampling frame to identify a sample for further investigation. We might be interested in how children of different ages in different schools experienced and managed their illness. We could use the survey data to identify a sample of children that was stratified according to age, school and gender and use this to invite children to a focus group or interview. The second qualitative phase of the research would explore the meaning of illness for these children – a very different type of research question than prevalence.

The ethnography and case study approach

Some research approaches such as ethnography and case studies are dependent on using mixed methods. Ethnography relies on observation as an essential aspect of its methods toolkit, but this is typically augmented by interviews, focus groups and sometimes surveys. Similarly, case study research is premised on collecting multiple forms of data. This may include a critical review of organizational literature, observation and interviews. For both of these instances, the convergence of multiple sources of evidence is the key to obtaining more rounded and, arguably, more valid findings – as increasingly endorsed in the multitude of recent research texts on mixed and multidisciplinary methods (see, for example, Pope et al. 2007; Tashakkori and Teddlie 2010; Cresswell and Plano Clark 2011).

Research design and mixed methods

The various ways that different kinds of research methods can be combined have been outlined. The order and combination of methods must be planned carefully to accrue maximum benefit. Simply applying a range of methods to a research problem – a shotgun approach – is likely to yield little additional benefit. The particular research problem or question must be determined first. It is only after such decisions are made that actual methods and research instruments can be defined, evaluated and adopted.

An important consideration in a mixed-method research design is the intended relationship between the types of data to be collected. Most designs rely on data collected in an early research phase to influence later phases, through the definition of a sample or the development of a research instrument. A further vital issue is how different kinds of data collected from different sources can be integrated analytically. Furthermore, it is important to consider at an early stage how research findings that draw on different forms of data will be presented in a final report.

Triangulation

The use of multiple sources of data is one of the principles behind the notion of triangulation. Triangulation, a navigational term based on using two bearings to locate an object, has been used in two ways in the social sciences. In the first, the term has been used to imply that the aggregation of data from different sources can validate a particular truth, account or finding (see Denzin 1970). In the second, multiple methods can be used in order to gain a greater understanding of a particular phenomenon – it can be seen from a number of different perspectives, each of which is defined by a particular method. Triangulation is used in the latter sense here. Collecting different kinds of data (for example, first-person accounts of an experience, observational video, survey data from participants and focus groups with participants) provides the opportunity to build a holistic understanding of the object of study. It does not attempt to privilege one account over another. The account given of a phenomenon through different methods will be based on a particular theory and the structure and meaning provided by that perspective (see Silverman 2011).

The application of a coordinated analysis of a common data set using a range of different analytical perspectives is another aspect of triangulation. This might involve a series of interview transcripts being analysed independently from a sociological, political science and psychological perspective. The findings from the three different analyses of the same data set, when brought together, reveal more than the application of any single analytical framework. Similarly, a number of analysts who agree a common coding framework can then independently apply this to all of the data before meeting to reach a consensus on interpretation and findings can also lead to far more robust results.

Another variation is where a research team includes a number of researchers from more diverse disciplinary backgrounds who independently analyse and interpret different types of data, quantitative and qualitative, and thereby gain a far more in-depth understanding of phenomena being studied which is then seen from different perspectives (Patton 2002; Yin 2009). The challenge posed of writing up results is discussed in the next chapter.

The Value of Multidisciplinary Research in Health Care

Towards a more holistic approach to health

The impact of lifestyle and the importance of patient participation in decisions about health care are now recognized as key aspects in ensuring good health. It is also acknowledged that chronic conditions and recovery from trauma or illness can be managed more successfully with patient and carer participation. No longer can health outcomes be simply understood as the product of medical intervention or pharmaceutical treatment alone. How patients access services, the ways they participate in decisions about treatment and the social context in which they are treated, live and work are all important to health outcomes. The implication of this 'holistic' model of health for research is that a number of different disciplines and research methods are required to study the impact of health and illness.

For instance, smoking is associated with many millions of deaths worldwide annually. Smoking changes the metabolism and retards healing. Therefore, smoking cessation is important from a public health perspective, and is also recommended as part of the 'treatment' for many medical conditions from asthma to coronary heart disease (Mackay and

Eriksen 2002). But there is no way to 'prescribe' smoking cessation, or to understand the meaning of smoking, without considering the social context and the lifestyle of the patient (Copeland 2003).

Another factor leading to a more holistic view of health and, inter alia, the importance of research using mixed methods and a multidisciplinary approach, is the recognition of the impact of long-term, chronic conditions on health expenditure. This has placed greater emphasis on the possibilities for professional/patient partnership and on day-to-day self-management. The adoption of the Expert Patient Programme by the NHS is one example of this (Department of Health 2001). The programme is a development from an earlier initiative developed at Stanford University in the USA and now covers an estimated 13,000 patients, providing support and training for patients to manage their own condition.

This broader view of health has in turn contributed to an interest in, and acceptance of, patient narratives as an important method and type of data in designing health services. Patient narratives take many forms, but in general they provide a temporal framework for the patient experience and help people to explore the impact, meaning and understanding of their illness experience and how this affects broader social networks and lived experience (Kleinman 1988; Frid et al. 2000; Bury 2001). The use of patient narratives and the study of patient pathways or journeys through the illness and treatment process put further pressure on health care to be more human and holistic (Carlick and Biley 2004). Furthermore, acknowledging the value of qualitative research in health in terms of providing access to the patient experience is potentially an effective mechanism for increasing patient satisfaction and their willingness to follow medical advice. This may be one factor behind the increasing acceptance of qualitative methods among physicians.

At a more macro policy level, the Wanless report (2004) on future health strategy in the UK urges the government and the NHS to pursue a 'fully engaged scenario' in order to mitigate the impact of chronic illness, and to ensure that all members of the public feel responsible for their health and are encouraged to act in ways that work with, rather than against, clinicians. This is a challenge for the researcher as it implies a reconceptualization of 'health work' as an activity that takes place both outside and inside clinical settings.

The consequences for researchers of a holistic approach

The implication for researchers is that research methods suited to exploring lifestyle and the experiential aspects of health care, as well as classic epidemiological data about incidence, morbidity and mortality, are required. Researchers must also consider various types of theoretical and conceptual frameworks to explain their findings. Clinical knowledge must be integrated with social science expertise as well as other disciplines, such as history and statistics, in order to explore and understand contemporary health care. Multidisciplinary research in health care is challenging as it goes against historical hierarchies of knowledge in medical care. Researchers must now attempt to draw in the range of health professionals who are concerned with diagnosing, treating and caring for people. These factors indicate increased complexity in the research process and underline the importance of good research management if high quality work is to be undertaken (O'Cathain et al. 2008).

Research credibility

For research to have an impact on policy, on practice and on the thinking of professionals and academics, the findings must be credible. Many factors affect credibility, such as the research methods used; the findings and outcomes from research; the reputation of researchers; the status of the funding body; and the peer review process. The most fundamental factor is the first: the logic of the design, the management and process of the research, the methods used to collect data and their link to research questions, and acceptance of the analytical framework adopted. These will all affect the perceived validity of the findings. The degree of fit or triangulation between the findings when using different methods is an important mechanism for ensuring acceptance of research findings.

Multiple forms of data derived from different methods, but analysed and interpreted in an integrated fashion, are now seen to yield greater validity. However, in biomedical circles, as noted elsewhere in this volume, the randomized controlled trial (RCT) is still seen as representing the most powerful form of research evidence. The RCT yields quantitative statistically validated results but, as suggested in Chapter 2, it constructs physiological and social factors in a very particular way. The lack of recognition of epistemological differences is at the heart of some of the difficulties in integrating qualitative and quantitative data.

The credibility accorded different kinds of data is a reflection of different disciplinary cultures. The dominance of quantitative data and the RCT is in part a consequence of their centrality to epidemiology and medical training that draws on bioscience. This creates a culture in which issues of sampling, the representativeness of a sample and generalization are central to the evaluation of research findings. These criteria are antithetical to qualitative methods and interpretive data analysis. It is worth noting that in health care many of the decisions are made by a managerial or policy elite who may not be clinically trained. In the past, the longstanding bias of decision makers for 'hard' quantitative data with numerical measures of outcomes and effects is well known (Bowling 2009). This has undermined the opportunity for qualitative and mixed-method research to make a significant impact on health planning and policy, although it is worth noting that there were significant exceptions – for example, the work of Stacey on the care of children in hospitals (Stacey et al. 1970; Hall and Stacey 1979).

Despite this dominant tradition, there is growing appreciation of the value of other methods and multiple-methods research. Dixon-Woods et al. (2001) and Donovan et al. (2002) argue that qualitative, and quality of life, measures should be integrated into RCTs. It is also apparent that, increasingly, articles published in health journals adopt a mix of methods. Similarly, it has been recognized that multiple methods employed by a multidisciplinary research team are likely to maximize the opportunities to present a study and research findings as legitimate and valid. One of the values of a multidisciplinary research team is the familiarity with a range of audiences and dissemination routes. This will enable a tailoring of the findings and a presentation of the research design that is more appropriate and acceptable to different kinds of research consumers. Indeed, many research funders actively encourage multidisciplinarity (for example, the National Institute of Health Research in the UK, the Wellcome Trust and the National Institutes of Health in the US). The definition of multidisciplinary research teams varies for funders and maybe centres on the inclusion of health economists and epidemiologists with clinical researchers, but increasingly recognizes the strength of research collaborations between the social and medical sciences (see, for instance, Øvretveit 2009).

CASE STUDY

Mixed methods and multidisciplinary research in practice

An example of a project highlighting the benefits of mixed methods and multidisciplinary research is *Developing and Evaluating Best Practice in User Involvement in Cancer Services*, which was part of the UK Health in Partnership initiative that the author led between 2000 and 2003. It provides a good example of a collaborative project that used a variety of methods and relied on the participation of a range of organizations, as well as managers, health professionals, service users and academic researchers from a number of disciplinary backgrounds. The project was funded by the Department of Health over a three-year period, and was based at Avon, Somerset and Wiltshire Cancer Services. Two universities, the West of England and Warwick, and two voluntary organizations, the Bristol Cancer Help Centre and Cancerlink Macmillan, collaborated in the project as did a number of NHS Trusts. Drawing on the different expertise of the academic, voluntary sector and health service partners, the project aimed to identify how user involvement was understood and practised within one cancer network. Specifically, it aimed to:

- Identify the variety of definitions of user involvement and methods that had been used by different health organizations and multidisciplinary cancer teams.
- Develop a consensus statement on user involvement in cancer services that could be supported by a range of stakeholders.
- Explore the impact of user involvement on both providers and users.
- Document the influence of user involvement in training and support programmes.
- Identify facilitators and barriers to success in user involvement activities and find examples of good practice.

The research team adopted different research methods to fulfil these aims and research tasks were disaggregated into five phases that are described below.

Mapping user involvement activities across the network

The first task was to undertake a mapping exercise of existing mechanisms for user involvement in cancer services in the region. We focused on activity in the health

(Continued)

(Continued)

service and the cancer voluntary sector, but also collected data from hospices and local government. Focus group discussions were used to construct two question-naires: one for the voluntary and one for the statutory sector. These were then piloted extensively. In late 2000, the statutory questionnaire was administered to 65 individuals with a 68 per cent response rate. In early 2001, 70 local voluntary organizations providing support services were sampled from a database and the questionnaire administered in January 2001. The response rate was 57 per cent. From the data, a range of different definitions of user involvement was identified. The analysis also showed the scope of user involvement and provided examples of implementation across the cancer network.

Consensus development around user involvement

In the second phase, we undertook a formal consensus development exercise apply-ing both a two-stage Delphi exercise and the Nominal Group Technique to obtain information. Bowling (2009) describes these techniques (see also Daykin et al. 2002). She sees the Delphi technique as an efficient way of getting information from a large number of people. A postal questionnaire asking open-ended questions on a topic is sent to a range of experts who give answers anonymously. Their responses are recycled into a questionnaire and participants are asked to rank their level of agreement with the ranking. In the nominal group, or expert panel, process a small number of experts (around 12) decide their individual views on a topic or health inter-vention by ranking factors on a Likert scale from 0 (never use) to 9 (always use). At a subsequent meeting and sometimes after reading additional literature, the results are summarized, discussion takes place and panel members re-rank their views. In the cancer project, the techniques were used to agree a consensus statement on best practice in user involvement in cancer care. We drew on the expertise of 367 individuals from key stakeholder groups such as cancer doctors, managers, general practitioners, cancer nurses, users, cancer voluntary organizations and academic researchers. Our final statement identified nine key aspects that all participants agreed were central to user involvement.

Interviews with users about their experience of involvement

In the third phase, we undertook interviews with users about their understanding, experience and satisfaction with user involvement. Our sample of 37 users of cancer services included three groups: those with experience of user involvement; those who had taken part in a training programme alongside health professionals; and those with no experience. The interviews allowed us to explore factors that contributed to users' conceptions of what it meant to be involved and their level of satisfaction.

A survey of users' willingness to be involved

In the fourth phase based on the above interviews, a questionnaire was developed to survey users' attitudes towards involvement and their willingness to contribute to the evaluation and development of cancer services in the future. A random sample of 700 users that met particular inclusion/exclusion criteria was extracted from cancer registry data. The accuracy of the data was checked against patient records and, with approval from clinicians, 388 users were surveyed in the summer of 2002. The response rate was 67 per cent. The survey was the first to give an indication of the proportion of cancer patients who were willing to be involved in service development, and the factors that affect willingness to participate, such as demographic characteristics, cancer type and the level of satisfaction with care received. Based on a verified random sample of 388 surviving cancer patients drawn from the Regional Cancer Registry database in January 2002, 19 per cent had some experience of contributing to service development. Of these, 71 per cent said they would be willing to be involved again. Almost half (49%) of those who had no experience said they would be willing to participate in the future (Evans et al. 2003).

Selected case studies of a cancer multidisciplinary team in three Trusts

The fifth phase of the study aimed to understand the differences in the interpretation, attitude and experience of user involvement within different trusts, and within the multidisciplinary teams responsible for treating different types of cancer. We conducted case studies in three trusts, one in each of the health authorities covered by the cancer network and with varying levels of user involvement. In each setting, we looked at the multidisciplinary teams delivering services to people with the same range of cancers – breast, colorectal, lung and prostate cancer – as well as palliative care. Key providers and managers were interviewed to establish policy, rationale and practice and those data were used to evaluate the user involvement system against criteria developed in the earlier stages of the project and from the literature.

Project management

This project also highlights the importance of project management in mixed methods and multidisciplinary research. Members of the team came from different disciplines and were employed by different organizations outside of the project. Specific roles were established within the team to ensure appropriate management and support for researchers and administrative staff associated with the project. We set up a steering group to include service users. Following advertisements in local media and surgeries and clinics, two users agreed to serve although only one stayed throughout the project. We paid a monthly fee to users to cover reading and preparation, and an additional fee for attending the steering group and associated travel costs. Time was allowed for discussion with cancer service users before and after meetings to keep them well briefed.

Much of the research in health necessarily involves working in a clinical context and with clinical colleagues. A major benefit of working in a clinical setting with a multidisciplinary team is the virtually open access it brings to health care professionals and to patients and patient data that would otherwise require lengthy negotiation. In particular, access to medical staff and medical networks can bring great benefits to the research process. From negotiating research ethics committees to gaining agreement from staff to participate in interviews or identify potential respondents, medical personnel add legitimacy to a research team. These benefits are often

(Continued)

(Continued)

directly related to the seniority as well as the discipline of the staff member. In health care settings, status differentiation still runs along professional lines. For example, having the senior cancer consultant and ex-director of the Oncology Centre working in one of our projects helped to identify the names and location of key clinical managers within the eight area hospitals in the study. His experience of working in the local area for 20 years and his high profile in cancer care nationally helped to ensure that the team were well prepared when seeking access, as well as providing credibility to the project.

The Challenges of, and Strategies for, Multidisciplinary Working

The experience of working on a multidisciplinary project suggests that a number of common difficulties and challenges arise when working across different institutional and disciplinary cultures.

Workplace style and culture

A culture may be so embedded in a workplace that members of a work team may be unaware that their working lives are governed by particular norms until these norms are breached. There were a number of occasions when this occurred on the cancer project. For example, the research team were based in local health authority accommodation provided for cancer network administrative staff. Researchers had access to a 'hot-desk' in a large room shared by the administrative staff. Local researchers spent considerable time out of the office collecting data or attending meetings. The administrative staff kept to health service working hours, arriving at 8.30 a.m. and leaving at 5.00 p.m. Researchers were accustomed to looser academic timetables. One team member, anxious to meet a writing deadline, completed a report at 8.00 p.m., only to find all the lights turned off in the building and the main entrance locked. They were only released after contacting the off-site security company.

Differences in the work cultures of academe and the public sector were evident in the case of whether employees were required to have a physical presence in the workplace or not. For example, in the health service, people were only deemed to be working if they were visibly present at the desk or clinic. In academe, more emphasis is placed on work outputs and there is a greater degree of flexibility on where and when work is done. Management styles between the health service and academe also differed. Initially on the project, there was pressure for a directive and bureaucratic form of project management, in which critical dialogue about the direction and progress of the research was seen as rebellion. It was also expected that reports and potential publications would be vetted – possibly because there was fear of repercussions from above in response to negative comments on findings or process. Conversely, the academic culture tends to be based on a high degree of autonomy and less hierarchical colleague relationships. Critical comment is expected and valued.

Over time, team members became aware of different expectations and sensitivities and sufficient trust was built to reach accommodation on the requirements of the various cultures of employment. However, multidisciplinary projects need to anticipate and allow for such learning.

Balancing the research team

In developing a research proposal, balancing the composition of the project team with the requirements of the research design is one of the primary objectives. Projects that adopt mixed methods are likely to incorporate researchers from a range of disciplines. The specialization of individuals in particular methods may be a key justification for their inclusion in a research team. However, this can lead to a series of separate mini-research projects, each of which has been conducted independently. Such an approach may serve as a barrier to a common conceptualization of the research problem and the opportunity to adopt an integrated approach to the analysis and the interpretation of data. The benefits of using different methods and data through triangulation may be lost and this in turn may undermine the validity of the research findings.

The challenge for research management

The difficulties of research management are likely to be increased when research teams come from different institutions and/or there is a separation of research responsibilities. Inevitably, members of research teams who have had little history of working together and are drawn from different disciplinary backgrounds and work contexts will have different experiences and expectations of how to conduct research. Furthermore, applied research may be based on collaboration with staff who have little experience of research. Their expectations may be very different from those of the project team and funders. Lack of knowledge about work cultures, responsibilities and styles of working can lead to confusion, disagreements and inefficiency. Good project management, regular team meetings and investment of time in creating a common conceptualization of the whole project, the contribution of each objective to the project as a whole and their relationship to each other, are the best way to avoid fragmentation.

Many projects establish an advisory group as an aid to project management. Typically, such groups include representatives of stakeholders such as user groups, funding bodies, statutory authorities or independent experts with particular skills. These can be useful sources of advice and data for a project but can also add layers of communication that increase the administrative workload and may slow down decision making. It is important to establish roles and responsibilities at the start. Furthermore, the research team should be clear on what they want from an advisory group and prepare well for meetings.

Writing up results in multidisciplinary teams

The process of writing up and the attribution of authorship vary significantly between disciplines. For example, it is common in scientific disciplines for authorship to include the entire research team, while in the social sciences team members are credited in the text but do not necessarily appear as authors. As other chapters in this book point out, issues of authorship can cause unhappiness and conflict, so they are best tackled early. For a long-term project, items written late in the life of a project may cause particular difficulties. Junior members of the team may have left to take up other posts. Certain kinds of funding may not include time to write up findings for publication. Wherever possible, this should be costed and written into research proposals – as discussed further in Chapter 23.

Moving from multidisciplinary to interdisciplinary research

The issues raised above highlight the different forms of collaboration in research and also suggest the distinction between multidisciplinary, interdisciplinary and trans-disciplinary projects (see Rosenfield 1992). Both interdisciplinary and trans-disciplinary research are premised on working through differences in perspective and arriving at a consensus on an approach that is acceptable methodologically to all team members. The resulting research will be far more integrated and coherent and have greater potential to yield methodologically interesting results. However, interdisciplinary research requires a great deal of time and contact early on in the project, in order to learn about and from the different members of the research team. Multidisciplinary research will yield important results but they will be different from those emerging from interdisciplinary work.

Research that has an international aspect, because the study either draws data from different countries or involves researchers from different national backgrounds, presents particular challenges. Language differences themselves may make communication or comprehension difficult. If data are sourced in different languages, the costs of translation must be taken into account. Translation may hide rather than reveal different underlying cultural assumptions. The example in Box 22.1 describes an international project and provides an illustration of some of the cross-cultural and cross-national issues that arise.

Box 22.1   Example: Globalization and citizens in health care

Exploring the role of users, choice and markets in European health systems

This project aimed to explore the impact of health care reforms in Finland, Britain and Sweden on competition, marketization, patient choice and user involvement within the context of the European Union and international legal regulation, as reflected in the policies promoted by the Organization for Economic Cooperation and Development, the World Health Organization and the World Trade Organization. The project was funded by the Academy of Finland.

The majority of the research team were fluent in three languages: Finnish, Swedish and English. The language used within the team was English, but reports to the funder needed to be made in Finnish. The Advisory Group included Finnish, Swedish and British experts. The approach to policy making differed between the three countries and so did the scope of publicly available documentation. Furthermore, the same pieces of European Union legislation had been implemented at different rates and with different outcomes and effects.

Cultural differences added to the complexity. For example, August tends to be a public sector holiday month in Britain. In Finland and other Nordic countries, however, this is considered early autumn and July is the main summer holiday month. The scheduling of interviews at the same time over the summer period was therefore difficult.

Conclusion

The use of a range of methods in a single research project is becoming more common, as indeed is the multidisciplinary and international research explored in this chapter. Indeed, many of the chapters in this book illustrate these themes and Chapter 21 is devoted to the challenge of comparative research. Using mixed methods and working with colleagues both nationally and internationally can be achieved in small-scale as well as larger projects. There are both benefits and pitfalls and, as the research process becomes more complex, managing and planning the process becomes a major task.

In terms of using a number of methods in a single project, as argued in this chapter, it is extremely important to consider the purpose and value of employing particular methods when planning a project. The epistemological status of the data collected, that is the nature of data and the kind of knowledge produced, should also be considered. Where different methods are used, the purpose and added value to understanding should be examined carefully. A crucial decision to be made is the order of data collection using different methods. As has been demonstrated here and in other chapters, there may be an argument for first using a qualitative method such as a focus group or in-depth interviews, to explore the concepts and understandings of the research participants. The insights gained may then be incorporated into a questionnaire to test the generalizability of a hypothesis or frequency of occurrence. However, there may also be an argument for an initial questionnaire to explore the frequency of a particular phenomenon, followed by, for example, in-depth interviews to investigate a different aspect of the phenomenon. A variety of combinations is possible, but it is vital that the reason for using a particular combination of methods and the associated value added are clear and that they fall within the available budget. An exercise follows to facilitate further understanding of some of the issues raised in this chapter.

Exercise: Mixed methods and multidisciplinary research application to develop support for people with coronary heart disease

You want to apply to a regional government office to consider how the experience of carers could be used to develop support for people who have coronary heart disease.

The exercise is designed to make you think about how to design research using mixed methods and drawing on multidisciplinary expertise. While the material contained in this chapter may help you consider many of the issues, you may wish to access additional material from a library or the Internet. If you want to prepare a formal answer, then write a research proposal or protocol.

1 What sort of methods will you use?

Consider the range of possible respondents and sources of information (this will include patients, carers, voluntary organizations, health professionals and information leaflets).

Consider the patient pathway and how you will ensure that your data reflect the needs of people at different points in their journey through the illness and care process.

2 How will you select the sources of data that are relevant?

Consider what sort of methods you want to use.

How will you manage generalizability?

3 How will you bring together the analysis of different kinds of data?

What forms of coding and analysis will be appropriate for each?

What mechanisms will you use to create a common analytical framework and the opportunity for joint interpretation of the findings?

4 What sort of resources will you need?

Can you plot the different activities over time and in relation to resources?

How do various types of project meetings fit into this timetable?

5 How will you present your findings and to whom?

What would be your plan for dissemination?

What are the implications for authorship?

How would you begin to cost your proposal?

Recommended Further Reading

Dixon-Woods, M., Fitzpatrick, R. and Roberts, K. (2001) 'Including qualitative research in systematic reviews: opportunities and problems', *Journal of Evaluation in Clinical Practice*, 7: 125–33.
This is an interesting consideration of how qualitative and quantitative evidence can be synthesized together and influence clinical practice.

Strauss, A. and Corbin, J. (eds) (1997) *Grounded Theory in Practice*. London: Sage.
This book engages explicitly with the issues of integrating the analysis of different kinds of data – exemplified by different research projects with diverse designs and objects of study.

Yin, R. (2009) *Case Study Research: Design and Methods*, 4th edition. London: Sage.
This definitive book on the case study as a form of research usefully illustrates how to bring together a range of methods to generate a holistic understanding of specific areas.

Online Readings

Mayoh, J., Bond, C. and Todres, L. (2012) 'An innovative mixed methods approach to studying the online health information seeking experiences of adults with chronic health conditions', *Journal of Mixed Methods Research*, 6: 21–33.
Why was a mixed methods approach appropriate in this context? What are the key elements of the approach as outlined in this paper?

Austin, W., Park, C. and Goble, E. (2008) 'From interdisciplinary to transdisciplinary research: A case study', *Qualitative Health Research*, 18: 557–64.
Why was a transdisciplinary approach appropriate in this context? What are the key elements of the approach as outlined in this paper? What barriers did the authors face? How did they overcome them?

References

Bowling, A. (2009) *Research Methods in Health: Investigating Health and Health Services*, 3rd edition. Buckingham: Open University Press.

Bury, M. (2001) 'Illness narratives: fact or fiction?', *Sociology of Health and Illness*, 23: 263–85.

Carlick, A. and Biley, F.C. (2004) 'Thoughts on the therapeutic use of narrative in the promotion of coping in cancer care', *European Journal of Cancer Care*, 13(4): 308–17.

Copeland, L. (2003) 'An exploration of the problems faced by young women living in disadvantaged circumstances if they want to give up smoking: can more be done at general practice level?', *Family Practice*, 20(4): 393–400.

Cresswell, J. and Plano Clark, V.L. (2011) *Conducting and Designing Mixed Methods Research*, 2nd edition. Thousand Oaks, CA: Sage.

Daykin, N., Sanidas, M., Barley, V., Evans, S., McNeill, J., Palmer, N. et al. (2002) 'Developing consensus and interprofessional working in cancer services: the case of user involvement', *Journal of Interprofessional Care*, 16(4): 405–6.

Denzin, N. (1970) *The Research Act*. Chicago, IL: Aldine.

Department of Health (2001) *The Expert Patient: A New Approach to Chronic Disease Management in the Twenty-first Century*. London: HMSO. (Progress updates available at: www.expertpatients.nhs.uk/about_progress.shtml)

Dixon-Woods, M., Fitzpatrick, R. and Roberts, K. (2001) 'Including qualitative research in systematic reviews: opportunities and problems', *Journal of Evaluation in Clinical Practice*, 7: 125–33.

Donovan, J., Brindle, L. and Mills, N. (2002) 'Capturing users' experiences of participating in cancer trials', *European Journal of Cancer Care*, 11(3): 210–14.

Evans, S., Tritter, J., Barley, V., Daykin, N., Sanidas, M., McNeill, J. et al. (2003) 'User involvement in UK cancer services: bridging the policy gap', *European Journal of Cancer Care*, 12(4): 331–8.

Frid, I., Ohlen, J. and Bergbom, I. (2000) 'On the use of narrative in nursing research', *Journal of Advanced Nursing*, 32: 695–703.

Hall, D. and Stacey, M. (eds) (1979) *Beyond Separation: Further Studies of Children in Hospital*. London: Routledge & Kegan Paul.

Kleinman, A. (1988) *The Illness Narratives*. New York: Basic Books.

Lowes, L. and Hulatt, I. (eds) (2005) *Involving Service Users in Health and Social Care Research*. London: Routledge.

Mackay, J. and Eriksen, M. (2002) *The Tobacco Atlas*. Geneva: World Health Organization.

O'Cathain, A., Murphy, E. and Nicholl, J. (2008) 'The quality of mixed methods studies in health services research', *Journal of Health Services Research and Policy*, 13: 92–8.

Øvretveit, J. (2009) 'The contribution of new social science research to patient safety', *Social Science and Medicine*, 69(12): 1780–3.

Patton, M. (2002) *Qualitative Research and Evaluation Methods*, 3rd edition. London: Sage.

Pope, C., Mays, N. and Popay, J. (2007) *Synthesizing Qualitative and Quantitative Health Research: A Guide to Methods*. Maidenhead: Open University Press.

Rosenfield, P. (1992) The potential of transdisciplinary research for sustaining and extending linkages between the health and social sciences', *Social Science and Medicine*, 35(11): 1343–57.

Silverman, D. (2011) *Interpreting Qualitative Data: Methods for Analysing Talk, Text and Interaction*, 3rd edition. London: Sage.

Stacey, M., Dearden, R., Pill, R. and Robinson, S. (1970) *Hospitals, Children and their Families*. London: Routledge and Kegan Paul.

Tashakkori, A. and Teddlie, C. (2010) *Handbook of Mixed Methods in Social and Behavioural Research*, 2nd edition. Los Angeles, CA: Sage.

Tritter, J. and McCallum, A. (2006) 'The snakes and ladders of user involvement: moving beyond Arnstein', *Health Policy*, 76(2): 156–68.

Wanless, D. (2004) *Securing Good Health for the Whole Population*. London: HMSO.

Yin, R. (2009) *Case Study Research: Design and Methods*, 4th edition. London: Sage.

23

The Research Process and Writing up Health Research

JUDITH ALLSOP AND MIKE SAKS

Introduction

- In this chapter, we aim to give practical advice on the different stages of the research process and writing up research for publication. The first part of this chapter focuses on the research process from the point that a proposal has been agreed to presenting the completed text for a research-based essay, thesis or doctoral dissertation – or a grander piece of funded research. The process is similar even if the scale and complexity of the tasks differ. The key to carrying out a research project is to see it as a series of stages where decisions have to be made in order to progress. We examine these stages and the choices to be made at each stage and the typical problems that can occur. Reference can be made to previous chapters for more detailed explanations of particular methods and their application. In the first section, the stages used in qualitative and quantitative research will be addressed in turn. Any study using mixed methods will have to account for both.

- The second part of the chapter looks at writing up research reports and publication in journals. This examines the conventions for writing up quantitative methods, qualitative methods and mixed method research. There is some overlap here between the two sections as writing in order to gain an academic qualification is similar to writing for publication. However, there are different

(Continued)

(Continued)

conventions and constraints. In our view, as noted in Chapter 2, completing a research project successfully is as much about good project management skills as intellectual ability. In any project, unexpected difficulties occur from personal life events to barriers to data collection. Flexibility, optimism and seeking help from supervisors or colleagues where appropriate and circumventing sticking points are essential. A clear plan provides a guide and road map to anchor the project. Perseverance is a key factor in writing up. The chapter concludes by again considering questions of ethics in research.

The Research Process

Starting a research essay, dissertation or thesis

You will first need to develop a proposal for your health project (see Offredy and Vickers 2010 for a practical guide for so doing). As will be apparent from this book and other sources, this should be done as effectively as possible (see, among others, Punch 2006; Dawson 2009). Once a proposal has been agreed, you need to put it into operation. This requires foresight and the construction of a plan. A first step is the drawing up of a timetable with an end point – whether this is for a period of two or three months or three or four years for a Masters or PhD (see, for instance, Dunleavy 2003). A timetable will give an outline of what tasks will have to be completed when. This means breaking your research into parts to construct a work programme with a logical structure leading to an end point – the presentation of a written document. It is best to have the timetable on paper and always in view. It will drive production and can be revised during the process of the research as necessary. Your research question should also be on view to prevent straying into areas that are interesting but not relevant. The various chapters in this book and other research texts will provide guidance on particular methods (for example, Green and Thorogood 2004; Bruce et al. 2008). The structure of a long essay, dissertation or thesis is predictable and, perhaps surprisingly, there is little difference in the basic structure of a work that uses quantitative or qualitative methods, although the time devoted to each phase may differ, as discussed below.

The importance of a timetable

As the timescale of projects differs, it is not possible to construct a standard timetable in terms of months and years, but this can be done in the form of a flow chart with the weeks and months along a horizontal axis and the tasks to be completed along the vertical axis. Further recommendations are included in Box 23.1.

Box 23.1   Recommendations for the project timetable

- A quarter of the time could be allocated to carrying out a literature review, refining the research question(s), drawing up a plan and establishing access to respondents and participants.
- About half of the time may need to be devoted to setting up the project in terms of access to respondents or participants, developing research instruments and collecting and analysing data.
- The final quarter of the time could usefully be spent on writing up the final draft. Writing should be continuous throughout with draft memoranda.

Writing up the results of research for an academic qualification is a particular challenge, as it is at the same time a learning exercise. Unexpected problems will arise even in the best planned project. These must be solved pragmatically and quickly with the help of colleagues and supervisors. A comment made frequently by both students and researchers is that not enough time was set aside for writing up.

Once the research question is refined, this then guides the research process. It should be displayed in a prominent place on a wall next to the timetable or on your computer. The other essential piece of equipment at this stage is a research diary and a research notebook. The diary may record, at a minimum, decisions about research design and methods, meetings held and targets met by date. The notebook is for thoughts, comments and references. This is particularly important when using qualitative methods where the research question is less clear. It can be used to record observations and impressions at meetings, libraries visited and sources of data. Both sources will be useful for writing up during, or in the final stages of, a project.

Supervision and identifying gaps in knowledge

As noted above, undertaking research for an extended essay or postgraduate degree is a problem-solving exercise. It is also an exercise in learning from experience and acquiring techniques through research training (see Ramkalawan 2005). Regular supervision and discussion of problems is essential. It is important to write drafts of the sections in the literature review and discuss these with your supervisor. This not only charts what you have done, but also helps you to reflect on the strengths and limitations of your approach. Drawing up a plan to operationalize the methods you decide to use can also be a useful exercise. It may be that you identify a gap in your skills. Either seek help from an expert or set aside time to learn a new skill. Statisticians are usually prepared to help researchers, and time may be taken out to learn how to use SPSS or NVivo computer packages to manage and analyse quantitative or qualitative data. It is also useful to review the sections or chapter outline on a regular basis to provide a foundation for the final writing up. This helps to keep the research question in mind and assists in developing an argument.

It is always useful to keep a draft list of chapters close at hand and to revise these periodically. It is vital to keep your research question in mind as you progress through the various stages of your project. A generic outline of the structure for a dissertation or thesis is shown below in Box 23.2.

Box 23.2   The structure of a dissertation/thesis: an outline

- *Title*: this should be suitably descriptive
- *Abstract:* this should include aims and objectives
- *List of contents*: sections or chapters
- *Introduction:* a brief statement of the research question and the rationale for the research – including what it will add to our understanding
- *Literature review*: what others have said, including key concepts and theories, ideally identifying a gap in the literature
- *Research method*: how data were collected and analysed, with comments on the rationale and research process, including dilemmas and solutions, ethics and how your own position may have influenced your interpretation (reflexive thinking)
- *Results, findings and analyses*: this should including data sections/chapters
- *Discussion*: this should relate to aims, objectives, existing studies, concepts and theories
- *Conclusion*: a summary of what the research has added to knowledge.

Stages in the research process

There are several stages in the research process, as variously outlined in research texts both generally (see, for instance, Cresswell 2009) and in the health field specifically (see, for example, Polgar and Thomas 2008), which will now be considered in turn. These include: literature review, data collection, access to participants and respondents, data analysis, findings, interpretation and discussion. Each one of these is now covered in more detail and is followed by a section on the final stage of the process – writing up.

The literature review

Chapter 3 discusses how to carry out a systematic literature review. Here, the aim is to show with examples, how a literature review contributes to the research process and the part it plays in the final essay, dissertation or thesis. Taraborrelli (1993) reports on how doing a literature review allowed her to develop her research questions. She proposed to do a dissertation on the impact that caring for a relative with dementia had on the lives of women who became informal carers. Her literature review identified various sources of information from large-scale national studies of the demographics and costs of informal care in the UK – studies of how and why people became carers. She noticed a gap in the literature. She did not find any study of the dynamics of caring and how the carer's experiences changed over time as a consequence of the changing level of dependency of those for whom they cared. From her studies in medical sociology, she came across the concept of 'career' – that is, the way in which a movement from one position to another brought different tasks and responsibilities that shaped individuals' motivations and perspectives sequentially. She then reviewed studies using the concept of career and theories of career progression. The aim of the project was to study the career of those who were informal carers of people suffering from Alzheimer's disease, and to explore the objective factors and subjective responses that brought about a 'career' change.

A different kind of literature review would be undertaken by a student who wished to assess the outcome for patients following a heart transplant. One aspect of this would be to review the various instruments for measuring quality of life. Bowling (2001) conducted such a review and commented that there are a wide range of domains of health-related quality of life, including emotional well-being, measured with indicators of life satisfaction and self-esteem; psychological well-being, measured with indicators of anxiety and depression; physical well-being, measured by physical status and physical functioning; and social well-being, measured by social networking and support, community integration and social roles. She concluded that while there was considerable overlap between the different measures available, there was disagreement about what the content should be. A researcher aiming to use these measures would have to assess which measure was most suitable for their project. Bowling suggests that measures are more developed in relation to satisfaction with life among older people, but not younger people.

In summary, students should use the literature review to undertake a critical and analytic investigation against which they can test and refine their ideas. It should help them to sharpen their research question, suggest appropriate methodologies and may even change the direction of their research. A target to aim for is a written commentary on the literature a quarter of the way into a project. This provides a base for additions and revisions during the course of the research. The literature review is a continuous process through the life of a project. It will not include everything, but in the final draft should be structured in a way that provides an explanation of the research question addressed; the logic of the design and methods; and the argument that will be carried through in the substantive chapters on findings/results.

Data collection

Data collection is the core of any research project (Sapsford and Jupp 2006). It may be desk-based or in the field. Three critical decisions must be made during this stage of the project. First, a plan must be devised for establishing access to research subjects. Second, any instruments used for data collection must be designed in advance: examples are schedules for collecting standard information from research participants, drawing up questionnaires and preparing patient information sheets. Any instrument designed should be piloted to test for efficacy. Third, particular equipment may be needed, such as a tape-recorder, and arrangements made for transcription. The various methods of data collection are described in the chapters in Parts II and III of the book and will not be discussed further. Instead, illustrative examples will be given in this chapter of the decisions to be made in different kinds of research.

Access to participants and respondents

Once a research question has been defined with sufficient clarity, the next step is to organize access to participants and respondents, including the institutions of which they are part. If the research method is qualitative, a range of other techniques may be used, such as snowballing, key informants and advertising, as considered in Chapters 4 to 8. In the case of Taraborrelli (1993) cited above, the challenge was to identify a 'rare population' of informal carers of people with Alzheimer's disease. Their domain is a private one. She tried to access people through the local social services department who did not keep a list. Access through the local psychiatric hospital unit would have required approval through the local research ethics committee, a time-consuming process ruled out by the scope of the project. She then tried the Alzheimer's Society, a national voluntary group with local branches. They identified two local support groups for carers who were happy for her to attend meetings. This allowed overt observation of matters relating to the research question and eventually led to identifying a sample of 23 carers to interview. This included both existing carers and ex-carers whose relative had died or had moved to a residential home.

In quantitative research, a researcher carrying out an experiment must determine the criteria for selection or exclusion, as variously explored in Chapters 9 to 14. If the study is an RCT, then a matching control group must be recruited. If human subjects are involved, this will require ethical review, as discussed in Chapter 15. In a study with a cross-sectional design, the sample population to be studied will also have to be identified on the basis of what characteristics or variables the researcher wants to represent and compare – such as sex/gender, age, ethnicity, class and geographical area. The research question will determine selection of the primary and, if necessary, secondary sample. Chapters 9 and 10 consider issues of sampling and sampling frames. If a project has a case study design, the criteria for selection should be stated (Yin 2009). Is it chosen as representative, unique or exemplifying a particular characteristic? For a cross-sectional study, a population with particular characteristics must be identified and a sample drawn. See Box 23.3 below for an example.

Box 23.3 Example: Selecting a sample on satisfaction with health care

The following is an example taken from a study of dissatisfaction with health care undertaken by Mulcahy and Tritter for the Department of Health. The authors rejected accessing a sample through health agencies as they wanted to interview a cross-section of the population. In the first sample, they selected five 'typical' areas on the basis of census data: two from the inner city, two suburban and one rural. A second sampling frame identified zones and clusters of streets within these areas to represent the socio-demographic characteristics of the local population. Representativeness was checked on a weekly basis as the interviews took place. This example illustrates the process of obtaining access and also how the process of deductive and inductive reasoning works. A quantitative researcher is likely to argue for a very clear, simple primary question. Mulcahy and Tritter wanted to identify the incidence of dissatisfaction with health care, the reasons for dissatisfaction and the action taken in response, if any. The method chosen was to undertake a house-to-house survey as it was known from previous research that making a formal complaint is a rare event.

Source: Mulcahy and Tritter (1998)

It is worth noting that in quantitative research designing research instruments is time-consuming and critical to the success of the project. For example, the questionnaire must be designed and a pilot carried out to ensure external validity. In qualitative research, there is more exploratory research, access may pose problems and the question and theoretical framework for analysis may shift during the course of a study, as was the case with the study by Taraborrelli (1993) of informal carers. Data collection in either form of research can also pose problems for which solutions must be found. At this stage, diary entries and note taking are particularly useful for recall. It is strongly recommended that a written draft of the methods is produced at this point. This should cover how access was negotiated, how instruments were designed and how these were fit for purpose in addressing the research question. This will provide a basis for the research methods section/chapter later.

Data analysis

With qualitative data, no matter which way observations are collected, they must be reproduced in written form in a way that can be manipulated. This is a time-consuming process. For example, interviews must be recorded and transcribed. It has been estimated that one hour of interviewing takes six hours to transcribe (Bryman 2012). For documentary analysis, selections of text must be made. Transcriptions are the basis for a thematic analysis of the data which also take time to develop through a process of trial and error.

Many qualitative researchers suggest that a thematic analysis can begin early with a small number of transcripts with modifications and adjustments in the light of subsequent transcripts. The aim is to identify core themes to develop a coding framework (Saldana 2009). The themes are related to the research questions and to theories that can explain recurring patterns. The coding framework is a method for breaking the text down into component parts that are then coded or labelled systematically so that links between codes can be identified within and between transcripts. This establishes recurrences of the ways in which phenomena are understood by participants. Thematic analysis is a way of managing a mass of data by reducing it to a number of interconnected themes to develop a structure that is credible. Systematic differences within themes can also be detected – for example, differences on the basis of gender, class, age or ethnicity.

The process of analysis is an aid to theory building. The literature review, observations and notes taken in the field and sources read contemporaneously will continue to inform the process of analysis until the researcher is satisfied with the coding framework. There is a zigzag between theory and data, during which themes arising from the data are identified (Denzin and Lincoln 2005). Strauss (1987), one of the founding members of the method of analytic induction, recommends analytic memoranda to aid interpretation during data analysis in qualitative research, by writing extended memos on concepts and theories and on themes as they develop during the data collection phase and analysis. For example, a memo on a theme arising in early interviews can be identified, theorized and used to test robustness at a later stage in the research. Memos on the theories used in a conceptual framework, and decisions on how to manage data analysis, should also be recorded.

At this point, a student will have to choose whether to use a data analysis package. There are a number of computer-assisted qualitative data analysis software (CAQDAS) packages which can help in data management by storing segments of data so solving some of the clerical problems in dealing with qualitative data. Coded sequences can be recovered and ordered into categories, making them easier to manipulate. This replaces the old-fashioned method of scissors and paste. In the opinion of Bryman (2012), there is no clear market leader for qualitative data analysis programs but nevertheless he provides a useful introduction to using NVivo.

The example set out in Box 23.3 illustrates the process of identifying a structure in one letter out of a data set of over 100 letters of complaint about general practitioners. The letters were conceptualized as narratives with a temporal structure. The letter below names the practitioner, allocates blame and makes a claim within the context of assumptions about the caring responsibilities of the doctor and carer. The example below shows the codes/labels that were identified and used to apply to the data set as a whole. The method did not fragment the data but maintained the narrative structure of each account. The example in Box 23.4 is included to demonstrate how data can be analysed.

Box 23.4 Example: Complaints about doctors

Theory:

Attribution theory suggests untoward/adverse events are explained by people who use various strategies to allocate responsibility and blame (Antaki and Fielding 1981). Felstiner, Abel and Sarat (1980–1) used the concepts of naming and claiming in their large-scale US study to investigate the trajectory of complaints in different settings. At the time of the study, general practitioners within the National Health Service had particular contractual responsibilities to provide a service.

Codes were used to label different types of allegation related to service obligations (technical breaches) and allegations related to a doctor's behaviour (normative breaches). It became apparent that carers and patients also saw themselves as having caring responsibilities so letters contained defences as well as allegations. These were also coded and theorized in terms of expectations of professional/patient relationships and protecting caring identities.

Example of a coding frame:

I wish to make a complaint about Dr X to Y *[the 'Trust' as the authoritative body]* … my son Matthew (3 years old) *[complainant kin relationship to patient]* … complained of earache … he was holding both ears … a severe headache and crying bitterly *[lay knowledge of mother that the child was ill]*. I tried to … comfort him … [he became] more upset and became hysterical *[good mother, limits of lay knowledge]*. He was … rolling on the floor and holding his head and crying. I rang the surgery and Dr X was speaking on an answerphone service giving an emergency number, which I then rang *[competent lay action taken]*.

Later:

I took Matthew to Dr X's surgery *[lay action to seek medical help]* and Dr X was most annoyed *[allegation of poor social skills]* and said that I had cost him/her £24 by calling the emergency number three times … *[not providing a service, breaking NHS norms]*. I asked him to examine Matthew but he refused saying there was no need *[lay action through request/allegation that help refused]*.

On the basis of the large number of letters, frequencies and deviant cases could be calculated as a way of reducing the data. Both tables and selected typical quotations were used to support the argument (see Bryman 2012 on how to select quotations).

Source: Allsop (1998)

In a research design using quantitative methods, many of the decisions about data analysis are pre-determined as they are integral to the design of an experiment, a sampling frame, a questionnaire and how the latter is pre-coded. The questions included in any structured questionnaire will already be based on implicit assumptions related to the research question and the variables for cross-tabulation to test the hypothesis or research question. Questionnaires, telephone interviews and structured interviews must be logged with dates and responses and reminders. Response rates should be calculated.

Once the data are collected, the next step is to manage the data. In a cross-sectional study using a questionnaire, the data are checked for obvious errors, or 'cleaned' and entered into a data-processing program such as SPSS. Time should also be set aside to learn how to use SPSS or any other data analysis program. This form of research method aims to test the theory so that the way the data will be analysed is already implicit in the questionnaire design. The analysis will reduce the data to tables, figures and graphs showing the relationship between variables and the results of various statistical tests. Further explanation is given in Chapter 11 on how to present quantitative data.

Findings, interpretation and discussion

The presentation of findings and results may constitute a number of sections or chapters in a dissertation or thesis. These form the core of any project. As shown below, there are different conventions about how texts should be presented within the clinical sciences and the social sciences, as well as between quantitative and qualitative methods. Here, we make some general comments on writing for an academic qualification.

If you have already completed drafts of the literature review and the methods used for the research, you are moving towards completing a first draft. In these final sections, you need to be selective and structure the final sections around particular themes, provide descriptions of the research setting, and choose particular themes and extracts from the data to illustrate your argument. You will not be able to include everything so you will have to choose carefully.

In qualitative research, the writer is constructing a credible account that makes sense to the reader. It is better to choose a representative quotation rather than an outlier, unless you are trying to cite something as a deviant case. It is useful to indicate how strong patterns in the data are and how and why you have reached particular conclusions. It can be helpful to use grids or figures to sum up patterns of association. There may well be further theoretically based analysis introduced during the course of the writing up. As Richardson (1990) comments, writing is an aid to thinking and part of the process of discovery and communication. There may also have been adjustments to the initial research question and new theories to explore. One consequence is that the final structure the work will take is less predictable; changes will occur during the writing process; and the period over which drafting takes place is typically longer than with a quantitative study.

In quantitative research, findings will be discussed in relation to tables and graphs and be subject to tests of significance. Again, the challenge is one of selection. What should be included and what left out? A general guide for inclusion is the relevance of data to answering the research question and therefore of contributing to the argument to be made in the discussion and conclusion. It is important to summarize the content of a table, figure or graph and draw attention to the particular aspect of the content that is important for addressing the research question and supporting (or providing contrary evidence to) your argument. You must spell out for the reader what you want them to know and point out the association between variables.

How results or findings and analyses are discussed varies with the discipline, the research design and whether the methods were quantitative, qualitative or mixed. The chapters in this section of a research study should contain summaries and analyses of the data collected. When you are confident that most of the pieces of the jigsaw are in place, you can proceed to writing up a final draft – the last stage of the research process.

Writing Up Health Research

The basic task of writing up

When you are ready to move to a final draft of your research-based project, thesis or dissertation, find out what the requirements are for presenting your project and follow them exactly: the form of presentation, length, style of referencing, footnotes, endnotes, bibliography, appendices, time limits for presentation, viva arrangements, and so on. These will usually be available in written form (Schober and Farrington 2000). Conventions for presentation vary between the clinical and social sciences and also between disciplines in the health field. Those publishing in the clinical sciences are expected to undertake a systematic review to contextualize the study (Greenhalgh 2010). In the social sciences, where positivist methodologies and quantitative methods are used, reports may follow the scientific model of aims, methods, results and discussion but conventions differ between disciplines and journals. This is also the case for interpretivist methodologies and qualitative methods. The differences in presentation reflect different styles of thinking and language. A cautious student will check with their supervisor that the form of presentation reflects both the methods used and the orientation of their external examiners before writing up the final version of their thesis.

Preparing a final draft of a health research project usually involves an intensive period of thinking and writing and takes time, even for the most experienced writer. The quality of presentation and the succinctness of the writing are important and a number of drafts will be required to achieve clarity and intelligibility. The writer will need to persuade the reader that they have carried out the research in a thorough way and that their interpretation is well grounded in the data. As a narrative, a written output should aim to present a coherent and logical account, supporting an argument that runs through the work.

Bear in mind that in the final writing up, you are aiming to write a persuasive account of a project that began with a research question. You have gathered evidence and reached a conclusion on the basis of that evidence. When writing, you will be looking back objectively and justifying that conclusion and reporting how you got there. There is no need to refer to your problems along the way other than in the methods chapter. Remember that you are writing for an external audience which has not shared your experience or thinking, so you have to give a clear explanation of the development of your argument. In order to do this, all the sections or chapters of a dissertation or thesis should include an introduction, sub-headings and a summary of the content. Bear in mind that a final draft is about reducing the complexity of data, editing down, cutting out words, correcting typographical errors and ordering paragraphs.

The structure revisited

Box 23.1 above outlined the shape of a dissertation or thesis. Leaving aside the *Title*, *Abstract* and *List of contents*, the *Introduction* to a dissertation or thesis should provide a summary of the shape of the thesis: it is likely to contain a short account of the research question, the gap in knowledge and how you set about answering it and the argument you make. It is the key for the reader in understanding your work. It is likely the introduction will be reworked a number of times as you progress through the final draft.

You will need to say what your study is about, why the question you address is of interest and how you came to carry out the investigation. You may wish to refer to your values as a researcher. This has been a convention in some feminist and other forms of research (Letherby 2003). Do not be concerned about revealing some key findings. This is not a detective novel. You may say something about how the question addresses a gap in knowledge, and links to particular theories and to an area of scholarship. If relevant, you may also say how the evidence you found contributes to knowledge. This may be through increasing understanding of a health problem or findings that are useful to policy makers or health service providers. The introduction is the place where you have the opportunity to convince the reader that you are a serious and competent researcher. This can be done by writing precisely, confidently and above all persuasively.

The *Literature review* is where research questions can be discussed in greater detail, together with theories and substantive studies associated with these questions. The final draft is where you should include new studies or areas of literature that proved to be valuable in understanding the analysis or discussion in the substantive chapters of the study. You could conclude the literature review chapter by saying how the literature review shaped your choice of research method.

The *Research methods* section or chapter is the place in the thesis where you may discuss the process of doing the research from your own perspective. It can be an account of the decisions made in choosing the methods, why they were chosen and the design of research instruments. If the work is for an academic qualification, then you may want to say what you learnt from the process. You may make reference to problems encountered, changes of direction and additional skill training that proved necessary. Here you can draw on your records to check details. The section on quantitative analysis above gives details on what should be included. In qualitative research, a description of coding framework construction should be given, with an example of raw data.

The methods chapter should refer to decisions on ethical issues that arose during the research. Reference can be made to obtaining ethical committee approval within the university and/or the health service committee (Long and Johnson 2007). You should mention how you obtained the informed consent of research participants, what information you gave them about the project and the opportunities given for participants or respondents to raise questions. You should also describe how you kept data secure to maintain the anonymity of research participants.

The methods section is also the place to reflect on the research process and to discuss the shortcomings of the methods and research instruments used in a form of auto-critique. You may want to comment reflexively on the research process. Reflexivity is a concept that refers to the role the researcher plays in the construction of knowledge at all stages of the research process. Certain kinds of qualitative research have stressed the importance of being reflexive about your own position and values. This strategy has been popular in action research and in areas where identity politics are an important aspect of the research question. Here, to talk reflexively about one's own position is to acknowledge subjectivity and the way in which this may act as a filter in observation and interpretation. Bryman (2012: 394), in a fuller discussion of the concept, argues that it has been defined in various ways by scholars whose views vary.

The sections or chapters that deal with *Results, findings and analyses* and *Discussion* should be drafted and redrafted to bring out the argument. A way of doing this is to begin by restating the research question or hypothesis. Then move on to state the main findings or themes, and discuss these in turn, commenting on the extent to which the findings confirm (or not) the proposition put forward. Headings and sub-headings help to structure the argument. Not all results can be included so stick to the findings or interpretations that relate to the research question.

The *Conclusion* should not simply be a summary but taken as an opportunity to restate your starting point and draw out ways that your thesis has contributed to knowledge. You should take the opportunity here to look at the ways in which the research has been innovative or original. You may have shed light on a little known area or been able to question or confirm existing theories and/or methodologies. You may be able draw out the implications of your work for patients and patient groups, as well as for policy makers and service providers. The limitations of your study can also be highlighted, in addition to the possibilities for further research.

Some tips for writing up your essay, dissertation or thesis are included in Box 23.4 below.

Box 23.4 Tips for Writing

- Develop an argument that is sustained throughout the work.
- Present your work within a clear structure through sub-headings or chapters.
- If in doubt, it is better to assume a lower level of knowledge.
- Avoid sexist and racist language and statements that are patronising to research participants.
- Read your work aloud to establish the rhythm and flow of the language.
- Set aside your work for a while so you can take a fresh look at it later.
- Ask someone else – your supervisor or a colleague – to read your work through and make comments.

The final stage of preparing a project is to proofread it to check again for errors and ensure consistency. You will also need to check the footnotes or endnotes, references and bibliography to make sure that all the sources quoted are referenced. These should be internally consistent and also conform to any format recommended by your institution. It is important to check for word length, and add an abstract and any appendices that can provide information on your working methods, such as a questionnaire, a list of people interviewed with a sample letter or an information sheet for participants in your project. All this can be time-consuming and remember that a common regret among research students is that they did not leave enough time for writing.

Conventions for writing up research for reports and articles

In principle any piece of research, from an undergraduate or postgraduate, as well as an employed scholar or researcher, may be suitable for journal submission if it is original, well written and has a clear conclusion. To be publishable, a paper should be based on sound and well-articulated methods and data analysis; generate appropriate data; and follow through an argument that is plausible. As journal articles are generally short, between 4,000 and 8,000 words, emphasis should be given to one main research question to drive the argument through the paper. To indicate the openness of the process, one publication in a top international health journal, *Social Science and Medicine* – a study by Lovell (1983) of late miscarriage, stillbirth and perinatal death – began life as a Master's dissertation. The same is the case for the article by Taraborrelli (1993), quoted above.

In writing up research in health, it is very important to decide on which journal you wish to target before submitting, and to adjust the style of presentation by reading recent issues to understand the nature and formal guidelines of the journal. This point is accentuated by the distinction between natural and social scientific journals. As noted in the opening chapters, there are two basic forms of narrative: the biomedical scientific or quantitative and the naturalistic or qualitative. Although each has different conventions, methods and language, the actual structure of reports or articles in specialist journals is very similar.

Many journals in the health field accept articles from both the natural and social sciences, so there has been accommodation to the conventions of each.

Writing for a scientific journal or report using positivist methods

Biomedical scientific writing on matters related to health tends to operate within a very strictly defined set of conventions, of which a subset would be scientific research using an experimental or quantitative method (Greenhalgh 2010). The normal requirements for scientific journals are shown in Box 23.5, and provide one paradigm type.

Box 23.5   The structure of a scientific paper using positivist methods

- Introduction: the research question being addressed, including current gaps in research
- A review of the literature to put the research question in the context of existing knowledge
- A descriptive title and biographical details of author(s)
- An abstract of 100–200 words, including a summary of the research question, methods, findings and contribution to knowledge
- The hypothesis or null hypothesis being addressed
- The type of study being undertaken: either primary (experiment, clinical trial or survey) or secondary (overview, guideline study, decision analysis or economic analysis)
- The study design and method, such as experimental with an RCT, cohort study, case-control study, cross-sectional survey or single case report, inclusion and exclusion criteria and how the outcomes were measured
- The research results or findings
- A conclusion
- References
- A declaration of interests.

Source: Adapted from Greenhalgh (1997a, 1997b)

One characteristic of such writing is that the voice of the writer is absent from the text. The researcher presents the work as a series of facts. This serves to underline the scientific nature of the writing, although actually the author still structures, shapes and selects what is written, what constitutes evidence and how this is presented. The form of writing aims to minimize the likelihood of bias and error, but also preserves the way in which knowledge is structured by scientists. The research protocol identifies a narrow and specific hypothesis that is to be tested in a study, most often an experiment. The structure of any scientific paper is reinforced by publication norms and adherence to a particular format is expected. Data are likely to be presented in a formal manner with tables and with tests of statistical significance when analysing data sets.

Writing up qualitative research for a journal or report

Qualitative, descriptive or naturalistic methods within an interpretivist framework study phenomena in their natural setting. The objective is to capture the meanings and understandings of people in everyday life. The authoritative voice of the author can be present and explicit in terms of structuring the text, analysing and interpreting data. For example, when writing about methods, some authors follow a style that emphasizes the authorial presence by using the first-person singular ('I analysed the data in the following way ...') or plural ('After completing the fieldwork, we developed a framework to code the data ...'). This indicates that the interpretation of data was their own. However, there is considerable variation between authors in how qualitative findings are used to support an interpretation or theme. Some authors present qualitative data formally in a table form with illustrative quotations representing particular themes. Others give verbatim quotations as they were spoken and recorded in a transcript with pauses. Between these extremes, there is variation. When writing a journal article or report, it is sensible to give your criteria for selection and to check the style followed by a journal before submitting an article. A number of texts provide useful guides on writing up qualitative research (Lincoln and Guba 1985; Becker 1986; Strauss 1987; Richardson 1990; Wolcott 1990).

Although less predictable than the structure of a quantitative piece, the final product, whether in the form of a report, a thesis or paper, will usually require the elements shown in Box 23.6 below.

Box 23.6   The structure of a qualitative study

- The title should be short, descriptive of the study and attract the reader.
- The name of the author with full biographical details should be given.
- Abstract and keywords: abstracts may be published in an abstracting journal, while keywords are used for insertion in bibliographic indexes.
- Introduction: this locates the topic, indicating why it is important and introducing controversies – stating the research question, aims and objectives and the research gap filled.
- Literature review: this locates the research in existing theoretical and empirical literature. It should draw only on material relevant to the research question. References to any quantitative research should be included.
- The research strategy and process which includes the context of the study, for example the research site, the selection of respondents, data collection recording methods – in sum, sufficient detail to replicate the study.
- The data and the interpretation of the data.
- A concluding section and, in the case of reports, recommendations: these need to be geared to the particular audience.
- References and appendices.

Source: Adapted from Greenhalgh and Taylor (1997)

Writing up research using mixed methods

As previously noted, health researchers on funded projects may now employ a mix of quantitative and qualitative methods in their research. In this volume, a number of contributors have referred to mixed methods in terms of using methods within the same paradigm or across the positivist/interpretivist divide through multidisciplinary research. The advantages for doing so are discussed in Chapter 2 and more fully in Chapter 22.

Using a mix of methods poses additional challenges for writing up results (see Cresswell and Tashakkori 2007). There is no set of conventions, as the use of mixed methods is relatively new. So authors must make their own decisions on the basis of what they think will make the study comprehensible to readers. In writing up projects that use mixed methods, the rationale for so doing should be explained in terms of the relevance to addressing the research question and the anticipated benefits (Bryman 2008). The logic of combining two different methods should be reflected in the design of the research instruments, and an account of whether the anticipated benefits were realized should be given in the project.

It should be explained why a particular mix was chosen, and why this was used in a particular sequence. When describing the methods, an account should be given of the methods for each arm of the study. When discussing the findings, the aim may be to show the different aspects of the research question that the methods address or to use the findings of each method to corroborate the findings of one with the other. Alternatively, it may be that one method is a stepping stone to another. If the findings or results can be integrated around particular themes, this then can be a way forward. Bryman (2012: 659) concludes that the use of mixed methods may lead to a better understanding of a phenomenon by triangulation, as discussed in the previous chapter, but this adds to complexity and can have increased resource costs.

Leaving the balance of benefit and cost on one side, in reading using mixed methods, authors may therefore be subject to the following questions, amongst others: Has a justification been given for using a mix of methods in the research design? Have each/all of the methods and the strategies for data collection and analysis been described in full? Have the findings from each analysis been given? Has the data been integrated in the paper and, if so, how? Is this appropriate to the study? Since the user is often at the centre of mixed methods research, there may also be subsidiary questions about the stages at which users have been involved, their level of engagement, how they were selected, recruited and trained/supported – and indeed themselves informed about the research findings through publication and other means (Wright et al. 2010).

Conclusion

In conclusion, it is worth reiterating that writing up research, like other stages of research, has a moral aspect. The researcher has an obligation to follow a rigorous and systematic process in data collection, analysis and writing up. In the case of health research, there is an obligation, particularly on field researchers, to publish findings even if these are negative. Research subjects will have given their opinions, their time and sometimes access to their bodies for additional procedures, interventions and medications because they believe a project is worthwhile and may help others. Given that being a research participant may have emotional and physical costs, researchers have an ethical obligation to carry out research as rigorously as they can, and then make the results available. There has long been concern that there is a publication bias in clinical trials; that there is a long time lag between a trial and publication; that drug trials are over-represented; and that negative results are hard to publish (see Chalmers 1990; Chalmers and Matthews 2006; Godlee 2012). This may be for many reasons, including that neither journal editors nor researchers think it worthwhile to publish negative results. Yet these also add to knowledge, along with the positive findings that come out of health research, and can help to save lives.

Recommended Further Reading

Becker, H.S. (1986) *Writing for Social Scientists: How to Start and Finish Your Thesis, Book, or Article.* Chicago, IL: University of Chicago Press.
In this book, Becker, a master of research and pioneer in qualitative methods, provides a readable and stimulating account of the writing process based on long experience of teaching doctoral students at universities in the US.

Bryman, A. (2012) *Social Research Methods*, 4th edition. Oxford: Oxford University Press.
This book provides a guide to the research process and examples of how to write up research using examples. It gives practical solutions based on student experience.

Dunleavy, P. (2003) *Authoring a PhD: How To Plan, Draft, Write and Finish a Doctoral Thesis or Dissertation.* London: Palgrave.
This is a useful practical book to assist those completing their doctoral dissertations.

Johnson, M. (2004) *Effective Writing for Health Professionals: A Practical Guide to Getting Published.* London: Routledge.
This book provides insights and strategies for publishing and has the advantage of being specifically directed towards a health professional audience.

companion
website

Online Readings

Hemingway, H., Angell, C., Hartwell, H., and Heller, R. (2011) 'An emerging model for publishing and using open educational resources in public health', *Perspectives in Public Health*, 131: 38–43.
Write an outline plan for the key sections of the above paper, discussing the utility of the approach.

Gardner, W. and Heck, K. (2009) 'Ethical requirements in the instructions for authors in journals publishing randomized clinical trials, *Research Ethics Review*, 5:131–37.

What are the key ethical issues that authors face in writing up research? How might these be managed during the research process?

References

Allsop, J. (1998) 'Complaints and disputes in the family practitioner committee setting: an empirical and theoretical analysis', PhD thesis, University of London.

Antaki, C. and Fielding, G. (1981) 'Research on ordinary explanations', in C. Antaki (ed.), *The Psychology of Ordinary Explanations in Social Behaviour*. London: Academic Press.

Becker, H.S. (1986) *Writing for Social Scientists: How to Start and Finish Your Thesis, Book, or Article*. Chicago, IL: University of Chicago Press.

Bowling, A. (2001) *A Review of Disease Specific Quality of Life Measurement Scales*, 2nd edition. Buckingham: Open University Press.

Bruce, N., Pope, D. and Stanistreet, D. (2008) *Quantitative Methods for Health Research: A Practical Interactive Guide to Epidemiology and Statistics*. Chichester: Wiley & Sons.

Bryman, A. (2008) 'Why do researchers integrate/combine/mesh/blend/mix/merge/fuse quantitative and qualitative research?', in M.M. Bergman (ed.), *Advances in Mixed Methods Research*. London: Sage.

Bryman, A. (2012) *Social Research Methods*, 4th edition. Oxford: Oxford University Press.

Chalmers, I. (1990) 'Under reporting research is scientific misconduct', *Journal of the American Medical Association*, 236: 1405–8.

Chalmers, I. and Matthews, R. (2006) 'What are the implications of optimism bias in clinical research?', *Lancet*, 367: 449–50.

Cresswell, J. (2009) *Research Design: Qualitative, Quantitative and Mixed Methods Approaches*, 3rd edition. London: Sage.

Cresswell, J. and Tashakkori, A. (2007) 'Developing publishable mixed methods manuscripts', *Journal of Mixed Methods Research*, 1: 107–11.

Dawson, C. (2009) *Introduction to Research Methods: A Practical Guide for Anyone Undertaking a Research Project*. Oxford: How To Do Books.

Denzin, N. and Lincoln, Y.S. (eds) (2005) *Handbook of Qualitative Research*, 3rd edition. Thousand Oaks, CA: Sage.

Dunleavy, P. (2003) *Authoring a PhD: How To Plan, Draft, Write and Finish a Doctoral Thesis or Dissertation*. London: Palgrave.

Felstiner, W., Abel, R. and Sarat, A. (1980–1) 'The emergence and transformation of disputes: naming, blaming and claiming', *Law and Society Review*, 15(3–4): 631–54.

Godlee, F. (2012) 'Research misconduct is widespread and harms patients', *British Medical Journal*, 344: e14.

Green, J. and Thorogood, N. (2004) *Qualitative Methods for Health Researchers*. London: Sage.

Greenhalgh, T. (1997a) 'How to read a paper: getting your bearings (deciding what the paper is about)', *British Medical Journal*, 315: 243–6.

Greenhalgh, T. (1997b) 'How to read a paper: assessing the methodological quality of published papers', *British Medical Journal*, 315: 305–8.

Greenhalgh, T. (2010) *How To Read a Paper: The Basics of Evidence-based Medicine*, 4th edition. Chichester: Wiley-Blackwell.

Greenhalgh, T. and Taylor, R. (1997) 'How to read a qualitative paper: papers that go beyond numbers (qualitative research)', *British Medical Journal*, 315: 740–3.

Letherby, G. (2003) *Feminist Research in Theory and Practice*. Buckingham: Open University Press.

Lincoln, Y.S. and Guba, E.G. (1985) *Naturalistic Inquiry*. Newbury Park, CA: Sage.

Long, T. and Johnson, M. (2007) *Research Ethics in the Real World: Issues and Solutions for Health and Social Care Professionals*. Philadelphia, PA: Elsevier Health Sciences.

Lovell, A. (1983) 'Some questions of identity: late miscarriage, stillbirth and perinatal loss', *Social Science and Medicine*, 17(11): 755–61.

Mulcahy, L. and Tritter, J. (1998) 'Pathways, pyramids and icebergs? Mapping the links between satisfaction and complaints', *Sociology of Health and Illness*, 20(6): 823–45.

Offredy, M. and Vickers, P. (2010) *Developing a Healthcare Research Proposal: An Interactive Student Guide*. Chichester: Wiley-Blackwell.

Polgar, S. and Thomas, S.A. (2008) *Introduction to Research in the Health Sciences*, 5th edition. Philadelphia, PA: Churchill Livingstone.

Punch, S. (2006) *Developing Effective Research Proposals*. London: Sage.

Ramkalawan, T. (2005) 'Training for research', in A. Bowling and S. Ebrahim (eds), *Handbook of Health Research Methods: Investigation, Measurement and Analysis*. Maidenhead: Open University Press.

Richardson, L. (1990) *Writing Strategies: Reaching Diverse Audiences*. London: Sage.

Sapsford, R. and Jupp, V. (eds) (2006) *Data Collection and Analysis*, 2nd edition. London: Sage.

Saldana, J. (2009) *The Coding Manual for Qualitative Researchers*. London: Sage.

Schober, J. and Farrington, A. (2000) 'Presenting and disseminating research', in M. Saks, M. Williams and B. Hancock (eds), *Developing Research in Primary Care*. Abingdon: Radcliffe Medical Press.

Strauss, A.L. (1987) *Qualitative Analysis for Social Scientists*. Cambridge: Cambridge University Press.

Taraborrelli, P. (1993) 'Exemplar A: becoming a carer', in N. Gilbert (ed.), *Researching Social Life*. London: Sage.

Wolcott, H.F. (1990) *Writing up Qualitative Research*. London: Sage.

Wright, D., Faster, C., Amir, Z., Elliott, J. and Wilson, R. (2010) 'Critical appraisal guidelines for assessing the quality and impact of user involvement in research', *Health Expectations*, 13: 359–68.

Yin, R.K. (2009) *Case Study Research: Design and Methods*, 4th edition. Los Angeles, CA: Sage.

24

Disseminating and Using Health Research

MIKE SAKS AND JUDITH ALLSOP

Introduction

- The previous chapter focused on the research process and the challenge of writing up health research findings for both quantitative and qualitative studies and those employing mixed methods. Despite the expansion of visual media and the use of electronic devices, writing, whether in journals, reports or books, is still the main means of communication for scholarship in health research. A research degree will not normally be awarded without being written up and, if research does not get published in some form, it will not inform other scholars or reach a wider audience. While there are other means of disseminating health research, including PowerPoint and other presentations at conference and workshop events, these are in turn often translated into published form. Parallel reports feeding back to commissioners of research to fulfil contractual commitment to sponsors of research in government and commercial circles, as well as to users to fulfil our ethical obligations to those participating in research, also typically take written form. Increasingly, though, dissemination is taking place through e-sources, including e-journals and websites. A major focus of this final chapter, therefore, is on how health research is communicated in its many forms.

- In covering the area of dissemination of health research, this concluding chapter also considers the important question of how health researchers can make the greatest impact on health policy and practice at a local, regional, national

(Continued)

(Continued)

and international level. One of the biggest challenges faced in applying health research is in translating promising research work into action, whether based on qualitative, quantitative or mixed methods. Without the initial dissemination, the opportunity to influence policy and practice may be lost. Here, we examine in more detail this and other factors that may encourage or inhibit the implementation of health and health-related research in ways that benefit users and other stakeholders and advance the public interest.

The Health Research Project

As has been seen in this book, the road to completing a successful health research project is a long but intriguing one. The journey starts with the formulation and refinement of an interesting research question in the health field based on a favoured paradigmatic position that will provide a methodological framework for further study. This may be formulated in a variety of contexts from an extended undergraduate essay to a postgraduate thesis and a doctoral dissertation in higher education. The project may also be formulated either individually or as part of a team at postdoctoral level and beyond, and may be funded at local, national or international level – through sponsoring bodies like local health providers, pharmaceutical companies, national research bodies and international funders of research, such as through the European Union.

Typically following a literature review, a health research project develops from a base of qualitative or quantitative research methods, as outlined in Part II and Part III of this book, or a combination of these. As readers of this text will appreciate, such research should be ethically sensitive and suitably inclusive of users as appropriate. It may or may not be focused on one or more of the contemporary issues flagged up in Part IV of this volume – spanning from minority groups in health and user involvement to public health and comparative health research. However, the culmination of following the various stages of the research process outlined in the preceding chapter should, following analysis, lead to results or findings with greater or lesser relevance to the outside world.

As indicated in Chapter 23, the next step in this process is writing up health research for publication in a range of outlets from work for postgraduate higher education qualifications that may go into university libraries or other repositories and research reports to more formally published journals. Publication also extends to books which may take the form of small circulation, but high prestige, scholarly monographs directed at the academic community to wider-selling texts building on the research undertaken and oriented towards professional practitioners and/or the lay public.

In this process, feedback will be variously received from key audiences, ranging from internal and external examiners and research commissioners to journal and book reviewers. If a response other than a straight acceptance or rejection is received from a journal editor, requests for minor or major amendments should be responded to calmly, politely and systematically, if you wish to follow through to publication. This also applies in parallel to feedback on relevant pieces of student work, including university PhD dissertations, following the conducting of a viva, if a pass is to be achieved (Dunleavy 2003). This leads on to the next section of this final chapter which focuses on different aspects of the dissemination of health research – before concluding by assessing how health research may be translated most effectively into practice.

The Art of Disseminating Health Research

Publishing health research

The chapter now looks more specifically at the art of presenting health research findings in published and other work as part of the process of dissemination. There are many hurdles to be overcome in this area, including ethical considerations about what to say and what not to say. Writing for health and other fields is a time-consuming and often difficult business. Moreover, turning research reports, dissertations, theses and other research into publications can be a hit-and-miss affair, as a would-be author is in the hands of editors. Nonetheless, as well as luck, shrewd judgement and persistence are often rewarded (on this process, see, for example, Johnson 2004 and Lang 2010). The remainder of this section aims to be of assistance in taking forward the research journey to its final 'impact' stage.

As well as adding to the general body of knowledge about a particular area on which others can build, health research that is written up, disseminated and published brings a number of benefits. First, for the researcher there may be positive personal benefits on publication in terms of public prestige; income streams from book sales; further research funding; and career development. Conversely, future funding may be jeopardized by poor outputs and a failure to publish. For funders, research consumes considerable resources in terms of time and money. Researchers making a bid for funding in health and other fields are often now required to include proposals for dissemination, and to show they have considered the utility of their research, as well as who will benefit from the findings and at what point in the process. Outputs are also frequently subsequently audited (Berry 2010).

Funding bodies themselves are monitored and audited as research grants are awarded by public bodies, commercial organizations and charitable institutions, which are accountable for ensuring value for money. Research-funding bodies may specify interim reports or targets to be achieved during a project. For them, outputs signal a return on investment and reporting on these – not least through journal and other forms of publication – is typically a requirement. The wider community of scholars, as well as professionals, policy makers and the general public, can benefit from research findings, but only if they are accessible. Examples of bodies to which health researchers can bid for funding in the UK are listed in Box 24.1 below.

Box 24.1   Examples of bodies funding health research in the UK

Those in need of funds for health research can apply to the following:

- The Department of Health (e.g. Research for Patient Benefit, Programme Development Grants).
- The European Union (e.g. Framework 8 Programme).
- Research councils (e.g. Medical Research Council, Economic and Social Sciences Research Council, Engineering and Physical Sciences Research Council).
- Charities (e.g. Cancer Research UK, Diabetes UK, Mental Health Research UK).
- Pharmaceutical companies (e.g. Wellcome Trust, GlaxoSmithKline).

Herein too lies the ethical obligation to provide access to key findings to both research participants and the funding body – which in all likelihood will have expectations regarding dissemination. Separate summaries which convey to the reader as clearly, concisely and convincingly as possible the aims and outcome of the research (Schober and Farrington 2000) may also be useful in other contexts – including, as we shall see later in this chapter, providing the basis for press releases to the media and at dissemination events such as conferences and workshops where health research presentations can be made.

Styles and authorship

This example of dissemination to patients and other health care users reminds us that written outputs are of varying styles and lengths. In a thesis or dissertation, the methods chapter is a critical part of the work (Dunleavy 2003). In a report or article, though, a detailed explanation of methods may interrupt the flow of the narrative and findings, and may be of less interest to the reader. One device in a report or scholarly monograph is to give a short explanation in the main text, and add a methodological appendix. In an article or conference paper, a table or short footnote giving essential details may suffice. An account of methods should always be presented in a way that shows the approach as logical in relation to the research question. It should not normally focus on the actual process experienced by the researcher, which may include false starts and the pursuit of issues that were later abandoned.

In dissemination, therefore, it is crucial that, if publication is intended, the paper or other output is designed accordingly (Huff 2009). In this regard, the style of writing in terms of language and presentation will vary according to the audience. Any would-be author should take time to find out, and think through, what is expected of them and tailor their account accordingly – whether it is for a published research paper, thesis or dissertation (see, for instance, Turabian 2007). After a period immersed in a research project, the minutiae of the findings and the task of interpretation, it is all too easy to forget that an account must be comprehensible to the reader. In some cases in the health field, knowledge of specialized requisites is important, as in health services research (Thomas 2000). In others, an understanding of technical language cannot be assumed. This is illustrated by the difficulty that many researchers have in writing consent forms that are comprehensible to participants, who may, for example, be children or have a terminal illness or some form of learning disability (Brazier and Lobjoit 1991).

Health researchers should also appreciate the dilemmas posed by multi-authored works, as well as by those intended for a diverse audience (Richardson 1990). In health research projects where there is more than one researcher, issues of authorship – such as whose names should appear on publications and in what order – should be discussed openly. Ideally, this should be determined early on to avoid potential disputes at a later stage. In this respect, the conventions between scientific and social scientific disciplines differ. In the former, senior academics may be included in the list of authors, even though they have had only a nominal part in a project. In this case, the current convention is that their name appears last. In social science research, however, distant help from supervisors or senior academics is more likely to simply be acknowledged in a footnote or elsewhere.

In a health research project where there are a number of authors, the lead author is generally the author who has played the major part in obtaining funding, in leading a project and in the analysis and writing. In writing with colleagues, one convention is that the lead author is the one who has produced the first draft. However, all the above are informal guidelines and the issue of designated authorship, like many other aspects of health research, remains open to the influence of power and politics (Pierce 2008). Such specific influences may be particularly apparent when senior academics involved in research have particular career incentives to be first authors – and their interests are pursued at the expense of more junior researchers, whatever the ethics involved. At the other end of the spectrum, there may also be incentives when this increases opportunities for publication, especially in situations where the review process for articles and books is not blinded.

Writers disseminating their work in all these different guises do their writing in very different ways depending on personality, lifestyle and life stage. So, it is important to be aware of what works best for you – early mornings, late nights, short bursts or long sessions. Setting a word target or a time target is a possible strategy for getting work completed. Setting aside a period of time of days, weeks or months, depending on the length, probably works best. The shifting and sorting process often continues overnight. A problem that seems insurmountable in the evening may be resolved by the following morning. Herein lays the art of presenting and disseminating health research in published and other forms.

Dissemination Strategies for Health Research

Dissemination outlets

As previously noted, in terms of strategies for dissemination, the main outlets for publication in health research are books, monographs and reports, articles in scholarly, professional and popular journals, and conference papers – the abstracts of which may be published in conference proceedings. The health researcher should be clear that these are not mutually exclusive means of dissemination. For example, part of a research report can be published as a conference paper that may be turned into a journal article. It should also be noted that a number of these outlets are now available on the Internet – with a profusion of e-journals and e-books, as well as the availability of conference records online.

Having produced a dissertation, thesis or research report for a funding body, there is usually an expectation of further dissemination to reach a wider audience through publications or other presentations. However, while researchers are typically required to publish, avenues to publication are controlled by a variety of producers who apply filters and can block access. Journal editors may apply restrictions on publication. Funding bodies may embargo research. Researchers should therefore ensure that a funding contract includes the proviso that permission to publish must not be unreasonably withheld (in relation to gate-keeping roles, see, for instance, the account by Hannaway 2008 on the politics of biomedical research).

As writing is a time-consuming process, researchers should plan their strategy carefully and be prepared to switch, if opportunities arise unexpectedly. For example, although publication in a high-ranking journal may be the ultimate objective, preparing a paper for a conference or giving a presentation to a group of professionals may be good preparation and offer opportunities for learning. Any form of presentation is better than none. If choices have to be made between competing offers, then ask the questions: Will this further my career? Does it pay well? Will I enjoy it? When two or more of these criteria apply, you may wish to choose the option concerned.

Offering to give a conference paper is a way of focusing on a particular aspect of a research project. It can allow for reflection and feedback on a paper that may later be refined as a book chapter or submitted to a journal. Care should be taken in writing a conference abstract, which is usually limited to around 200–300 words. This should fit with the conference theme and aim to make one major point. The abstract is important not only because it will need to pass through the conference filtering process for selection, but because it may be published in conference proceedings. Selected papers or presentations may also be published on the Web. However, it is as well to remember that, once this happens, such work, and the ideas behind it, enter the public domain and may be used by others – raising potential intellectual property issues in a globalizing world (Bennett and Tomossy 2010).

Presentations to policy makers, users and practitioners are particularly important for publicly funded policy research in health and indeed may be a requirement of funding. The cost of such presentations should be included in research proposals. Press releases, radio and television presentations may also be part of publicizing a research project. For all these forms of dissemination, the target audience must be carefully considered, and any output carefully prepared and tailored to suit that audience. Generally, such presentations should also focus on a key theme – although flexibility is of course often required in responding to questions, which may not always be predictable.

Book publication

For a researcher in health, a book or scholarly monograph offers the best opportunity to present a full account of the research findings and reach a wide audience, with a publisher bearing the costs of publicity. However, there are some disadvantages, as even if a book is based on a research report, it is likely to take at least a further year to produce, and still longer to get into print. Moreover, although a book may help to enhance a researcher's reputation under the UK's periodic Research Excellence Framework (formerly the Research Assessment Exercise) – and similar systems in other countries for rating academic research – it has historically not been the most highly rated form of publication. This is the refereed article in high-impact journals in particular subject fields. There are also specific barriers to publication in both these potential outlets.

Publishers are largely driven by market factors and will normally only publish books that will have sufficient sales to make a profit, or at least cover their costs. It has in fact become increasingly difficult to obtain a publisher for research-based books as sales may be low. In the first instance, it is as well to discuss an idea for a book with a publisher to find out if the idea is attractive and has a fit with their publishing strategy. If there is a positive response, the researcher will be asked to write an outline of the book and its constituent chapters and indicate the likely market for the publication. The most significant sector is the student market and the optimum length is usually around 70–90,000 words. There may be a request for sample chapters as well. Typically, the proposal will be sent to one or more reviewers who will give their opinion, and the editorial team at the publishers will make a final decision.

A rejection by a publisher should not necessarily be taken as an indication of the scholarly quality of the work as there are other factors, such as topicality and appeal to a wider audience, that a publisher will take into account in deciding whether to proceed.

As well as commercial publishers, there are a range of specialist academic and university-based publishers who provide outlets for more scholarly works, particularly for those with a connection to a university. Examples of these are the university presses of Cambridge, Manchester and Oxford in the UK and Cornell, Harvard and Yale in the USA. There are specialist presses such as the Radcliffe Medical Press for works in health and medicine and the Policy Press for social policy monographs. A number of university departments also publish monographs or have occasional paper series, which have limited circulation. These tend to be shorter and may be an edited-down version of a research report for a funding body. While getting into print may be easier through this outlet, such publications may form part of the grey literature referred to in Chapter 3, especially in so far as they are not official publications and publicity and marketing are restricted.

A more recent dissemination outlet is Internet publishing through websites, blogs and such like, which provide the facility for downloads. This parallels the growing use of the Internet in research itself, including facilitating the application of research methods such as surveys and focus groups in the health field (Fielding et al. 2008). Publication through this medium has advantages and disadvantages. A wide range of organizations, such as scholarly and charitable foundations, government departments, university departments, research centres and professional associations now have websites that publish research reports and working papers. In health, this includes elite research-funding bodies such as the Economic and Social Sciences Research Council and the Medical Research Council in the UK. A major benefit of publishing on the Web is that research becomes available quickly and at a low cost. One drawback, though, is that, without publicity, the 'hit' rate of such sites may be low and publications may only be kept on websites for a limited period.

Journal publication

Reports and articles in a scholarly journal are, for most disciplines, the most highly rated form of research output in health and other areas. The requirements for publication are also relatively transparent. However, the filtering process, particularly in highly rated journals, is rigorous. Hargens (1988) estimated that between 50 and 80 per cent of articles submitted in the social sciences were rejected. Some journals give information on their rejection rate on their website. Box 24.2 shows that the commonest reasons for rejection of quantitative and qualitative articles are broadly similar. These could be grouped into two main areas. First, authors were not giving enough information on the methods used and, second, they were not giving sufficient explanation of how data were analysed.

Box 24.2   Why papers were rejected by journals

Quantitative research paper The study:	Qualitative research paper The study:
Did not address an important scientific issue	Did not address an important social scientific issue
Was not original	Was not original
Did not test the author's hypothesis	Did not test a research question
Research design was not appropriate for answering the research question	The method was not appropriate for answering the research question
Was compromised by practical difficulties	Was compromised by practical difficulties
The sample size was too small	Had no rationale for numbers (interviews/observations/choice of sites etc.)
Was not adequately controlled	Had no rationale for the selection of respondents/groups
The statistical analysis was incorrect	The basis of the data analysis was not explained
Conclusions did not relate to the data	Conclusions did not relate to the data
Indicated a significant conflict of interest	Indicated a significant conflict of interest
Was incomprehensible due to poor writing and presentation	Was incomprehensible due to poor writing and presentation

Sources: Adapted from Greenhalgh (1997a, b); Belgrave et al. (2002)

Final reports and journal articles should provide sufficient detail of research design and methods to demonstrate the internal and external validity and reliability of the research findings. In a qualitative study, they must show how the research question is linked to data analysis and the theoretical underpinning of the interpretation made so that the account is plausible. For articles based on the research, it is wise in terms of output to only choose some of the data and to write a number of papers.

Aspiring authors wishing to have a paper in the health field accepted for publication should identify the most appropriate journal early on. Each journal aims at a given audience and subject coverage and takes a particular line on methodological approaches. There will be specific requirements as to how a paper should be presented, which should be precisely followed. When a paper is received, it will generally be sent to two reviewers for comment. Typically, a reviewer, who will have some knowledge of the topic but will not necessarily be an expert, will be asked whether the paper should be accepted (with minor amendments if necessary), returned for major revision or rejected outright. A final decision is made by the editorial board. Editors and reviewers act as the final gatekeepers in this process.

In this respect, a rejection by one journal should not be taken as the end for an article. It is an opportunity to revise and resubmit to the same or a different academic journal with the benefits of comments from reviewers. External events such as the topicality of the content of the paper and academic contacts will play some part in its subsequent placement. An article may, for example, be published as a book chapter or adapted for a professional journal where the style is necessarily more accessible and applied. Publication does not just have to be in high-level academic journals. There are other outlets for health research, such as presentations for health care practitioners or other groups – as well as articles for popular magazines or newspapers.

Finally, it should be noted that the dissemination of research findings in the health field may not be an unequivocal benefit. Once in the public domain, a work can take on a life of its own. It can be misinterpreted, misquoted or misapplied. There is little the researcher can do to prevent this. There is also the question of the ownership of ideas and attribution to be considered. It is true that publication in a scholarly journal or book for fellow scholars who understand the conventions of citation and attribution may limit circulation, but safeguard ownership. However, Morse (2000) comments from personal experience that, having placed a presentation on the Internet, her ideas were very rapidly colonized and distorted in a way that she did not intend. Perhaps the message is that the dissemination of ideas operates within a free market. The best that a health researcher can do is to aim for the more secure forms of dissemination or, alternatively, accept that their ideas and research will percolate down and influence the thinking of others – even if it is in unintended fashion.

However, rigour is vital, particularly when reporting health research, as publication in certain journals itself gives legitimacy to the research results and status to the author(s). This is of critical importance, as poorly constructed or unethical research may risk damage to patients and can lead to setbacks in public policy, as highlighted by the example in Box 24.3, which underlines the need to understand how research is used in practice.

Box 24.3 Example highlighting the need for care in journal publication

A paper by Wakefield and colleagues published by *The Lancet* on the measles, mumps and rubella vaccine (MMR) highlights the need for care in journal publication. The article was taken to suggest that there might be a link between this vaccine, bowel disease and autism, even though this idea is now largely discredited. As this information was in tune with certain contemporary beliefs and attitudes, it had a significant effect on the number of children presenting for the vaccine – with a consequent detrimental impact on the level of population immunity. In this instance, the review process did not screen out the article and it was left to subsequent research to refute the claims.

Source: Wakefield et al. (1998)

Using Health Research

This leads neatly on to the final section of this chapter on using health research in order to maximize the chances of the findings of particular research publications and other outputs translating into policy and practice for public benefit. While publication is likely to have the most positive translational impact, this is not the whole story. Much depends too, of course, on the quality and nature of the research itself and its applicability to stakeholders in the health field. This is illustrated by the willingness of doctors to embrace innovations in the health sciences, such as the introduction of transplantation and cholesterol-lowering drugs underwritten by research (Le Fanu 2011).

Much also hinges on the motivation of natural and social scientists themselves in bringing their ideas to market. There has certainly been resistance among some social scientists to moving beyond the ivory tower in researching health and other areas, either because of a commitment to 'value freedom' as an ideology or to academic values not resonant with commercialization or the more general operationalization of their ideas (Saks 2012). This can have knock-on effects for, as Chalmers (2003) argues, professionals can do more harm than good in medicine and other fields when their policy and practice is not based on rigorous evaluation. Although Chalmers' own preference in terms of methods is for randomized controlled trials (RCTs), much the same comment could equally apply to the implementation of the analysis of qualitative data, not to mention assessments based on mixed methods.

Nonetheless, it is possible to incentivize the behaviour of individuals, groups and institutions over and above an appeal to humanitarian values. As Bowling (2009) notes, in the promotion of change, dissemination may need to be complemented by associated interventions, such as education, audit, interpersonal contact from respected people and financial incentives. The role of incentivization is also well exemplified at institutional level by the 2014 Research Excellence Framework in the UK, where universities making submissions for background research funding in health and other subject units are now, for the first time, required to present 'impact analyses' as part of the assessment of research quality. These require the mobilization of evidence demonstrating 'impact' defined by the Higher Education Funding Council for England in terms of 'an effect on, change or benefit to the economy, society, culture, public policy or services, health, the environment or quality of life, beyond academia' (HEFCE 2011: 26).

This is an important incentive for universities to encourage staff to work to apply their findings to health and other areas, as impact analysis includes benefits to policy and practice as well as the reduction or prevention of harm, risk and cost. Interestingly, though, while the Research Excellence Framework still tends to foster expertise in specific subjects in health-related areas like the natural and social sciences, there is increasing international evidence that problem-based interdisciplinary work can lead to greater utilization of research in practice (see, for example, Landry et al. 2001). This is particularly so when the results from this and other forms of research work are communicated concisely and effectively to both non-academic and academic audiences, with practical recommendations for action providing a bridge to policy (Court and Young 2006).

The implementation of research findings in health and other areas also seems to be contingent on the standing of the researcher and the nature and policies of the funding body, whether in the private or public domain (Tang and Sinclair 2001). It has been found that the timescale for, and degree of responsiveness of, governments to health policy research in the social sciences may depend on whether they operate through an approach based more on consensus or centralization (Orosz 1994) – or indeed have sponsored the research themselves (Hammersley 2005). Either way, there is always the possibility of health research being embargoed if the recommendations of even commissioned work pose financial or other challenges to sponsors, be these governments or other bodies – as in the case of a study of the regulation of health support workers for the Department of Health in the UK, where publication was delayed for several years despite pressure from the media and health unions (Saks and Allsop 2007).

As we have seen in this volume, users are becoming much more engaged with the research process across Europe and beyond (Wickham and Collins 2006). Their involvement in health research spans from being advisory members of research steering groups to being active lobbyists against unethical health practices (Scambler 2002). It also extends to the role of patients and carers at a group level in the policy process (Baggott et al. 2005). As a result in part of their growing influence on governance arrangements, citizens are now themselves more decisively influencing the response of governments in health care, including research, along with other stakeholders (Kuhlmann and Saks 2008). All this places an ever greater premium on ensuring that research in health care, based on the methods considered in this book, is responded to appropriately and, notwithstanding the interests that may be involved in the politics of health, serves the public interest (Saks 1995).

Conclusion

In this concluding chapter, we initially summarized some of the common issues emerging from the various chapters of the book in relation to setting up and conducting health research projects. It is vital that this task is undertaken on the most sound and rigorous basis, if a strong platform for dissemination is to be established. We have also drawn on the advice given by those who have been involved in getting research results published and implemented, as well as on our own experience in so doing in the health field. We have highlighted the importance of disseminating research findings, but also pointed out that publication is not necessarily straightforward. Having said this, the dissemination of health research can be a most rewarding process. Disseminating research and getting published are exciting for researchers as they have the potential to make an impression on the wider community, whether from a scholarly or applied perspective. Although there is no guarantee of results being implemented, there is a real opportunity – assuming that the research findings are robust and accessed by appropriate players – of making an impact on thinking, policy and practice in the health arena (Becker and Bryman 2004). Whatever the outcome, the expertise contained in the previous chapters of this edited collection will not itself be fully utilized unless the reader is prepared to publicize the research being carried out. Therein perhaps lies the ultimate fulfilment for those involved in the fascinating task of researching health, employing qualitative, quantitative and mixed methods.

Recommended Further Reading

Becker, S. and Bryman, A. (eds) (2004) *Understanding Research for Policy and Practice: Themes, Methods and Approaches*. Bristol: Policy Press.
This text helps students, policy makers and practitioners to understand the importance and place of research in health and related areas, and how to use research findings.

Fielding, N., Lee, R.M. and Blank, G. (eds) (2008) *The SAGE Handbook of Online Research Methods*. London: Sage.
This book addresses the increasing propagation of research on the Internet.

Schober, J. and Farrington, A. (2000) 'Presenting and disseminating research', in M. Saks, M. Williams and B. Hancock (eds), *Developing Research in Primary Care*. Abingdon: Radcliffe Medical Press.
This chapter provides concisely expressed advice on writing up a research project, as well as on presenting and disseminating research in the health field.

 ## Online Readings

Al-alawy, K., Roche, T. and Alwali, W. (2011) 'Implementing public health in secondary care: A Rotherham perspective on strategy development and implementation', *Perspectives in Public Health*, 131:137–43.
Ask students to access the author guidelines from *Perspectives in Public Health* and consider how they would meet them – including headings; page numbering; abbreviations; references; and setting out a bibliography. Consider too how far the findings of this particular article have influenced practice in public health – or may do so in future.

Taub, A., Gilmore, G. and Olsen, L. (2011) 'Workforce development: Using role delineation research findings for policy-making and professional practice', *Global Health Promotion*, 18: 55–58.

Discuss how the research described in the paper may help to influence policy and professional practice. Are there any lessons to be learned?

References

Baggott, R., Allsop, J. and Jones, K. (2005) *Speaking for Patients and Carers: User Groups and the Policy Process*. Basingstoke: Palgrave Macmillan.

Becker, S. and Bryman, A. (eds) (2004) *Understanding Research for Policy and Practice: Themes, Methods and Approaches*. Bristol: Policy Press.

Belgrave, L., Zablotsky, D. and Guadango, M.A. (2002) 'How do we talk to each other? Writing qualitative research for quantitative readers', *Qualitative Health Research*, 12(10): 1427–39.

Bennett, B. and Tomossy, G.F. (eds) (2010) *Globalization and Health: Challenges for Health Law and Bioethics*. Dordrecht: Springer.

Berry, D. (2010) *Gaining Funding for Research: A Guide for Academics and Institutions*. Maidenhead: Open University Press.

Bowling, A. (2009) *Research Methods in Health: Investigating Health and Health Services*, 3rd edition. Buckingham: Open University Press.

Brazier, M. and Lobjoit, M. (eds) (1991) *Protecting the Vulnerable: Autonomy and Consent in Health Care*. London: Routledge.

Chalmers, I. (2003) 'Trying to do more harm than good in policy and practice: the role of rigorous, transparent, up-to-date evaluations', *Annals of the American Academy of Political and Social Science*, 589: 22–40.

Court, J. and Young, J. (2006) 'Bridging research and policy: insights from 50 case studies', *Evidence and Policy*, 2(4): 439–62.

Dunleavy, P. (2003) *Authoring a PhD: How To Plan, Draft, Write and Finish a Doctoral Thesis or Dissertation*. London: Palgrave.

Fielding, N., Lee, R.M. and Blank, G. (eds) (2008) *The SAGE Handbook of Online Research Methods*. London: Sage.

Greenhalgh, T. (1997a) 'How to read a paper: getting your bearings (deciding what the paper is about)', *British Medical Journal*, 315: 243–6.

Greenhalgh, T. (1997b) 'How to read a paper: assessing the methodological quality of published papers', *British Medical Journal*, 315: 305–8.

Hammersley, M. (2005) 'Is the evidence-based practice movement doing more good than harm? Reflections on Iain Chalmers' case for research-based policymaking and practice', *Evidence and Policy*, 1(1): 85–100.

Hannaway, C. (2008) *Biomedicine in the Twentieth Century: Practices, Policies, and Politics*. Fairfax, VA: IOS Press.

Hargens, L.L. (1988) 'Scholarly consensus and rejection rates', *American Sociological Review*, 53: 139–51.

HEFCE (2011) *REF 2014: Assessment Framework and Guidance on Submissions*. Bristol: HEFCE.

Huff, A.S. (2009) *Designing Research for Publication*. Thousand Oaks, CA: Sage.

Johnson, M. (2004) *Effective Writing for Health Professionals: A Practical Guide to Getting Published*. London: Routledge.

Kuhlmann, E. and Saks, M. (eds) (2008) *Rethinking Professional Governance: International Directions in Healthcare*. Bristol: Policy Press.

Landry, R., Amara, N. and Lamari, M. (2001) 'Utilization of social science research knowledge in Canada', *Research Policy*, 30: 333–49.

Lang, T.A. (2010) *How to Write, Publish, and Present in the Health Sciences: A Guide for Clinicians and Laboratory Researchers*. Washington, DC: American College of Physicians.

Le Fanu, J. (2011) *The Rise and Fall of Modern Medicine*, 2nd edition. London: Abacus.

Morse, J. (2000) 'The downside of dissemination', *Qualitative Health Research*, 10(3): 291–2.

Orosz, E. (1994) 'The impact of social science research on health policy', *Social Science and Medicine*, 39: 1287–93.

Pierce, R. (2008) *Research Methods in Politics: A Practical Guide*. London: Sage.

Richardson, L. (1990) *Writing Strategies: Reaching Diverse Audiences*. London: Sage.

Saks, M. (1995) *Professions and the Public Interest: Medical Power, Altruism and Alternative Medicine*. London: Routledge.

Saks, M. (2012) 'The challenge of implementing social science research', *Portuguese Journal of Social Science*, 11: 71–84.

Saks, M. and Allsop, J. (2007) 'Social policy, professional regulation and health support work in the UK', *Social Policy and Society*, 6(2): 165–77.

Scambler, G. (2002) *Health and Social Change: A Critical Theory*. Buckingham: Open University Press.

Schober, J. and Farrington, A. (2000) 'Presenting and disseminating research', in M. Saks, M. Williams and B. Hancock (eds), *Developing Research in Primary Care*. Abingdon: Radcliffe Medical Press.

Tang, P. and Sinclair, T. (2001) 'Exploitation practice in social science research', *Science and Public Policy*, 28(2): 131–8.

Thomas, S.A. (2000) *How To Write Health Services Papers, Dissertations and Theses*. Edinburgh: Churchill-Livingstone.

Turabian, K.L. (2007) *A Manual for Writers of Research Papers, Theses and Dissertations*, 7th edition. Chicago, IL: University of Chicago Press.

Wakefield, A.J., Murch, S.H., Anthony, A., Linnell, J., Casson, D.M., Malik, M. et al. (1998) 'Ileal-lymphoid-modular hyperplasia, non-specific colitis and pervasive developmental disorder in children', *Lancet*, 351: 637–41.

Wickham, J. and Collins, G. (2006) 'Involving users in social science research: a new European paradigm?', *European Journal of Education*, 41(2): 269–80.

Glossary

Action research A participative method that engages people in the research to gain knowledge for action and change.

Analytical induction A method for systematic qualitative data analysis where the researcher identifies themes that provide an explanation for a phenomenon with the progressive refinement of theory until no disconfirming evidence can be found.

Bias Research data may be skewed for known or unknown reasons leading to false estimates of the effect of an intervention. Common sources of bias lie in recruitment, selection, performance, detection, attrition or actions by researchers or participants.

Bivariate analysis. An analysis that addresses the possible relationship between two variables.

Boolean operators The refining words 'and', 'or', 'not', which are used to combine search terms to retrieve the most relevant articles in a literature review.

Case-control study Compares the characteristics of a particular phenomenon in the group of interest to a control or reference group.

Case study design The selection of one or more examples of a phenomenon as a unit of analysis (an organization, place or person) where the focus is on their circumstances, dynamics and complexity.

Coding frame A list of codes used to analyse data in a structured questionnaire. In **open coding** the researcher must break down, compare, conceptualize and categorize data. In **closed coding** this is usually pre-coded so data are translated from the respondent's answer to the survey questions and to a database where aggregate data can be analysed.

Cohort studies A selected population is studied over time to investigate the effect of a particular factor on health outcomes.

Comparative design A design where the same phenomenon, an institution, custom, tradition or culture is compared within two or more contrasting socio-cultural settings.

Confounding variable A third variable – an unknown factor – that intervenes between two variables which then appear to be associated, but the relationship between them is false.

Convenience sample A technique for obtaining a sample by contacting known, rather than randomly selected informants.

Conversational analysis A detailed analysis of recorded talk collected in a naturalistic setting.

Covert research Research data collected without the subject or participant's knowledge and consent.

Cross-over study A type of trial design that involves one treatment in a first phase, a wash-out period with no treatment and then a second randomized treatment with a control group.

Cross-sectional design A study that requires the collection of data from a number of subjects/objects over a specified time with the aim of establishing an association between variables.

Deductive reasoning An approach where the researcher draws on a body of theory and knowledge to deduce a hypothesis or proposition that can be tested through empirical research.

Descriptive statistics The numerical, graphical and tabular techniques for organizing, analysing and presenting data.

Discourse analysis An approach that analyses talk in natural settings to identify the rules of talk in context to show how social phenomena are constructed through language exchange.

Double-blind trial A type of randomized controlled trial where neither the investigators nor the trial participants (volunteers/patients) are aware of who is receiving the active or placebo treatment. A **single-blind trial** is where the therapist knows which arm has the placebo and the active treatment.

Epidemiology The study of variations in the pattern of disease and well-being in populations and their causes.

Epistemology The nature of knowledge or how we come to know certain things about the world.

Equipoise A term used in clinical trials to indicate where researchers and research participants have an equal belief in the likely outcomes of the two active treatments being compared.

Ethnography A method for collecting data from communities and groups through observation, interview and the analysis of cultural artefacts to develop theories and explanations.

Ethnomethodology An approach based on taking informants' stories and interactions as accounts of how social order is accomplished.

Experiment A research design based on the scientific method to test changes by having a treatment and control group and aiming to establish a relationship between cause and effect.

Experimental method An umbrella term including a variety of techniques used to maintain scientific rigour by testing a hypothesis, reducing bias and ruling out alternative explanations.

Focus group A specific research technique derived from market research where a number of people (usually strangers) are brought together to discuss a topic in a 'focused' way.

Frequency table This captures the number of times each value of a variable appears in a distribution – enabling a more precise understanding of data than can be gleaned from a chart.

Generalizability The external validity of research findings, based on extrapolating findings from a smaller to a larger population.

Grounded theory Research begins with a general area of interest rather than a hypothesis and moves on to identify the concepts and theoretical connections emerging from the data.

Hawthorne effect The possibility that the researcher's presence influences the behaviour observed.

Health needs assessment Assessing one or more of the following in relation to health: expressed needs, normative needs (defined by experts), comparative needs (in relation to other groups) or felt needs.

Health technology assessment Evaluating evidence in order to identify what medical technologies or care pathways work best.

Hypothesis A proposition that underpins a research question to be tested by further research.

Incidence A measure used to assess new cases of a disease, lifestyle behaviour or exposure to a risk factor that occur in a defined period of time.

Incidence rate The number of cases (for example, deaths) occurring in a given period of time in a defined population.

Inductive reasoning A process that begins with observation and/or data collection, finds patterns or associations and builds theory or explanations, on the basis of the evidence.

Informed consent A participant freely agrees to participate in research and fully understands the consequences of this agreement.

Interpretivism A theory that knowledge about social phenomena is constructed by research subjects and is embedded in society and culture. It is sometimes also referred to as **constructivism**.

Interval/ratio scale A scale which ranks results from highest to lowest but also measures the differences, or intervals, between them.

Lay epidemiology A set of beliefs in the population about illness, its causes and distribution.

Longitudinal design The study of a phenomenon or phenomena over time.

Measures of central tendency A term used to indicate the typical or average value for a distribution. Three common measures are the **mode, median** and **mean**.

Methodology A set of guidelines and principles used to gather information and assess evidence in order to address a particular problem. This is to be distinguished from **methods**, which are techniques used to collect data such as experiments, surveys, observation and interviewing.

Narrative analysis A method that explores the structure of texts and the ways in which the narrator uses the narrative.

Narrative review A literature review that identifies key concepts, specific terms and the theoretical approaches adopted by different authors to understand a phenomenon.

Naturalism In the social sciences the term refers to a research technique that collects data in everyday settings with a minimum use of intrusive methods. In the sciences it can refer to the use of the scientific method.

Nominal scale Classifies cases into categories that have no quantitative ordering.

Ordinalcale A ranking of cases according to the quantity or intensity of the variable expressed by each case.

Paradigm A cluster of beliefs or set of assumptions about the nature of knowledge that influences what should be studied and how research should be conducted.

Participant observation A research method where the researcher spends an extended period of time in a natural setting participating in, and observing, particular classes of activity.

Patient narratives Accounts of the patient pathway through the illness and treatment process.

Phenomenology An interpretivist methodology that aims to study how individuals themselves make sense of their world.

Placebo A non-active treatment used in a trial.

Positivism An epistemological position favouring methods drawn from the natural sciences in conducting research, which aims to identify general laws and objective facts in the natural and social world.

Pragmatic study A study that investigates what happens in practice.

Pragmatic trial A trial undertaken to assess whether a therapy will work in everyday practice.

Prevalence A measure of the burden of disease or lifestyle choice of a population, which indicates the number of cases of disease in a population at a given time.

Probability sampling A sample where each unit or element of the population has a specifiable chance of being selected.

Protocol A written plan of a clinical research project to cover aims and process to justify a proposal for peer review.

Public involvement A term used to promote research that is carried out 'with' or 'by' members of the public, rather than 'about' or 'for' them'.

Purposeful sampling A method where informants are selected with specific knowledge about the research question.

QALY A measure of a benefit in terms of one added year of perfect health. This measure is set against the costs of treatment to assess clinical cost-effectiveness.

Quasi-experimental design A research design that includes a non-randomized control group, a before and after study and an interrupted time series design.

Quota sampling A non-probability technique for sampling commonly used in market research. It involves selecting sample elements according to a pre-determined distribution across certain defined categories.

Randomized controlled trial This evaluates the effects of a particular treatment or management strategy in a population by comparing the outcome with a control group where no intervention has been made.

Reflexivity This refers to the 'tacit' or assumed knowledge of researchers when undertaking a project, who should be aware of their role in the construction of knowledge at all stages of the research process and not make unwarranted assumptions about their informants' views.

Reliability The extent to which research instruments and concepts are stable and able to yield an unvarying measurement. This is termed **synchronic reliability** when observations are consistent in the same time period.

Replicability The extent to which the results of a study can be reproduced by a trained researcher.

Research governance A term referring to the arrangements to set assess and monitor standards to safeguard the quality of research and promote good practice.

Sampling The practice of selecting information from a population to allow defensible inferences to be drawn from data applying to populations.

Sampling frame A list of units or elements that are assumed best to define the target or survey population.

Snowball sampling A sample drawn by asking one informant to suggest another.

Social marketing The psychological and organizational techniques used to promote behaviour change for the social good.

Stratified sample A method to ensure the desired distribution of a sample across certain groups in the population.

Survey A quantitative method to collect data from a population sample at one point in time. The cases or units of analysis provide a structured data set. Surveys can be ad hoc, cross-sectional, national or longitudinal.

Systematic review A synthesis of what is known, and not known, about the efficacy of a particular intervention based on the most robust evidence available for critical appraisal.

Target population The population 'of interest' for a proposed investigation.

Theoretic sampling A method by which the analyst jointly collects, codes, and analyses data and decides what data to collect next and where to find them, in order to develop theory. It is a term used in grounded theory, where sampling continues until no new information is generated.

Triangulation A navigational term based on using two bearings to locate an object used in two ways in the social sciences: to imply that the aggregation of data from different sources can validate a particular truth, account or finding; and to argue that more than one method provides different perspectives on a phenomenon and can lead to greater understanding.

Validity The 'truthfulness' or accuracy of research findings used to test whether an indicator is measuring the concept it is intended to measure.

Index